D0298104

Epidemiology
Principles and Methods

Epidemiology
Principles and Methods

Second Edition

Brian MacMahon, M.D., Ph.D., D.Sc.(hon)
Henry Pickering Walcott Professor of Epidemiology, Emeritus,
Harvard School of Public Health, Boston

Dimitrios Trichopoulos, M.D., M.S., M.D.(hon)
Vincent L. Gregory Professor of Cancer Prevention and
Professor of Epidemiology, Harvard School of Public Health,
Boston

MEDICAL LIBRARY
QUEENS MEDICAL CENTRE

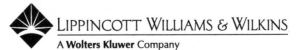
LIPPINCOTT WILLIAMS & WILKINS
A **Wolters Kluwer** Company
Philadelphia · Baltimore · New York · London
Buenos Aires · Hong Kong · Sydney · Tokyo

Copyright © 1996 by Brian MacMahon

Second Edition

Previous edition copyright © 1970 by Brian MacMahon

All rights reserved. No part of this book may be
reproduced in any form or by any electronic or
mechanical means, including information storage
and retrieval systems, without permission in
writing from the publisher, except by a reviewer
who may quote brief passages in a review.

1005414144

Library of Congress Cataloging-in-Publication Data
MacMahon, Brian, 1923–
    Epidemiology : principles and methods / Brian MacMahon,
    Dimitrios Trichopoulos. — 2nd ed.
        p. cm.
    Includes bibliographical references and index.
    ISBN 0-316-54222-9
    1. Epidemiology. I. Trichopoulos, Dimitrios. II. Title.
    [DNLM: 1. Epidemiologic Methods. 2. Epidemiology.
WA 950 M167e 1996]
RA651.M24   1996
614.4—dc20
DNLM/DLC
for Library of Congress   96-5095
                                                              CIP

Printed in the United States of America

MV-NY

2 3 4 5 6 78 9

LIPPINCOTT WILLIAMS & WILKINS
530 Walnut St.
Philadelphia, PA 19106 USA
LWW.com

Editorial: Jo-Ann T. Strangis, Deeth K. Ellis
Production Editor: Marie A. Salter
Composition and Production Services: Spectrum Publisher
    Services, Inc.
Designer: Louis C. Bruno, Jr.
Cover Designer: Deborah Azerrad Savona

To Heidi Marie MacMahon-Graber

Contents

Preface

The beginnings of the mid-twentieth century renaissance of epidemiology resembled to a remarkable degree developments during the second half of the nineteenth century. In both periods, resurgence of interest in the field was stimulated by a major discovery—recognition of the method of spread of cholera in the 1850s and demonstration in the 1950s of the disastrous effects of cigarette smoking on health. However, subsequent to these initial events, the patterns of development in the two centuries diverged.

In the nineteenth century, with notable exceptions, there was little concern for the refinement of epidemiological methods or for the understanding of the principles that led to the new discoveries. Rather, major work was concerned with the application of existing methods to the solution of practical problems, primarily the control of the major infectious diseases, which at that time were the most serious health problems facing countries in both the developed and developing worlds. Collaboration of epidemiology with the newly developing microbiological sciences led ultimately to remarkable accomplishments—worldwide eradication of smallpox, virtual elimination of poliomyelitis, and control of the major enteric diseases, at least in the developed world.

Following the widespread recognition in the 1950s that epidemiologic methods also may have utility in application to noninfectious diseases, or, more accurately, to diseases not known to be associated with microbiological agents, there was a greatly increased effort to apply these methods to cancers, cardiovascular diseases, neurologic diseases, and other conditions not yet known to be associated with microbiologic organisms. There of course had been individual efforts of this nature prior to 1950, notably the geographic studies of coronary disease by Ancel Keys and the studies of migrants by William Haenszel and others, but the flow of such work increased swiftly after the 1950s. In addition—and what was not seen to the same extent in the nineteenth century—epidemiologists came to recognize with increasing frequency the importance of statistical methodology to their discipline. Paralleling this recognition, there arose considerable interest in understanding and articulating the underlying premises and philosophy of epidemiology that lie within the bounds of scientific inference and that are not subsumed by statistics and related sciences but are specific to epidemiology.

A number of relevant texts have been written by current or past members of the Department of Epidemiology, Harvard School of Public Health; some focus on theory,[a] some on specific substantive areas,[b-d] and others are of a more general nature.[e,f] This text is the third in a series of books meant to introduce epidemiology at an introductory level and bring the reader to the point of understanding the prevailing major concepts and methods of contemporary epidemiology. The first of these books was published in 1960[g] and was, we believe, the first systematic account of mid-twentieth-century epidemiology. An extensively revised version of the text was published in 1970.[h] Although planned as a second edition of the 1960 book, it was judged sufficiently different from its predecessor to be considered a new book. Since 1970, the face of epidemiology has so changed that one may question the feasibility of "updating" a book written that long ago. In fact, we have omitted a great deal of material that might be considered relevant to such an update: for example, specialized methods in psychiatric epidemiology, occupational epidemiology, nutritional epidemiology, and others (several of these topics are subjects of their own specialized texts). Many, although not all, of the enormous changes in the discipline of epidemiology are at least touched on here, and it is hoped that the reader will come away with a general sense of epidemiology as it exists currently and will have a sufficient base from which to explore, in other sources, the areas with which we have dealt lightly. Although the changes between the 1970 and 1996 versions are at least as great as those between the 1960 and 1970 versions, the publisher has chosen to characterize this volume as a second edition of the 1970 text; we have no objection.

The objective of this book remains the same: to provide an introduction to epidemiology that will be understood by the novice and to present some mid-level material. The reader who is looking only for an introduction may find some of the material in Chapters 9 and 10 more than he or she needs. However, for the student who intends to proceed to mid- and advanced-level courses, this material may serve as a useful bridge.

B.M.

D.T.

References

a. Miettinen OS. *Theoretical Epidemiology: Principles of Occurrence Research in Medicine.* New York: Wiley, 1985.
b. Monson RR. *Occupational Epidemiology,* 2nd Ed. Boca Raton, FL: CRC Press, 1990.
c. Willett W. *Nutritional Epidemiology.* New York: Oxford University Press, 1990.
d. Weiss NS. *Clinical Epidemiology: The Study of the Outcome of Illness.* New York: Oxford University Press, 1986. (Monographs in Epidemiology and Biostatistics, Vol 11.)
e. Rothman KJ. *Modern Epidemiology.* Boston: Little, Brown, 1986.
f. Walker AM. *Observation and Inference: An Introduction to the Methods of Epidemiology.* Boston: Epidemiology Resources, Inc., 1991.
g. MacMahon B, Pugh TF, Ipsen J. *Epidemiologic Methods.* Boston: Little, Brown, 1960.
h. MacMahon B, Pugh TF. *Epidemiology: Principles and Methods.* Boston: Little, Brown, 1970.

Acknowledgments

We are greatly indebted to Dr. Chung-cheng Hsieh and Dr. Murray Mittleman, who reviewed Chapters 9 and 10 in considerable detail and made many useful suggestions and corrections. Dr. Chung was also very helpful in the organization of the book in general and in reading other sections. Dr. Lucien R. Karhausen and Dr. Neil Pearce made useful comments on the section on "Refutation in Epidemiology" in Chapter 5, and we have made free use of our local colleagues for similar purposes throughout the book.

Dr. Loren Lipworth and Sandra Chinn were very helpful in literature research, and we thank, in particular, Dr. Lipworth and Dr. Anastasia Tzonou, who organized and checked the references for this edition. Dr. Tzonou also helped respond to copyeditors' comments and made corrections in page proofs.

We thank our editors at Little, Brown—Evan R. Schnittman, Jo-Ann T. Strangis, and Deeth K. Ellis—and the production staff at Spectrum Publisher Services, Inc.—Kristin Miller and Kelly Ricci—for their prompt responses to our requests for assistance and for their patience and advice.

Epidemiology
Principles and Methods

1 Epidemiology

Definition

Epidemiology is the study of the distribution and determinants of disease frequency in human populations.

Two main areas of investigation are indicated in this definition—the study of the *distribution* of disease and the search for the *determinants* (causes) of the disease and its observed distribution. The first area, describing the distribution of health status in terms of age, gender, race, geography, time, and so on, might be considered an expansion of the discipline of demography to health and disease. The second area involves explanation of the patterns of disease distribution in terms of causal factors. Many disciplines seek to learn about the causes of disease; the special contributions of epidemiology are its search for concordance between the known or suspected causes of a disease and the known patterns of the distribution of the disease, *or* the use of these patterns to postulate elements of the environment that should be investigated for possible causal roles.

Like many sciences, epidemiology has developed from the study of the exotic or the unusual into the formulation of general principles. Epidemiology is now no more restricted to the study of disease outbreaks than meteorology is to the study of hurricanes or astronomy is to the study of solar eclipses. Yet an epidemiologist today might still consider his or her concerns to be primarily the study of epidemics, if a broad view is taken as to what constitutes an epidemic, and if it is recognized that research to explain epidemics cannot be restricted to periods during which epidemics prevail.

1

Concept of an Epidemic

In the past the term *epidemic* was used almost exclusively to describe an acute outbreak, usually of an infectious disease. More current usage stresses the concept of *excessive frequency*, rather than *acuteness*, as the basic implication of the word "epidemic." Excessive frequency is a feature of many noninfectious diseases as well as diseases known to be associated with microorganisms. Indeed, as the role of viruses in human cancer and neurological disease becomes more clear, the distinction between infectious and noninfectious diseases becomes even less distinct. The United States, for example, is currently in the grip of two seemingly noninfectious diseases—coronary heart disease and lung cancer—and the characterization of these two diseases as being epidemic in this country and in some other parts of the world is noncontroversial. The idea that the frequency of a particular disease is excessive may be developed by following its frequency over time, by comparing its frequency in different places, or by comparing its frequency among subgroups of a single population at a particular time. For example, lung cancer is now 30 times more common in the United States than it was in the mid-1920s; ischemic heart disease accounts for one-third of all deaths in the United States, although there are countries in which it is relatively infrequent; and many diseases are much more common in certain ethnic and nationality groups within the United States than in the country as a whole. That the excessive frequency must come about within a short period, or in a narrowly defined geographic area, is no longer an essential implication of the term "epidemic."

The term *pandemic* should be mentioned. It is used to refer to an epidemic that is without geographic bounds (i.e., is worldwide). The 1918–1919 pandemic of influenza is a well-known example. However, even that pandemic was epidemic in the sense that it was time limited. The term "pandemic" carries no specificity and is not referred to further in this text.

Study of Nonepidemic Disease Frequency

Even if our predominant concern is the explanation of epidemics, knowledge of disease frequency and distribution during nonepidemic times is useful. There are several reasons for this:

1. Without knowledge of nonepidemic frequency, how can the existence of an epidemic be recognized? How can it be determined that the frequency of a particular disease in a particular population at a particular time is excessive?

Sometimes the existence of an epidemic is obvious. This is so

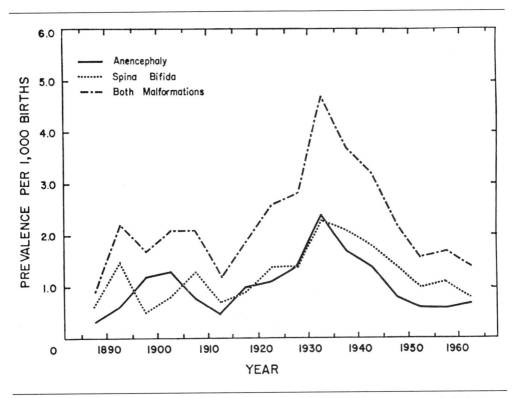

Figure 1-1. An unrecognized epidemic. Prevalence at birth of neural tube defects in two New England hospitals, 1885–1965. (From B MacMahon, S Yen. Unrecognized epidemic of anencephaly and spina bifida. *Lancet* 1971;i : 31–33, © by The Lancet Ltd, 1971.)

when the epidemic involves a large number of persons (or a few persons with a very rare disease), produces a distinctive illness, and occurs over a short period of time. Thus, there is little difficulty in detecting epidemics of cholera, plague, smallpox, or the common infections of childhood. The features of these diseases are characteristic, the difference between epidemic and nonepidemic frequency is large, and the transition from the nonepidemic to the epidemic is swift. However, even when the disease is familiar, less dramatic epidemics occurring over longer periods may be missed. For example, an epidemic of babies born with severe neural tube defects occurred during the 1930s in the northeastern United States (Figure 1-1). At its peak (1929–1932), the occurrence of these defects was three times what it was earlier in the century and what it is today. The neural tube defect epidemic went unrecognized for 40 years until revealed by a systematic study of hospital birth records.[318] The slow development of this epidemic concealed its size, as also for many years did that of the epidemic of ischemic heart disease.

Even acute and large-scale epidemics may pass unnoticed if they appear in unfamiliar form. For example, during the intense London fog of 1952, there was little realization of the full effects of the fog on the population's health. Only when deaths were counted and compared with the numbers in the periods preceding and following the fog during the same year and during similar periods in other years were the effects realized. It then became apparent that the fog had been responsible for more than 4,000 deaths in a period of about 10 days.[362]

2. An unusually low disease frequency in a population may be just as significant in understanding the causes of an epidemic as a high disease frequency. For example, the very low disease rates from cholera observed among two groups of people (workers in a brewery and inmates of a workhouse), who lived in the center of an otherwise epidemic area, led to a strengthening of the belief that the general water supply was responsible for the epidemic. Both the brewery workers and workhouse inmates had water supplies independent of the neighborhood supply.[508] Another example is the virtual absence of cancer of the uterine cervix among nuns was an important piece of evidence which linked the disease to some aspect of sexual activity.

3. In the chronic diseases, in which frequency changes generally extend over long periods of time, it may be difficult to decide whether a given frequency qualifies as epidemic (or excessively frequent) even if all necessary comparative information is available. It is common to find a gradient in the frequencies of disease in different populations. While the disease may be considered definitely epidemic when the highest frequency populations are compared with the lowest, the populations in between may present semantic difficulty. In such circumstances, attempts to correlate quantitative statements of the disease frequency with the frequency of suspected factors are more revealing than simple association of the dichotomy of the epidemic or nonepidemic with the dichotomy of the presence or absence of these factors.

Historical Background

Some of the basic concepts underlying the practice of epidemiology can be illustrated through references to historical episodes and personalities. A few episodes that seem particularly relevant to the development of current concepts and methods—as distinct from substantive knowledge of the epidemiology of particular diseases—are outlined in this section. While in one sense epidemiology is almost as old as medicine itself, in another sense it is a very young discipline. Although Hippocrates spoke in terms that have meaning to epidemiologists today, only in the last few decades has epidemiology become recognizable as a named discipline with which research groups and academic departments are identified. Since the 1960s, the discipline has been featured regularly in the media and in legal and regulatory settings.

The history of epidemiologic methodology is largely the history of the development of five ideas: (1) human disease is related to the environment in which we live; (2) the counting of natural phenomena may be even more instructive than the observation of them; (3) "natural experiments" can be utilized to investigate disease etiology; (4) natural experiments occur more frequently than we think and reflect the tremendous heterogeneity of human experience; and (5) "true experiments" can be conducted on human populations in some circumstances.

Disease and Environment

The idea that disease risk may be connected with the human environment was expressed by Hippocrates almost 2,400 years ago. Today the concept seems self-evident, but the clarity of Hippocrates' statement and its relevance to the objectives of epidemiology today deserve recognition. In *On Airs, Waters, and Places*, he states:

> Whoever wishes to investigate medicine properly should proceed thus: in the first place to consider the seasons of the year, and what effects each of them produces. Then the winds, the hot and the cold, especially such as are common to all countries, and then such as are peculiar to each locality. In the same manner, when one comes into a city to which he is a stranger, he should consider its situation, how it lies as to the winds and the rising of the sun; for its influence is not the same whether it lies to the north or the south, to the rising or to the setting sun. One should consider most attentively the waters which the inhabitants use, whether they be marshy and soft, or hard and running from elevated and rocky situations, and then if saltish and unfit for cooking; and the ground, whether it be naked and deficient in water, or wooded and well watered, and whether it lies in a hollow, confined situation, or is elevated and cold; and the mode in which the inhabitants live, and what are their pursuits, whether they are fond of drinking and eating to excess, and given to indolence, or are fond of exercise and labor.[210]

In light of such clear instruction from this influential teacher, it is remarkable that virtually nothing was discovered about the specific natures of unhealthy environments during the subsequent 2,000 years. Greenwood attributes this to the fact that the operative word in Hippocrates' statement is *consider*, not *count*.[185] However full of insight an investigator's considerings might be, if they are not supported by observations objectively recorded in quantitative terms, they are unlikely to form a basis for the considerings of successive generations of investigators.

Counting and Measurement

One of the first "counters" of health events was John Graunt, a London businessman and founding member of The Royal Society of London for Improving Natural Knowledge (now The Royal Society). In 1662, Graunt published his *Natural and Political Observations Made upon the Bills of Mortality*.[158] These bills, first appearing in 1592, were published weekly, although episodically, by the parish clerks of the City of London, and were stimulated largely by fear of the plague. Graunt described how they were assembled:

> When any one dies, then, either by tolling, or ringing of a Bell, or by bespeaking of a Grave of the Sexton, the same is known to the Searchers, corresponding with the said Sexton.
> The Searchers hereupon (who are antient Matrons, sworn to their Office) repair to the place, where the dead Corps lies, and by view of the same, and by other enquiries, they examine by what Disease, or Casualty the Corps died. Hereupon they make their Report to the Parish-Clerk, and he, every Tuesday night, carries in an Account of all the Burials, and Christenings, hapning that Week, to the Clerk of the Hall. On Wednesday the general Account is made up, and Printed, and on Thursdays published, and dispersed to the several Families, who will pay four shillings per Annum for them.[158]

Graunt assembled and analyzed the bills published between 1623 and 1660. His observations either foreshadowed or opened several quite distinct fields of endeavor. By showing the constancy of the ratio of males to females among newborns and deaths, that age-specific death rates were higher for males than for females, and that there were seasonal fluctuations in deaths from various causes, and by presenting a host of other new observations, he demonstrated the "uniformity and predictability of . . . biological phenomena taken in the mass"[592] and thus is widely regarded as a founder of the science of biostatistics. In developing methods to estimate the size of London's population, by showing that, although one-fifth of the population died during the great plague years, the city was fully repopulated within 2 years, and in attempting to create a life table that showed the age distribution of the population, he laid the foundation for the field of demography. In painting a systematic picture of the ebb and flow of various diseases and the characteristics of persons who became afflicted with them, and in using quantitative methods to test hypotheses, he led the way to epidemiology. Since the methods he used saw no further epidemiologic application for almost 200 years, Graunt might be more appropriately regarded as a forerunner, rather than a founder, of epidemiology.

The roots of today's epidemiology are more clearly detectable in the work of William Farr, a physician who was given responsibility for medical statistics in the Office of the Registrar General for England and Wales in 1839. The Annual Reports of the Registrar General during the subsequent 40 years established a tradition of the careful application of vital data (i.e., certificates of "vital events," such as birth, death, and marriage) to problems of public health and to other broad public concerns. Some of the matters that received Farr's attention were the mortality rates in the Cornish metal mines and other occupational settings, in prisons and other institutions, and among married and single persons. He also studied fluctuations in the marriage rate, which he believed were related to the price of bread (an index of the economy), the distribution of cholera, trends in the literacy rate, the life-time monetary value of a person, and the consequences of the nineteenth-century population movements in England and Wales. The thoroughness of Farr's analyses was illustrated by his attempt to ascertain the effect of imprisonment on mortality.[224] He determined the population at risk, as well as the number of deaths, to compute a mortality rate, compared the death rates in prison with those in the general population, took into account the age of the prisoners and the duration of their prison stay, and considered the fact that "prisoners rarely labour under any serious disease at the time of their committal," a circumstance that by analogy with today's terminology in occupational studies might be referred to as a "healthy prisoner effect." Finally, he computed what we call today an "attributable rate" (the difference between the death rates in prisons and the outside), concluding: "Only 8 criminals were executed (in) 1837, while . . . the average annual number of deaths due to imprisonment was 51." In considering the population at risk, the need to take into account differences in characteristics of compared groups (other than those by which they were defined), the biases involved in the selection of persons exposed to a suspected cause, and the ways of measuring risk, Farr identified some of the major concerns of epidemiologists today.

Natural Experiments

One of Farr's contemporaries was a physician who was most widely known for his administration of chloroform to Queen Victoria during childbirth, but who is remembered among epidemiologists for his demonstration of the spread of cholera by fecal contamination of drinking water. We shall refer to the work of John Snow in several contexts but, from the methodologic point of view, his most interesting investigation was the demonstration that cholera risk was related to the drinking water supplied by a particular commercial company in London and, by inference, to the source from which the company obtained its water.[508] (At that time, water was supplied to the inhabitants of London by a number of private companies.)

In 1849, Snow noted that cholera rates were particularly high in areas of London supplied with water by the Lambeth Company or the Southwark and Vauxhall Company, both of which drew their water from the Thames River at a point where it was heavily polluted with human sewage. Between 1849 and 1854, the Lambeth Company relocated its source to an upstream, less polluted part of the river; subsequent to the relocation, the incidence of cholera declined in the areas supplied by that company. During the same time period, there was no change in the disease incidence in the areas supplied by the Southwark and Vauxhall Company, which continued to "prescribe the mixture as before."[207] The situation in 1854 is illustrated in Table 1-1. The areas of London supplied solely by the Southwark and Vauxhall Company experienced 5.0 deaths from cholera per 1,000 population, whereas in the areas supplied entirely by the Lambeth Company the ratio was only 0.9 per 1,000. A large area supplied jointly by

Table 1-1. Mortality from Cholera in the Districts of London Supplied by the Southwark and Vauxhall Company and by the Lambeth Company, July 8 to August 26, 1854

Districts with water supplied by	Population, 1851	Deaths from cholera	Cholera deaths per 1,000 population
Southwark and Vauxhall Company only	167,654	844	5.0
Lambeth Company only	19,133	18	0.9
Both companies	300,149	652	2.2

Adapted from J. Snow. *On the Mode of Communication of Cholera* (2nd ed.). London: Churchill, 1855. Reproduced in J. Snow. *Snow on Cholera.* New York: Commonwealth Fund, 1936. Reprinted New York: Hafner, 1965.

both companies experienced 2.2 deaths per 1,000, a ratio midway between those for the areas supplied by either company alone.

Snow saw that, in the areas supplied by only one company, the observations were consistent with the hypothesis that persons drinking water supplied by the Southwark and Vauxhall Company were at greater risk of cholera than those drinking water supplied by the Lambeth Company. However, he also realized that many factors other than water supply could differ between these geographic areas and could explain the difference in cholera experience. Snow's genius lay in his recognition of a circumstance by which the hypothesis implicating the water of the Southwark and Vauxhall Company could be put to a crucial test. In his own words:

> . . . the intermixing of the water supply of the Southwark and Vaux-hall Company with that of the Lambeth Company, over an extensive part of London, admitted of the subject being sifted in such a way as to yield the most incontrovertible proof on one side or the other. In the sub-districts enumerated in the above table [Table 1-1, in this chapter] as being supplied by both Companies, the mixing of the supply is of the most intimate kind. The pipes of each Company go down all the streets, and into nearly all the courts and alleys. A few houses are supplied by one Company and a few by the other, according to the decision of the owner or occupier at that time when the Water Companies were in active competition. In many cases a single house has a supply different from that on either side. Each company supplies both rich and poor, both large houses and small; there is no difference either in the condition or occupation of the persons receiving the water of the different Companies. Now it must be evident that, if the diminution of cholera, in the districts partly supplied with the improved water, depended on this supply, the houses receiving it would be the houses enjoying the whole benefit of the diminution of the malady, whilst the houses supplied with the water from Battersea Fields would suffer the same mortality as they would if the improved supply did not exist at all. As there is no difference whatever, either in the houses or the people receiving the supply of the two Water Companies, or in any of the physical conditions with which they are surrounded, it is obvious that no experiment could have been devised which would more thoroughly test the effect of water supply on the progress of cholera than this, which circumstances placed ready made before the observer.
>
> The experiment, too, was on the grandest scale. No fewer than three hundred thousand people of both sexes, of every age and occupation, and of every rank and station, from gentlefolks down to the very poor, were divided into two groups without their choice, and, in most cases, without their knowledge; one group being supplied with water containing the sewage of London, and, amongst it, whatever might have come from the cholera patients, the other group having water quite free from such impurity.

Table 1-2. Mortality from Cholera in London, July 8 to August 26, 1854, Related to the Water Supply of Individual Houses in Districts Served by Both the Southwark and Vauxhall Company and the Lambeth Company

Water supply of individual houses	Population, 1851	Deaths from cholera	Cholera deaths per 1,000 population
Southwark and Vauxhall Company	98,862	419	4.2
Lambeth Company	154,615	80	0.5

Adapted from J. Snow. *On the Mode of Communication of Cholera* (2nd ed.). London: Churchill, 1855. Reproduced in J. Snow. *Snow on Cholera.* New York: Commonwealth Fund, 1936. Reprinted New York: Hafner, 1965.

> To turn this grand experiment to account, all that was required was to learn the supply of water to each individual house where a fatal attack of cholera might occur. (pp. 74–75)[508]

Within the subdistricts supplied by both companies, Snow inquired of relatives and others as to which company supplied the water to every house in which a death from cholera had occurred between July 8 and August 16, 1854. The results are shown in Table 1-2. The frequency of cholera deaths for customers of each company were similar to those of the same company's customers in subdistricts supplied exclusively by that company (see Table 1-1). Moreover, the risk of death for customers of the Lambeth Company was no higher than that for the rest of London, even though the majority of them were located in areas supplied also by the Southwark and Vauxhall Company, areas in which the epidemic raged severely. The hypothesis that the drinking of water supplied by the Southwark and Vauxhall Company was associated with death from cholera was therefore supported.

Although referred to as such by Snow, this was not an "experiment" in the sense used in this text and in the sense that the term is generally used today. An *experiment* refers to a study in which the circumstances are deliberately manipulated by the investigator *for the purpose of obtaining the desired information*. It can be argued whether the changing of the source of the Lambeth Company water was "deliberately manipulated," but it was certainly not done by the investigator or for the purpose of obtaining the information Snow derived.

Man-made circumstances, such as those Snow exploited, and natural calamities are not uncommon, but for many reasons, often because of the social disruption accompanying them, they have not been exploited as frequently as they should have been for the knowledge they can provide on disease causation. Notable exceptions are the opportunistic use of a major earthquake to study the effect of psychological stress on the frequency of fatal heart attacks[540] and the regular exploitation of excessive air pollution episodes to study their influence on overall mortality.[250,362,482] More long-term efforts to utilize environmental changes that were not produced for epidemiologic purposes include the Follow-Up Program of the Atomic Bomb Casualty Commission (now the Radiation Effects Research Foundation),[89,493] follow-up of patients treated with ionizing radiation for ankylosing spondylitis[77,83] or cervical cancer,[33,34] studies of morbidity and mortality among large populations that have migrated from one part of the world to another,[144,189,517] and a large number of investigations on the effects of occupational exposures to chemical and physical agents.[363] Many other opportunities have been lost or appear to be being underutilized, such as the radiation exposure of large populations following the nuclear accident at Chernobyl, the chemical explosion at Bhopal, and the respiratory effects of the exposure of thousands of persons to the extremely heavy air pollution caused by the oil fires in Kuwait following the Gulf War. While our first priority is always to deal with problems that will immediately benefit the exposed populations, we also should derive what knowledge we can from such disasters because experience tells us that not all health effects will be immediate and because of the possibility of such events recurring.

Frequency of Natural Experiments

There are many natural experiments, some of which we create ourselves, that are more subtle than those described in the previous section. These experiments are not obvious but are generated through the circumstances of birth, child-rearing, social environments and, subsequently, personal choice. The results are populations in which each individual is unique in his or her personal life, dietary habits, and environmental exposures. To derive any useful health information relating to such variables, we must group the unique individuals into categories classified around personal characteristics, such as cigarette smokers, lotus eaters, baseball players, and so on, recognizing that the individuals contained in the category are not homogeneous, except with respect to the characteristic that defines the category. Other behavioral and environmental characteristics may be quite different and the differences may be relevant to the health outcome being investigated. The extraction from these categories of valid information on the causes of human disease is the principal challenge and reward of epidemiology.

True Experiments

True experiments, in which human exposure is deliberately manipulated for the purpose of studying its effects, are assuming greater and greater roles in medicine in general (in the context of evaluation of therapeutic agents) and in epidemiology specifically (in the context of interfering with known or suspected causes of disease). The teachings of Sir Austin Bradford Hill in the mid-1900s were a major force leading to acceptance of the concept that *randomization* in the assignment of exposure is the unique tool that enhances the value of information obtained by experiment over that derived from passive observation. Note that randomization is not a feature of natural experiments. The major limitation of human experiment is that it ethically can be used only when the planned intervention is expected to be beneficial, or at the very least not harmful, in comparison to the expected course of events in the absence of the intervention.

Well-known early epidemiologic experiments include Lind's trial of fresh fruit against scurvy in 1747,[289] Jenner's experiments with cowpox vaccination in 1796,[236] the demonstration of the mosquito-borne nature of yellow fever by Finlay in 1881[125] and by Reed et al. in 1900,[431] and Goldberger and Wheeler's induction of pellagra by deficient diet in 1915.[152] In these instances, the interest of the experiments lies in the advances they produced in understanding the etiology of specific diseases, rather than in any contribution to new epidemiologic methods. Today, experimental epidemiology almost invariably encompasses the feature of randomization, predominantly features large numbers of subjects, often involves the collaboration of several groups of investigators, and tends to be multidisciplinary. The extensive resources required demand that all available expertise be brought to bear on the design, conduct, and analysis of such studies; epidemiology is only one of the disciplines involved and usually is not the major one. However, epidemiologic methods may play a special role in the exploration of the systematic bodies of carefully collected data, which are the products of many of these experiments.

In this context, the experiment of Fletcher assessing the protective effect of cured* rice against beriberi was ahead of its time,

---

*Cured rice is rice that is parboiled in its husk prior to milling. In the process of parboiling, the thiamine diffuses from the husk and germ and becomes fixed in the starchy kernel. Subsequent milling does not, therefore, remove the thiamine. "Indian" rice was prepared in this way; "Siamese" rice was milled without parboiling.

although the assignment of individuals was systematic rather than random.[129] In 1905, there was a severe epidemic of beriberi in the Kuala Lumpur Lunatic Asylum. Fletcher described his experiment as follows:

> The lunatics were housed in two exactly similar buildings on opposite sides of a quadrangle surrounded by a high wall. On Dec. 5th [1905] all the lunatics at that time in the hospital were drawn up in the dining shed and numbered off from the left. The odd numbers were subsequently domiciled in the ward on the east side of the courtyard and no alteration was made in their diet, they were still supplied with the same uncured (Siamese) rice as in 1905. The even numbers were quartered in the ward on the west of the quadrangle and received the same rations as the occupants of the other ward, with the exception that they were supplied with cured [Indian] rice. . . . On Dec. 5th there were 59 lunatics in the asylum; of these 29 were put on cured rice and 30 on Siamese rice. The next patient admitted to the asylum was admitted to the Bengal rice ward, and the one admitted after him to the uncured rice ward, the next to cured, and so on alternately to the end of the year. . . .
>
> By June 20th many cases of beri-beri had occurred amongst the patients in the east ward who were eating uncured rice, whereas no cases had occurred in the west ward, the inmates of which were dieted on cured [Indian] rice.
>
> In view of the theory so strongly advocated by Sir Patrick Manson that beri-beri is a place disease, it was thought possible that the east ward was infected. Therefore on June 20th the patients were transposed, those on uncured rice being moved to the west ward and those on cured (Indian) rice transferred to the east. From June 20th to Dec. 31st no beri-beri developed among the patients on cured rice although they were living in a ward were beri-beri had been rife amongst the lunatics who were fed on uncured (Siamese) rice.[129]

In all, among the 120 patients eating uncured rice, there were 34 cases of beriberi and 18 deaths; among the 123 patients assigned to cured rice, there were no deaths and only 2 cases, both of which had been manifest at the time of admission to the asylum.

Experiments of the U.S. Public Health Service, which evaluated the addition of fluoride to drinking water for the prevention of dental caries, should also figure prominently in any historical account of the development of experimental epidemiology. A good review of these experiments is found in Blayney and Hill.[31]

Since the 1970s, large-scale experiments that evaluate the health effects of changing dietary practices, reducing cigarette smoking, controlling blood pressure, and taking preventive medications have added a level of resource allocation and ambition to experimental epidemiology that itself still awaits full evaluation.

In these studies, the disease patterns that are hoped to be disrupted can be changed only slowly and the expected benefits from any given intervention to date have been, in relative terms, considerably smaller than those from some earlier epidemiologic experiments.

Observational Epidemiology in Recent Years

In addition to the large experiments just referred to, in the last few decades, there has been an extraordinary growth in observational epidemiology in general and in observations in large populations in particular, often followed prospectively over long periods of time. Without question, the stimulus that provoked this growth was the demonstration around the mid-1950s of the varied and serious effects cigarette smoking has on people's health. Although a tremendous volume of literature has been written on this problem, the landmark case-control and cohort studies of Doll and Hill[96,97] in 1952 and 1954, respectively, were turning points in society's expectation of what might be achieved by the application of sound epidemiologic methods to the study of chronic disease. The particular problem that these studies addressed turned out to be soluble. The hope that the application of similar methods to other major diseases will be equally fruitful fuels the growth of epidemiology and the support for it that still prevails.

Aims

Knowledge of the distribution of disease may be utilized to understand the causes of disease, explain local disease occurrence, describe the natural history of disease, or provide guidance in the administration and evaluation of health services.

Understanding the Causes of Disease

The most important purpose of epidemiology is to acquire knowledge of the causes of currently nonpreventable diseases. This aim encompasses a number of subsidiary objectives:

1. Develop hypotheses that explain patterns of disease distribution in terms of measurable human characteristics or experiences.
2. Test such hypotheses through specifically designed studies.
3. Aid in the classification of persons who are ill into groups that appear to have etiologic factors in common. Even if the etiologic factors are not identified in full detail, similarity of

epidemiologic behavior may point to etiologic commonalities, even of clinically dissimilar entities. Conversely, differences in the epidemiologic distributions of subgroups of a clinical entity may suggest that such subgroups should be regarded as separate disease entities for purposes of etiologic investigation.

Most frequently, epidemiologists are concerned with elucidating the causes of *disease occurrence.* However, the determinants of the *outcomes* of illness are also appropriate objects for epidemiologic study.[583] Other biologic processes, such as growth, multiple pregnancy, intelligence, and fertility, may also be studied by epidemiologic methods.

It is sometimes suggested that epidemiology should also be concerned with the positive components of health implicit in the definition used by the World Health Organization. According to this definition, "Health is a state of complete physical, mental and social well-being and not merely the absence of disease or infirmity."[605] However, the number of widespread and serious diseases for which the etiology is unknown is more than sufficient to occupy the world's epidemiologists for a long time. Concentration of effort on these diseases is appropriate because of the urgency of their reduction, as well as because of the difficulties of quantitative investigation of concepts that have not been defined in clinical, pathologic, or other terms.

Explaining Local Disease Patterns

Frequently the epidemiologist is concerned not so much with the acquisition of new knowledge about the origin of a disease as with using what is known already about the causes of the disease to understand the particular pattern it exhibits in a local area. For example, the epidemiologist may utilize what is already known about the etiology of typhoid fever to explain and deal with a particular outbreak, and to formulate preventive measures suitable to a particular community. This reasoning process is *deductive* rather than *inductive*, the latter attempting to utilize information from a single set of observations to derive principles that have a greater generality.

A rigid distinction cannot be drawn between deductive and inductive investigations since generalizable knowledge may be derived during the course of any routine study. Nevertheless, in a great deal of epidemiologic work, new generalizable knowledge of disease causation is not being sought. Investigations of localized outbreaks of food poisoning are typical. Currently, due to the limited knowledge of etiologic factors in most other disease, such practical or deductive uses of epidemiology are largely confined to infectious diseases, certain industrial intoxications, and contagion-like outbreaks of social behavior, such as hysteria and drug addiction.

Describing the Natural History of Disease

Although the majority of epidemiologic work is directed toward elucidating causal factors, many of the same methods are used in studies that seek to identify factors related to the course of the disease once established. Thus it is useful to know how the duration of a disease and the probability of various outcomes (e.g., recovery, death, complications) vary by age, gender, geography, and so on. Such information is useful not only for prognostic purposes but also for stimulating hypotheses as to what specific factors may be more directly involved in the patient's outcome and how the latter may be changed in a favorable way.

In addition, the relationships between various measures of disease frequency (discussed in Chapter 4) sometimes allow inferences about the course and duration of a disease when such measures cannot be derived by direct follow up of patients. For example, data on incidence and prevalence of cervical cancer have been used to estimate the average duration of the several stages of this disease.[109,247] Such estimates cannot be made by following patients because once the early disease is diagnosed, its natural course is interrupted by therapy. However, the volume of epidemiologic work in this field is still small.

Administrative Uses

Knowledge of the disease frequency in a population serves a number of administrative purposes. It is essential to the logical planning of facilities for medical care. For example, estimation of the number of hospital beds required for patients with specific diseases (e.g., chronic nephritis, mental illness) or for given segments of the population (e.g., prematurely born infants, the disabled elderly) requires knowledge of the frequency and natural history of the particular diseases or of all diseases in the affected segments of the population. The planning of efficient research, whether diagnostic, therapeutic, or preventive, also requires knowledge of how many cases of a particular disease are likely to be found in a given population during a given period.

Knowledge of the relative frequency of disease in population subgroups is also useful if it enables programs and studies to be directed toward the population segments manifesting the greatest concentrations of the disease. For example, if resources for screening are limited, epidemiologic information should assist in deciding which age, occupational, gender, geographic, or ethnic group should be the target for a program directed against, for example, tuberculosis, diabetes, or cervical cancer. Similar considerations apply to the choice of a population subgroup for any study that requires the maximum yield of cases for a given size of population studied.

Comparison of medical care costs under various systems of its administration and financing form an increasing component of societal activities devoted to the evaluation of medical services. Epidemiology has a role to play here, although it may be a minor one. The interpretation of the types of correlation seen in studies in these fields is often difficult and indeed treacherous, since many processes and features of the system are frequently changing contemporaneously. However, the information must be considered; at the time, it may be the only hard evidence available. For example, our assessment of the efficacy of the diphtheria vaccine still rests predominantly on the temporal correlation between the introduction of the vaccine and the dramatic decline in disease frequency. Such correlations are perhaps more informative when they do *not* exist; that is, when the introduction or presence of a particular medical procedure is *not* associated with the expected changes or differences in disease patterns. For instance, perceived improvements in the clinical management of several common cancers have not been accompanied by a decline in the population mortality, nor has it been established that the declines in mortality expected from putatively more efficacious treatment have been offset by increased incidence of the conditions.

Other Uses

Beyond these rather focused objectives, it behooves society, as a society, to keep accounts of its daily affairs—its numbers, business, experiences, and finances. Surely, among the matters on which society should keep an account is the health status of its members. John Graunt speculated as to the motives of the seventeenth-century parish clerks of London who published the *Bills of Mortality* and of the "several families" who purchased them. He concluded:

> . . . most of them who constantly took in the weekly Bills of Mortality, made little other use of them (than) to look at the foot, how the Burials increased or decreased; And, among the Casualties, what had hap-

pened rare, and extraordinary in the week currant: so as they might take the same as a Text to talk upon, in the next Company; and, withall, in the Plague-time, how the sickness increased, or decreased, that so the Rich might judge of the necessity of their removall, and Tradesmen might conjecture what doings they were like to have in their respective dealings: . . .[158]

Such things are appropriate matters for society to consider and foster. The *Bills of Mortality* have been replaced by an exquisitely refined power to detect antigens, the products of gene damage, the identification of substances found in the tissues and in the environment in only minute amounts, and a host of other technical miracles. These advances offer tremendous opportunities for the strengthening of epidemiologic studies but, as Graunt implied, one should keep an open mind as to what ultimate practical benefit may follow from the opening of a new source of knowledge.

2 Concepts of Cause

Definition

A principal objective in epidemiology is to identify alterable causes of disease. It is therefore necessary to understand, first, what we mean by *a cause*, and, second, what the basis is for forming categories of individuals who are said to have *a disease*. This chapter outlines concepts of cause that have particular relevance to epidemiology, and Chapter 3 deals with the creation of disease categories.

Certain events tend to follow others in time. Some of these temporal associations have qualities that lead the observer to think of them as cause and effect—the earlier event being denoted the cause of the later. The repeated observation of sequences of similar events gives confidence that a particular effect is likely to succeed a particular cause. However, as Hume noted: "We are never able, in a single instance, to discover any power or necessary connection, any quality which binds the effect to the cause, and renders the one an infallible consequence of the other. We only find that one does actually, in fact, follow the other."[223]

What, then, leads us to think of certain relationships as causal and others as noncausal? The word *cause* is an abstract noun and, like the word "truth," will have different meanings in different contexts. No definition will be equally appropriate in all branches of science. Epidemiology has the practical objective of discovering relationships that offer possibilities of disease prevention and, for this purpose, a causal association may usefully be defined as an association between categories of events or characteristics in which an alteration in the frequency or quality of one category is followed by a change in the other category. It may not always be possible to demonstrate this alteration, since a change in the supposed cause may be undesirable or impossible. This is the case, for example, of many presumed cause–effect relationships in the area of gender or age. Nevertheless, the belief that the presumed effect *would* change if the cause changed is the defining concept of the causal relationships that are meaningful in epidemiology.

Types of Association

To clarify the implications of the use of the term *causal association*, we describe some of the ways in which categories of events or circumstances may be related. A *category* of items means all those individual items that have the characteristics that define the category and that permit the individual items to be considered in those respects as a single entity. Associations can be studied only for categories or groups, not for individual items. With respect to each other, two categories of items may be:

A. Not statistically associated (independent)
B. Statistically associated
   1. Noncausal
   2. Causal
      a. Indirectly causal
      b. Directly causal

This classification illustrates a common progression in the investigation of a relationship—from demonstration of statistical association to demonstration that the association is causal, and then to evaluation of its directness.

Statistical Association

If one category of events occurs in a certain proportion, x, of a population and another category in another proportion, y, the two category-defining events will occur together among some members of the population by chance alone, in a proportion equal to the product of the separate proportions, xy.

When one of these categories is a disease and the other category is an attribute or experience of persons, there will be a number of individuals who exhibit both the disease and the experience by chance. While the disease and the experience are, in a nontechnical sense, *associated* in these individuals, this is not evidence of *statistical association*. Statistical association, or simply *association* in the epidemiological sense, means that the proportion of persons exhibiting both events is either higher or lower than the proportion predicted on the basis of the independent frequencies of the two categories, by a degree that is not likely due to chance.

While the content of the previous paragraph is obvious enough, its main implication, that statistical associations are determined for categories, not for individual persons, is not always heeded. For example, suppose that 100 persons are inoculated with a vaccine against an infectious disease and that 100 persons indistinguishable from the first group receive a placebo. During a subsequent epidemic in which the two groups have similar exposures to the disease, 20 of the vaccinated persons and 50 of the unvaccinated persons contract the disease. Because this difference is unlikely to be due to chance, we can conclude that a statistical association exists between vaccination and remaining free of disease. Because we assume that the two groups are in all respects (other than their vaccination) indistinguishable, we judge that this association is probably a causal one. However, it is not possible to say that the vaccination caused any individual person in the vaccinated set to remain disease free, because there were instances of vaccinated persons who contracted the disease and of unvaccinated persons who remained disease free. Within the framework of these results, it is even possible that there were persons who contracted the disease *because* they were vaccinated. This has occurred in the context of vaccines that were overall protective.[375]

However, information from the experience of a category of individuals may suggest the *likelihood* of causal association in an individual instance. The stronger the association between the two categories of events revealed by the group experience, the more likely the assumption of causal association in an individual instance is to be correct. Thus if the disease frequency was 99% in the unvaccinated series and was 1% in the vaccinated series, there would be a high probability that the absence of disease in any one vaccinated individual was a consequence of the vaccination. Therefore, the hypothesis that the absence of disease in any one vaccinated individual was causally related to his or her vaccination status most likely would be correct. The validity of the statement rests, however, on the total experience and not on observations made on that individual (other than that he or she was vaccinated and disease free).

Rizzi and Pedersen suggest a distinction between "singular causality," as in a specific patient, and "general causation," as in "disease etiology."[442] They state that "Knowledge of a causal connection of a general kind, may be the result of determining causality in an array of singular cases," and, noting Kassirer's view of the clinical context,[248] "we need and utilize knowledge of general causal relations to identify and explain causal relations between singular events." These comments appear to reflect the same principle expressed in the previous paragraph.

Causal and Noncausal Association

Only a minority of statistical associations are causal in the sense that change in one party to the association alters the other party. Leaving aside false associations that result from errors of information or selection (the latter are discussed later in the context of specific study designs), noncausal statistical associations usually result from the association of both categories with a third category. Thus, if A is causally associated with both B and C (i.e., A precedes and influences both B and C), B and C will also be associated. However, the association between B and C is noncausal, since there is no prospect of altering C by manipulating B, or vice versa. This type of association is common, and the role of C is said to be *confounding*. An example is provided by the facts that high serum cholesterol (A) is associated with coronary heart disease (CHD) (B) in a way that, although not fully understood, appears to be causal, and that persons with very high serum cholesterol levels tend to develop visible, protruding cholesterol deposits in the eyelids (xanthomata) (C). There is, therefore, an association between the presence of xanthomata and risk of CHD. However, the association between B and C is noncausal because removal of the xanthomata would not change the individuals' risk of CHD. The association between xanthoma and CHD is said to be *confounded* by the *confounder*, high serum cholesterol. Several other examples and the ways that confounding appears and can be dealt with in different types of epidemiologic study are described in several books and articles, as well as later in this text.

Once a statistical association has been demonstrated, how can it be determined whether it is causal; that is, whether B changes if A is altered. The most convincing evidence is obtained by experiment, by changing A alone and observing B. Although available to the laboratory worker, this method frequently is not possible in humans. Further, in certain associations, the presumed cause may not be susceptible to manipulation. Although knowledge of whether the relationship is causal in such a situation may be of little immediate value, it may nevertheless be important in identifying causal agents that *may* be manipulatable in other situations.

A number of researchers have suggested criteria for judging the likelihood of an association being causal in the absence of experimental evidence. A comprehensive review of these, along with illustrative examples has recently been offered by Evans.[120]

The early postulates of Koch[535] (more appropriately the Henle–Koch postulates), although well thought of for many decades, are limited in their application to the microbial determinants of disease and, as we show in Chapter 3, are in part tautologous. A list of nine criteria was presented by Bradford Hill in 1965.[208] According to Susser,[522] this list essentially summarizes the criteria used by various epidemiologists in the 1950s, but according to Morabia,[367] it bears some resemblances to rules that had been expressed by Hume some 225 years earlier.[223] The Bradford Hill criteria are much broader in their application than those of Henle–Koch, and they have been influential, indeed up to the present day.[437] However, some of Hill's criteria (e.g., specificity) were not well defined, one (biologic gradient) is often too strictly interpreted, and others (plausibility and coherence) seem to overlap. In the 1960 edition of this text,[316] we suggested that it is essential to consider three aspects when attempting to distinguish causal from noncausal associations: time sequence, strength of association, and consistency with existing knowledge.

Time Sequence
For a relationship to be causal, the events that are considered the causes must precede those thought to be the effects. When the sequence of events cannot be determined with certainty (a common situation in chronic diseases), there must be at least the possibility that such a sequence exists.

Strength of Association
The stronger the association between categories of events (specifically, the higher the ratio of the frequency of B following A to the frequency of B in the absence of A), the more likely is it that the association is causal. If the suspected cause is a quantitative variable, the existence of an exposure–response relationship—that is, an association in which the frequency of the effect increases (or decreases) as the exposure to the putative cause increases—is usually thought to favor a causal relationship, although even in a causal association, such a relationship may not exist over the whole range of exposure levels.[34] Further, there are many examples of well-established causal relationships (e.g., single major gene effects) in which the cause is dichotomous (e.g., present or absent) and in which exposure–response relationships are neither expected nor observed.

Consistency with Existing Knowledge
Here, several considerations come into play:

1. Evidence that the disease distribution in populations accords with the distribution of the supposed cause, particularly when such evidence is not part of the information that suggested the hypothesis in the first place, supports a causal hypothesis. Major discrepancies in the concordance that are not reconcilable in terms of other components of the causal picture weaken the hypothesis of causation.

2. The more extensive the efforts that have been made to identify noncausal explanations of the association, the more likely one is to believe that the association is causal.

3. A causal hypothesis is supported by invocation of cellular or subcellular mechanisms that make the hypothesis seem "reasonable" in light of current biological knowledge. The knowledge may be preexistent or it may come from attempts to reproduce the supposed effect in laboratory animals or other biological systems. Success in demonstrating the association in animals or in identifying a plausible micromechanism will usually profoundly increase the acceptance of an epidemiological hypothesis. However, failure to reproduce in another species an association noted in man may simply be a reflection of the uniqueness of the human in that respect. Similarly, failure to identify a biological mechanism for an observed relationship may be the result of limited available techniques or even knowledge. The process of contagion, the transmission of cholera and typhoid by the fecal–oral route, the origin of many diseases due to nutritional deficiency, the deleterious effects of cigarette smoke on health, and alterable risk factors for coronary artery disease were all identified as causal with sufficient certainty to provide means of prevention well before underlying micromechanisms were established.

Susser adds to the criteria discussed above "predictive performance" and "specificity."[521] Predictive performance is certainly a strong indicator of causal potential, and it is encompassed to some extent in the paragraph on Strength of Association, outlined above. With respect to specificity, however, one has to be careful how this term is used. It is probably true that the more specifically the cause is defined (e.g., hepatitis B virus rather than any hepatitis virus) and the more specific the supposed effect (e.g., hepatocellular carcinoma rather than cancer), the stronger is the hypothesis. This is essentially because the more specific the hypothesis, the easier it is to test and the better the opportunity for refutation. However, lack of specificity of the effect of a particular cause is not solid ground for doubting its causal relationship to any one of the effects it may produce. In fact, there are many important examples of substances that have effects on virtually every system of the human body, including cigarette smoke, alcohol, and endogenous estrogens, to name a few.

The evaluation of the causal nature of a relationship in the absence of direct experiment is neither easy nor entirely objective. Differences of opinion resulting from subjective assembly and interpretation of evidence, as well as differences in prior beliefs, are common. Caution in judging relationships to be causal is laudable. On occasion, however, such caution is carried to an unrealistic extreme and may indeed be simply a cover for dislike of the consequences of accepting a relationship as causal. When the derivation of experimental evidence is either impractical or unethical, there comes a point in the accumulation of observational evidence when it might be more prudent to act on the assumption that the association is causal rather than to await further evidence. If there is controversy, it should center around the question of whether that point has been reached and not on the unanswerable question of whether the causal hypothesis is proven.

This may be an appropriate place to take note of the concern expressed by Petitti that the word *effect* has at least two quite distinct meanings that should not be confused.[407] In the world of statistical modeling it means simply association, as in "the main effects" or "the effect estimate." It has no causal connotation. However, in less technical writing when we say A effects B there is a clear implication that A changes (and, therefore, causes) B. A breach of the need to distinguish statistical association from causal association was seen in a report prepared for the Government of Australia purporting to estimate the number of deaths in the population caused by alcohol consumption. The estimate was far too high because all associations between alcohol use and specific diseases were assumed to be causal.[309]

Direct and Indirect Causal Association

Causal associations may be direct or indirect. Thus, if A causes D and D causes B, there will be a causal relationship between A and B, but the association may be thought of as indirect since it operates via two other causal associations. The distinction between direct and indirect causal relationships is a relative one, perceived directness depending on the extent of current knowledge. For example, in prepenicillin days syphilis was treated by intravenous injection of neoarsphenamine (salvarsan). Jaundice was a common complication of this treatment and was known as "salvarsan icterus." It became evident, however, that the icterus was associated not with the salvarsan but with the use of inadequately cleaned syringes. Poor syringe hygiene then became the direct cause of the disease. However, since a certain number of icterus cases would presumably be prevented by failure to inject salvarsan, the association of syphilis treatment with icterus, in terms of our definition, was a causal one, although indirectly so. Further investigation revealed that the responsible agent was not simply the uncleanliness of the syringes but the presence in them of minute amounts of human serum remaining from previous use. The disease became known as serum hepatitis. Later, it became known that the hepatitis was associated directly not with the serum, but with the presence in the serum of hepatitis B virus. Thus the association with the virus became considered the direct one and that with the serum indirect, resulting in another name change, from serum to viral hepatitis B. Further studies may reveal what specific attributes or molecular components of the virus might be considered more direct causal factors of disease. Knowledge of causal mechanisms is rarely refined to the degree that makes it possible to state that *this* is the ultimate direct association and that no other associations intervene.

The practical significance of causal associations does not necessarily depend on their degree of directness. First, more direct associations may not yet have been identified and so there may be no choice but to make use of obviously indirect associations in preventive programs. For example, knowledge of the association of freedom from scurvy with diets containing fresh fruits and vegetables was put to use by Captain James Cook and others many decades before the identification of vitamin C, and prevention of smallpox antedates modern virology by almost 200 years. Second, more direct causes, although known, may not be susceptible to alteration for economic or other practical reasons, whereas the indirect ones may be. For example, preventive measures against viral hepatitis (as well as AIDS and other blood-related viruses) are still largely directed against poor syringe hygiene, as well as against contamination of the material to be injected. Decades after the discovery of the microorganisms associated with typhoid, cholera, and other enteric disease, preventive measures still focus, at least in the developed nations, on the provision of clean food and water, even though disease-specific vaccines of modest efficacy are available against many of these illnesses.

The Web of Causation

In this chapter, we discuss the types of association that can exist between two sets of events. In fact, effects are not dependent on single causes. The concept of chains of causation, although useful, has the defect of oversimplification. In Figure 2-1, some of the components that enter into the causal association between treatment for syphilis and viral hepatitis are shown. An equally complex picture could be drawn to illustrate the antecedents of infection with the virus of AIDS. When it is considered that only a few of the major components can be shown in such a chart, that these are indicated as broad classes of events rather than as multiple events that make up each class, that each component shown is itself the result of a complex genealogy of antecedents, and that the myriad effects of these components other than those contributing to the development of icterus are not shown, then it becomes evident that chains of causation represent only a fraction of reality, and the whole setting should be thought of more appropriately as a web, which in its complexity lies quite beyond our understanding.

Further, many such webs may exist for a given disease. There are many more ways in which to acquire viral hepatitis than by undergoing salvarsan treatment for syphilis—indeed today that would be one of the rarest ways of acquiring it—and several ways to acquire the AIDS virus other than by sexual intercourse with an infected person. Each of these ways has its own antecedents and its own causal web.

Necessary and Sufficient Causes

That diseases have multiple causes is a truism, and one that is frequently invoked as a synonym for ignorance. If a disease appears to have a single principal cause, it is for one of two reasons: Either we *know* of only one cause, or we have *defined* the disease in terms of a single cause, sometimes referred to as a *necessary* cause. The arbitrariness of defining necessary causes is discussed in Chapter 3. When using the term *multiple causation*, it is useful to consider which of its several implications it is being used: (1) the multitude of individual circumstances that must exist or occur in sequence such that the effect necessarily follows—this multiplicity of causes is sometimes referred to as the *sufficient* cause, a hypothetical concept of all the necessary elements, most of which are rarely, if ever, known to us; (2) the fact that each of these individual circumstances has its own causal web; or (3) the fact that a single disease (i.e., a category of which the members are currently indistinguishable to us in terms of pathological or chemical findings, symptoms, and prognosis) may result from several webs of sufficient causes that may or may not have components in common.

Rothman has proposed a theoretical framework within which

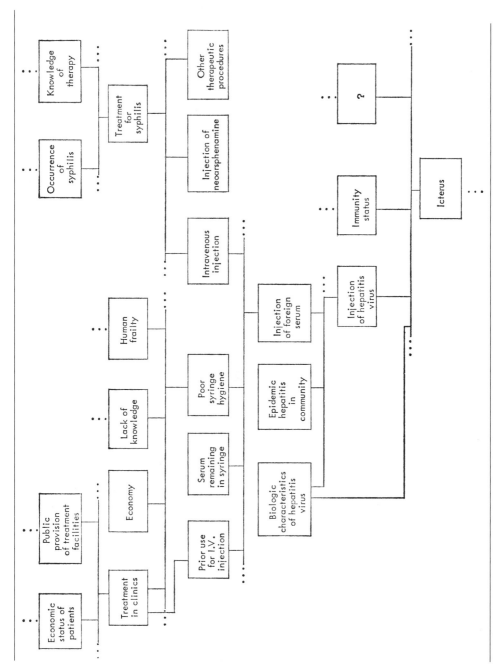

Figure 2-1. Some components of the association between icterus and the treatment of syphilis around 1940.

the terms sufficient and necessary causes are given more specific meanings than are indicated above.[463,466] In this model, a given disease is considered to have a finite number of constellations of sufficient causes. Each constellation is made up of a number of component causes, all of which must be present for the disease to occur. The component causes may be present in more than one of the constellations. If a component cause is a member of all the constellations that are sufficient causes for that disease, it would be a necessary cause of the disease. For example, for a woman, having a uterus would be a necessary cause of endometrial cancer. The construct may eventually be a useful one in thinking about the relationships between component causes; that is, in considering whether the joint effect of two component causes would be different if they were or were not members of the same causal constellation. However, currently, we have so little information about the different causes of any single disease that it is hard to evaluate the practical value of the intellectually appealing model. With regard to the term *necessary cause* in this context, we do not even know whether there is any disease for which we know of all the causal constellations, and it is hard to know how we would know when that goal was achieved, except when the word "necessary" is used in the defining sense referred to earlier.

Fortunately, it is not necessary to understand causal mechanisms in their entirety to effect preventive measures. Knowledge of even one small component may allow significant prevention. Thus in the days of salvarsan, and today in a different context, it is helpful to know that the sterilization of intravenous needles provides substantial, although not complete, protection against the acquisition of viral hepatitis. It is not necessary to know how the virus got onto the needle before it was sterilized or the immunologic status of the patient to be injected, even though these are important components of the causal web. Our knowledge of the causal web underlying lung cancer, of which cigarette smoke is one component, is extremely limited, but it is beyond question that lung cancer would be reduced to about one-tenth of its present frequency by the elimination of exposure to cigarette smoke.

3 Grouping of Ill Persons and Classification of Disease

As noted in Chapter 2, inferences that an association between two events or characteristics is more than random can be made only when the elements of the association are considered in groups or categories. Such inferences cannot be made from observation of individuals or specific events or circumstances. The grouping of events or individuals into categories is therefore essential to causal inference. The basic objective is to form groups that allow generalizations regarding the behavior of features of group members in some dimension other than that used in its formation.[204] This chapter considers specifically the creation of categories of ill persons for such purposes. Thus, a disease entity based on similarity of symptoms and signs would be useful if it allowed generalizations regarding its causes or its prognosis. Likewise, an entity based on identity or similarity of cause would be of service if it allowed prediction of the symptoms and signs that occurred in exposed persons or of the course of the illness.

The process of disease classification has two components. First, ill persons are grouped into categories such that the characteristics of the members of each category permit them to be distinguished from the members of another category. These categories are then viewed as being disease entities, and the members of a set are thought of as having *a* disease. This results in the creation of a terminology (*nosology*) or *nomenclature*. The second part of the process is the arrangement of the components of this nomenclature into groups thought to have common characteristics (*a classification*).

Grouping of Ill Persons

The creation of disease entities involves the grouping of ill persons into categories that are believed to have utility in the management of their illness or in understanding the circumstance that led to it. There is a common perception that the grouping of ill persons involves the search for categories that are in some sense *natural* (often thought of as carving nature "at the joints"), as distinct from *artificial* (categories that are created by man without regard to the natural features of the things being categorized). It is believed that artificial categories should be used only if natural ones are unclear. This is true to a very limited extent. Experts in different disciplines (e.g., anatomy, biochemistry, genetics) may take quite different views as to the "naturalness" of the boundaries of accepted disease categories, and categories that appear natural at one point may not appear so in light of new knowledge. All disease entities currently recognized represent artificial categories created by humans and constructed more for utility than for "naturalness."

Manifestational and Causal Entities

Two distinct types of criteria are used to categorize ill persons.

1. Manifestational criteria: Ill persons are grouped according to similarity of symptoms, signs, changes in body chemistry or tissues, behavior, prognosis, or some combination of these features. Examples of diseases defined by manifestational criteria are fractures, diabetes mellitus, mental retardation, the common cold, schizophrenia, and breast cancer.

2. Causal criteria: Causal grouping depends on the similarity of individuals with respect to one or more experiences believed to be the cause of their illness. Examples of diseases defined by causal criteria are birth trauma, silicosis, syphilis, lead poisoning, and, in principle, AIDS.

There is no logical reason to suppose that ill persons classified together by manifestational or causal criteria will remain as a group if the other type of criterion is used. For example, the identification of the tubercle bacillus by Koch[264] led to the belief, subsequently justified, that action against this particular component of the cause of the illness offered good prospects for both therapy and control of transmission. It consequently became the practice to group ill persons as having a disease of which this bacillus was one of the causes—*tuberculosis*. This led to a classification that grouped individuals from several of the manifestational entities in the nosologies of preceding times. In 1785, Cullen's classification of ill persons[79] consisted of the four manifestational cate-

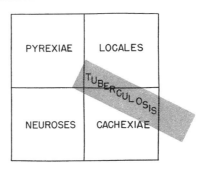

Figure 3-1. Classification of persons with active tuberculosis (an etiologic entity) according to the manifestational classification of Cullen.[79]

gories indicated in Figure 3-1. Each of the four categories included patients who today would be considered as having tuberculosis, including some outside the box in Figure 3-1 who might not be considered ill at all if the *bacillus* were not found in their sputum.

Examples can be found of close correspondence between the categories created by the two types of grouping. Thus, the gross manifestations of rubeola are so distinctive that a group of persons classified together on the basis of similarity of manifestations corresponds closely to the group of persons exposed to the rubeola virus in the absence of protective antibodies, and the manifestations of rabies are so characteristic that the causal and manifestational groupings would contain virtually the same individuals. Even when the gross manifestations of a causal entity seem heterogeneous, a more detailed examination of manifestations may be found that gives unity to the seemingly heterogeneous group. For example, the histologic lesion (tubercle) of tuberculosis is a manifestation common to *most* persons with illness caused by the tubercle bacillus. Therefore, the correspondence between the group of persons with illness presumed to be caused by the tubercle bacillus (causal criterion) and the group characterized by the histologic presence of tubercles (manifestational criterion) would be quite close. Such unifying manifestations are by no means common, however, and it is important to recognize that considerable disruption of existing disease categories may result from a decision to change the axis of definition for diseases currently based on manifestational criteria. This point is made by consideration of the variety of manifestational "diseases" that were combined to create the disease category *syphilis* when the role of the *Treponema pallidum* was discovered and utilized for categorization.

Appreciation of the lack of necessary congruence between the two ways of grouping ill persons is important to epidemiologists from the following points of view.

1. Polymorphous effects (manifestations) of newly isolated causal agents may be understood, indeed expected. For example, the fact that cigarette smoking is associated with several diseases other than lung cancer was used as an argument for several years against the acceptance of the association with lung cancer as causal; it was argued that truly causal agents would have more specific effects.[25] In fact, even if cigarette smoke contained only a single disease-causing agent, past experience would lead to the expectation of a diversity of effects.

2. It can be understood that an agent causally associated with a certain manifestational disease entity may not be causally involved with all of the ill persons with a particular manifestation. Following the identification of a causal association, the examination of disease subcategories may lead to refinement of the manifestational entity associated with the identified cause. For example, different pathologic varieties of lung cancer vary substantially in the strength of their association with cigarette smoking. Moreover, because of a lack of appropriate techniques, such subcategories may not be identifiable manifestationally even if they exist. For example, no particular manifestational category of coronary artery disease has been found to be associated with cigarette smoking, although the high frequency of the disease in nonsmokers indicates clearly that cigarette smoking is not involved in all cases of the disease.

3. The arbitrariness of the distinction between necessary causes, those without which the disease does not occur, and contributing causes will be realized. Thus, *Mycobacterium tuberculosis* is often spoken of as the necessary cause of tuberculosis, and other causal factors such as age, nutritional status, poverty, and genetic factors are considered contributing factors. Most commonly, the chosen factor is the necessary cause only by definition, in the same sense that automobiles are the necessary causes of automobile accidents. Thus, *M. tuberculosis* may be the necessary cause of tuberculosis as it is presently defined, but if medical knowledge had developed differently, many patients now categorized as having tuberculosis might have been included in a category defined on the basis of a specific nutritional defect. In this case, the nutritional factor would have been the necessary cause and the bacillus the contributing factor. It may be pointed out that one of the postulates attributed to Henle–Koch,[535] mentioned in Chapter 2 as a set of criteria to be used in establishing a causal association, is that the bacteriological causes of a disease should be found "in all cases of the disease in question." This is in fact an example of circular reasoning because the postulate implies that the microorganism is the cause of an already defined manifestational entity. In reality, however, the presence of the "disease in question" is defined in terms of the presence of the organism. As a corollary, the risk of disease among people exposed to the disease-defining factor is *infinitely* larger than the (null) risk among people not exposed.

4. It can be understood that not all persons experiencing the cause will acquire the disease. For example, although there is a definite causal association between the tubercle bacillus and tuberculosis, evidence of internalization of the bacillus is found in many persons who have no evidence of illness, just as many persons who smoke cigarettes do not develop lung cancer.

Selection of Criteria for Creation of New Disease Entities

As already suggested, the distinction between natural and artificial categories is rarely a useful one. Linnaeus' system of dividing plants into 24 classes according to the number of stamens and pistils in the flower is often cited as an example of an artificial system, whereas classifications that fit in with the current evidence on plant evolution are said to be natural. During a time not yet influenced by Darwinian theory it does not seem unnatural that differences between plants in the number of stamens were considered important; however, the usefulness of the Darwinian concept of species as the basis for a natural classification is itself now questioned.[114]

Furthermore, the particular interest of the observer determines to a large extent the kind of criteria selected. For example, for preventive purposes it is important to classify injuries by external cause, whereas manifestational aspects of injuries are essential for therapeutic and prognostic purposes. Usefulness for particular purposes is a major determinant of the type of criterion used for grouping of ill persons in medicine.

In the absence of knowledge of causal factors, manifestational criteria provide the only basis for categorization. In this case, setting limits of disease entities is a highly intuitive process, having as a governing principle the assumption that the greater the similarity of manifestations the more properly the illness may be considered an entity. The manifestational criteria are not limited to signs and symptoms but may include prognosis, as determined from previous subjects, and laboratory findings. Even when the basic criterion is manifestational, the definition of the disease may have experiential components. Thus, whereas Balkan nephropathy is primarily a manifestational entity, the adjective "Balkan" carries (unknown) etiologic implications, strengthened by the appearance of the disease in long-term residents of particular villages.[55] The manifestation "mesothelioma" has such strong correlation with a known etiology (asbestos exposure) that it also carries subliminal etiologic connotations that are sometimes strengthened by appropriate investigation.[475]

As causal factors are identified for manifestational entities, some are used to define new disease entities around etiologic factors. Predominant among these have been entities created around microbial agents because a great deal of experience and knowledge has been developed about ways of preventing and/or treating such entities. The acceptance of an agent as the basis for creation of a new disease entity stems from the perceived usefulness, for preventive or therapeutic purposes, of the categories created. Some newly discovered causal agents have not been used to develop new disease entities. For example, "cigarette smoker's disease," which could incorporate most cases of emphysema, carcinoma of the lung, and peripheral vascular disease, as well as some cases of coronary artery disease and bladder cancer, might be a useful entity from the preventive point of view. Yet, therapy remains the predominant purpose of medicine, and from that point of view it is much more useful to categorize the individuals with the various components of cigarette smoker's disease together with individuals with the same manifestations but different causal experiences. Because the objective of prevention is not seriously jeopardized in this instance by retaining the existing manifestational entities, it is unlikely that the concept of cigarette smoker's disease will replace the current manifestational entities shared by persons with a history of cigarette smoking.

Use of one way of grouping ill persons does not exclude concurrent use of another. Thus, the emergency department of a hospital may categorize injured persons into manifestational entities such as fractures, sprains, concussions, and cases of internal injury, whereas an accident prevention program is more likely to use causal criteria such as automobile accidents, fire, falls, and industrial accidents. Neither purpose is more correct or more natural than the other.

Role of Epidemiologic Observations

The epidemiologist frequently has no alternative but to undertake studies based on manifestational entities and to hope that the manifestations have strong enough ties to etiologic factors to allow for identification of such factors. The results of a successful study may reveal causal criteria from which revised groupings of ill persons can be made. Thus, creation of disease entities is not only a prerequisite for epidemiologic study but also one of its goals.

Even in the absence of identification of causal associations, epidemiologic criteria may be used to categorize groups of persons with specific manifestational diseases. For example, Caverly, describing an outbreak of paralytic disease in Vermont in the summer of 1894, included the season of the year during which the outbreak occurred[56] in his argument that it is a distinct disease (poliomyelitis). The classic distinction between typhus and typhoid fever by Lombard was based on differences between the disease he saw in Ireland and the one he saw in France and Switzerland.[294] In addition to differences in post-mortem findings, Lombard noted that the Irish disease (typhus) occasionally attacked breast-feeding infants, the elderly, and nurses and others attending the sick, whereas in France and Switzerland breast-feeding infants and the elderly were never attacked by the illness (typhoid) and hospital attendants were seldom attacked. These features attracted his attention to the existence of difference in the clinical manifestations of the two diseases, which up to that point had not been noted.

Epidemiologic observations may be sufficient to justify separation of disease entities, even in the absence of observable manifestational differences. For example, the 1909 edition of Osler's *The Principles and Practice of Medicine*[391] describes an entity known as infectious jaundice and notes that Weil had recently categorized a group of cases (Weil's disease) because "the cases occurred in groups, and in a very large proportion in butchers." This subgroup was subsequently shown to be caused by a specific spirochete. Other subgroups of the entity "infectious jaundice" that were identified on epidemiological grounds prior to the isolation of specific microbial agents, including "infectious hepatitis" and "serum hepatitis," are now attributed to specific viruses.[1]

Occasionally, epidemiological evidence suggests that two categories may usefully be merged, at least for the purpose of investigation of etiology. For example, similarities of anencephaly and spina bifida with respect to gender, socioeconomic status, ethnicity, and parity, as well as trends of frequency over time (see Figure 1-1) and the occurrence of both anomalies in the same sibships, provide a reasonable basis for considering them as one causal entity rather than two.[315] However, epidemiological evidence suggests less commonly that categories may be usefully merged than it suggests the separation of categories into subgroups. Furthermore, because categories that can be usefully merged for studies of etiology must still be considered as separate entities for the purpose of therapy, such evidence does not usually lead to revision of existing categories.

Classification of Disease Entities

As noted previously, creation of groups into which ill persons are categorized is followed by assigning names to the categories. This results in a *nomenclature* or *nosology*, a listing of disease names, and, beyond that, a *classification* of those disease names into categories that seem to bear some biological relationship to each other. The process of creating a classification is often even more arbitrary than that which led to the nomenclature. Nevertheless, agreement on some standard nosology and classification on a working basis, however arbitrary, is essential for communication between workers in a field.

Unlike the creation of entities of disease, the process of disease classification has little immediate relevance to the practitioner of medicine. Its usefulness lies primarily in efforts to achieve standardization and, therefore, comparability in the methods of presentation of mortality and morbidity data over time and across geographic and political boundaries.

Yet, similar to the process of defining disease entities, the process of classification is driven by the purposes of the classification. An *International Classification of Disease, Injuries and Causes of Death* (ICD), now the *International Statistical Classification of Diseases and Related Health Problems*, has been prepared and published by various international organizations since 1900. The ICD is now the responsibility of the World Health Organization (WHO); it is revised approximately decennially and is now in its tenth edition.[608] The difficulties and complexities of creating a classification that is intellectually satisfying is illustrated by the major groupings of the ICD-10 listed in Table 3-1. Most of the categories are based simply on the organ system affected by the disease (e.g., III: Diseases of the blood, VI: Diseases of the nervous system, XI: Diseases of the digestive system) with no implication that the disease entities within that category share any commonality of either manifestational or experiential criteria; largely, however, these categories are based on manifestational criteria because there are few causal criteria to follow. Two catego-

Table 3-1. Major Categories of the International Classification of Diseases and Related Health Problems (10th Revision)

Chapter	Title
I	Certain infectious and parasitic diseases
II	Neoplasms
III	Diseases of the blood
IV	Endocrine, nutritional, and metabolic disorders
V	Mental and behavioral disorders
VI	Diseases of the nervous system
VII	Diseases of the eye and adnexa
VIII	Diseases of the ear and mastoid process
IX	Diseases of the circulatory system
X	Diseases of the respiratory system
XI	Diseases of the digestive system
XII	Diseases of the skin and subcutaneous tissue
XIII	Diseases of the musculoskeletal system and connective tissue
XIV	Diseases of the genitourinary system
XV	Pregnancy, childbirth, and the puerperium
XVI	Certain conditions originating in the perinatal period
XVII	Congenital malformations, deformations, and chromosomal abnormalities
XVIII	Symptoms, signs, and abnormal clinical and laboratory findings, not elsewhere classified
XIX	Injury, poisoning, and certain other consequences of external causes
XX	External causes of morbidity and mortality
XXI	Factors influencing health status and contact with health services

Source: World Health Organization. International Statistical Classification of Diseases and Related Health Problems. Tenth Revision. Geneva: World Health Organization, 1992.

ries (I: Certain infectious and parasitic diseases and XX: External causes of morbidity and mortality) appear to be based primarily on experiential criteria, but some component of manifestational criteria is present in most of the members of the category. At least one category, II: Neoplasms, is based on an intuitive belief that there is a basic common pathway that underlies them all; however, this belief is wholly intuitive and there are many experiential and manifestational features that distinguish individual diseases within the neoplasm category. The predominance of manifestational categories reflects the ignorance of causes or the lack of ability to change causes that are known.

The individual components that make up the categories (chapters of the ICD) are also extremely heterogeneous; indeed, some of them appear to refer to conditions that one might hesitate to think of as either "diseases" or "related health problems." Chapter XV, for example, contains items as diverse as 080: Single spontaneous delivery, 030: Multiple gestation, and 088: Obstetric embolism. Although some of the chapters of the classification may be used to provide very crude estimates of the dimensions of certain problems in a community (e.g., infectious disease, reproductive problems, congenital malformations, external causes of injury), the ICD does not really serve the purpose of a classification but a nosology to provide a numerical identifier to facilitate for administrative or research purposes the compilation of groups of individuals for whom the same or similar diagnoses have been made.

Although used since its inception and now almost universally for the coding of causes of death for national and international statistics, the ICD lacks the detail that is often needed for morbidity statistics and for use by medical record librarians and by third party payers. In the mid-1970s, efforts led primarily by the United States were initiated to develop a nosology that would be compatible with the ICD in its topographical headings but that would provide the detail needed for clinical purposes, which to that point were served by various nosologies having no compatibility with the ICD. The *International Classification of Diseases, 9th Revision, Clinical Modification* (ICD9.CM) is published in the United States and is now in its fourth (1994) edition.[70] It is completely compatible with the ICD9 and is required for reporting diseases, diagnoses, and procedures to all Public Health Service and Health Care Financing Administration programs. It has greatly increased the value of such programs as sources of epidemiological data.

WHO has also published an *International Classification of Procedures in Medicine* (two volumes), covering diagnostic, preventive, surgical, and radiological procedures, as well as drugs and biological agents,[606] and an *International Classification of Impairments, Disabilities, and Handicaps*, a classification relating to the consequences of diseases, impairments, disabilities, and handicaps.[607]

Mental Disorders

Unprecedented efforts have been made in the last few decades to assemble a replicable nomenclature and classification for diseases of the mind. The American Psychiatric Association published the first edition of its *Diagnostic and Statistical Manual* (DSM) in 1952 and a fourth edition (DSM-IV) in 1994.[8] The classification is compatible with the corresponding section of the ICD but it is more detailed, and, because it indicates the clinical boundaries of the entities that it classifies, it is a nomenclature as well as a classification. Under the sponsorship of the National Institute of Mental Health (NIMH), a *Diagnostic Interview Schedule* (DIS) has been developed, widely tested, and broadly accepted. The responses to the DIS translate readily into the diagnostic categories of the DSM-IV. The DIS has been found to have high replicability whether administered by psychiatrists or laypersons with short training.[449] These two instruments, and the extensive scale on which they are being applied (e.g., in the Epidemiologic Catchment Area studies sponsored by NIMH[450]), offer the opportunity to substantially quicken the pace at which the knowledge of the epidemiology of mental illness has been growing.[550]

Neoplasms

In the same way that the ICD did not satisfy many clinical statistical purposes, the neoplasm section of the ICD was inadequate for clinical trials and other clinical statistics and research. The *International Classification of Disease for Oncology* (ICD-O) was first published in 1976 and is now in its second edition.[405] In a 10-digit code, the ICD-O provides for tumor categorization related to topography (four digits, adapted from and compatible with the categories of the ICD-10); morphology (four digits, adapted from the former Manual of Tumor Nomenclature and Coding of the American Cancer Society); "behavior" or degree of malignancy (e.g., benign or malignant [one digit]); and histologic grade and tumor differentiation (one digit). Although the neoplasms section of the ICD remains adequate for most epidemiological purposes, the ICD-O is increasingly used in clinical settings and in epidemiological studies involving morphology and other items not provided in the ICD.

4 Measures of Disease Frequency

This chapter describes some measures of disease frequency, particularly those that permit comparisons between populations or between subgroups within a population.

Incidence and Prevalence

Population measures of disease frequency are of one of two types, corresponding somewhat to the two ways in which one may judge the health of an individual. The first is evaluating the individual's state of health at a point in time by inquiring about symptoms and the results of a physical examination and biochemical tests, and by other means. The second is observing the number of health-related events that occur to that individual over a period of time. In the population context, the first of these types of measures is called measures of *prevalence*, that is what exists or prevails. In the second category are measures of *incidence*, that is the frequency of occurrence of events or incidents. For purposes of understanding disease etiology, measures of incidence are generally considered to be the more useful because they are proximal consequences of the coming together of the disease's determinants. Prevalence, however, is determined not only by the incidence of the disease but also by those factors that influence the fatality of the disease and by other determinants of the duration of the disease in affected individuals prior to death or recovery. Disease prevalence can therefore be expected to have a more complex set of antecedents than incidence.

Incidence and Incidence Rates

The incidence of a disease is the number of cases of the disease that come into being during a specified period of time. In practice it is usually not possible to measure incidence directly because the exact time of onset of an illness is uncertain and often a matter of definition (see Chapter 3). Instead, such events as onset of symptoms, time of diagnosis, date of notification or hospitalization, or even date of death are used. If two or more incidence frequencies are to be compared it is of course essential to use the same criteria for defining the point in its natural history at which the disease is said to be "incident." Changes in criteria for diagnosis over time or differences between populations must always be explored as possible reasons for variation in apparent incidence rates.

A simple statement of disease incidence might be "Six hundred persons have been diagnosed as having developed Acquired Immune Deficiency Syndrome (AIDS)." To have utility, any statement of disease frequency, including this one, must be accompanied by a specification of when and in what population the cases occurred or existed. For example, in this instance, the statement that "Among all residents of this city, in 1990, there were 600 persons known to have developed AIDS" might serve some purpose. For example, combined with knowledge of the natural history of the disease, it should facilitate the planning of medical facilities and economic resources for the treatment of the disease in that city because those responsible need to know how many cases they have to deal with. If, however, the purpose of the statement is to suggest that the inhabitants of one city have a greater or lesser probability of developing AIDS than do those of another city, such a statement has obvious limitations, the most obvious being that differences in the number of cases may be due simply to differences in population size. A second limitation is that the statement includes no indication of the length of the period of time during which these cases were observed, other than that it was in 1990. For comparative purposes, these two limitations must be accommodated. The variation in population size is taken into account by dividing the number of cases by the relevant population and multiplying by some convenient base number, usually some power of ten (1,000; 1,000,000; etc.). The "relevant population" is the population whose members would have been counted as incident cases if they had been affected, which in this example is the population of that particular city. The duration of observation is accommodated by dividing this fraction by the average duration of observation expressed in some standard unit of time, usually, although not necessarily, years. The units of population and time may be combined by multiplication into a single measure of *person-time*. If the units of time are years, these would be *person-years*. For example, if 1,200 cases had occurred in a city of 4 million people during a period of 3 years, the incidence rate would be as follows:

$$\frac{1,200}{3} \cdot \frac{1}{4 \cdot 10^6} \cdot 10^5 = 10.0 \text{ per } 100,000 \text{ per year}$$

This could also be stated as an *annual rate* of 10.0/100,000 or as a rate of 10.0 per 100,000 person-years. The person-years in this example are $4 \cdot 10^6 \cdot 3 = 12 \cdot 10^6$. This number of person-years could be accumulated by observing 4 million people for 3 years (as in this example), 2 million people for 6 years, or any other practical combination of number of persons and time.

Note that the unit of time is an integral component of the measure (the rate) and is quite distinct from any descriptive statement that might be made about the period of time during which the observations were made. In this terminology, a defining characteristic of a rate is that the denominator is person-*time*. The population size is the average number in the population during the period of observation, not, as in some measures we shall describe, the number alive at the beginning of the observation period. The incidence rate as defined here is in theory a measure of the density of events occurring during the observation period and has been referred to as the *incidence density*[358] or *hazard*. (Frequently, the term "incidence" is used when an incidence *rate* is being referred to, but the meaning can usually be inferred from the units used.) If the incident events being counted are deaths, or deaths from a specified disease, the incidence rate or incidence density corresponds to the *force of mortality* in life-table terminology. It should be noted that the *mortality rate* expressed as the number of deaths per person-time is a form of incidence rate—the incidence of death—and has the characteristics of a rate, which is in contrast to the *case fatality ratio* referred to later in this chapter.

Prevalence and Prevalence Proportions

As with incidence, the word *prevalence* refers to a *number* of cases. As noted previously, it is the number of cases that exist or existed at a point in time. The observations on which the number is based may not all be made at the same point in time; for example, information for the decennial U.S. censuses may be assembled during a period of several years, but the objective is to estimate the number of persons present (prevalent) on a specific day of the census year. In some older writings one may encounter the term *period prevalence*. It refers to the sum of the number of cases prevalent at a point in time (prevalence) plus the number that occur in a subsequent period (e.g., the subsequent year [incidence]). The measure has no administrative or scientific utility and is no longer used.

As with incidence, data on prevalent numbers may, and indeed do, serve useful purposes. Yet, if the objective is to compare prevalences in different populations, the numbers need to be related to the size of the population; however, unlike incidence, no time dimension is involved because the compared measures will each refer to a single specified point in time. Therefore, it will be sufficient for comparative purposes to express the prevalent number as a proportion of the relevant population. The relevant population is those persons who, if affected, would have been counted as prevalent cases.

The term *prevalence proportion* is cumbersome and unlikely to enter the vernacular. One frequently finds such proportions referred to as prevalence *rates*, but such terminology is not consistent with recent usage because the measure includes no dimension of time, and it is important to retain the strict definition of rates for reasons that will be discussed in Chapters 9 and 10. Use of the term *prevalence proportion* may usually be avoided by giving the referent; for example, in the phrase "a prevalence of 10 per thousand," the word prevalence clearly refers to a prevalence proportion rather than a prevalence number.

Other Proportions

The denominators of proportions and rates may not be populations in the usual demographic sense. For example, a hospital may express its maternal mortality rate as the number of maternal deaths per thousand deliveries. (Strictly, of course, this is a proportion, but the use of the term *rate* is common.) The women do not form a geographic population, but they do constitute the group within which the deaths occurred. Such a population, as with a demographic population, is often referred to as the *population at risk*. Similarly, the *case fatality ratio* has as its numerator the number of deaths attributed to a disease and as its denominator the number of patients with the disease, among whom those deaths occurred. In this instance, the patients constitute the population at risk.

The word *risk* is often used synonymously with rate, but it should not be. A *risk* is the accumulated effect of a rate operating during some specified period of time. For example, the *life-time* risk of dying of cancer is about 25 percent. This is a proportion, and it is the result of the *rates* of cancer that have prevailed during that lifetime. There are a number of situations in which a risk is an appropriate descriptive measure; for example, the lifetime risks (usually censored at age 70 or so) of being affected by or dying from specified diseases, or group of diseases, give a good overall impression of the contribution of those diseases to the total burden of morbidity or mortality. It may be useful to calculate such risks for individuals of specified ages (e.g., lifetime risk after age 40). There are some diseases that occur over a limited age range, such as congenital malformations, and it might be appropriate to speak of the risk of malformation associated with exposure to a teratogen. We should note, however, that this risk is usually incompletely measured because many malformed embryos die and would not be counted. What we observe in the context of malformations is usually the *prevalence* of the malformation at the time of birth. It is also useful to use the concept of risk in describing the cumulative incidence of a disease during the course of a transient epidemic or outbreak—often called an *attack rate*—although, again, this is strictly speaking not a rate. The *secondary attack rate* of an infectious disease, which is the proportion of individuals exposed to a primary case, such as the siblings or classmates of a primary case, who themselves develop the disease, is also not a rate but a proportion and may appropriately be referred to as a risk. Risks differ from rates in two important respects. First, risks have no time dimension as a fundamental component (other than descriptively, indicating the time period of an epidemic or an age limitation). Second, the reference population is the population unaffected at the beginning of the period of observation, as distinct from the average population during the observation period.

An Example

To illustrate the calculation of some of the measures described so far in this chapter we will refer to data from the Hypertension Detection and Follow-up Program (HDFP) of the National Heart, Lung and Blood Institute. This program was a multicenter collaborative study in 14 communities across the United States to determine, primarily, whether systematic drug treatment of hypertension would reduce mortality overall and, secondarily, to evaluate the effect of the treatment on mortality from cerebrovascular disease (stroke).[228] Screening for hypertension was offered to 178,009 individuals in the 14 communities and 158,906 (89%) completed the first medical examination. Of these, 22,978 (14%) had blood pressure high enough to suggest the presence of hypertension and were referred to a second screening examination. Among the 17,476 (76%) who completed this second exam there were 10,940 who satisfied the study's criteria for a diagnosis of hypertension and were entered into the trial. Approximately half of these (5,485) were chosen at random to receive Stepped Care (SC) in special study centers where drug dosage was increased stepwise to reduce blood pressure to or below set goals. The other half (5,455) received Referred Care (RC), in which participants were referred to their usual sources of medical care. During the 5 years after entry into the study, there were 349 deaths in the SC group and 419 in the RC group. Of these, 29 and 52, respectively, were due to cerebrovascular disease. During the 5 years of the study, 23 of the SC group and 38 of the RC group were lost to follow up and their status was unknown.

Before using these data for illustration, we should note that we are estimating rates and ratios only for the special populations involved in the study, not for the United States as a whole, or even for the 14 communities represented, because there was considerable self-selection of participants within the selected communities. Furthermore, we accept for this purpose the study definition of hypertension.

First, we estimate the prevalence of hypertension in this population. The estimate must be confined to the 89 percent of the population who completed the first screening. It may underestimate or overestimate the prevalence in the whole community, according to whether the nonparticipants were more or less likely to have hypertension than those who participated. Among the 158,906 who completed the first screening, we know that there were at least 10,940 who satisfied the criteria for hypertension. The minimum estimate of prevalence is, therefore, as follows:

$$\frac{10,940}{158,906} \cdot 100 = 6.9 \text{ percent}$$

We can also estimate a maximum estimate by assuming that all of the 5,502 suspected hypertensives who did not complete the second exam did indeed have hypertension. This gives a numerator of 16,442 and a prevalence of 10.3 percent. The range is therefore 6.9 to 10.3 percent. Perhaps the best estimate is obtained by assuming that the frequency of verification was the same among the 5,502 who did not participate in the second exam as in the 17,476 who did. This gives a numerator of 14,384 and a prevalence of 9.1 percent.

Next, we measure the incidence of the study outcome—death. The most useful type of incidence measure in this study, as in

most clinical follow-up studies, is the cumulative incidence during the 5 years of the study. This is the proportion of entered
patients who manifested the study outcome, and it is appropriately referred to as a "risk." We have this information only on the
two groups of patients enrolled in the two study cohorts (i.e.,
those already known to have hypertension). The possibility of
generalizing from these estimates, therefore, is limited; however,
the purpose of the study was not to derive generalizable frequencies, but to compare frequencies in the two groups. We will present
only the mortality data (i.e., data on the incidence of death). Crude
mortality risks over the 5-year period are derived by dividing the
number of events by the entry population and multiplying the
dividend by a suitable base, in this case 100. The 5-year risks are:

$$\text{SC:} \quad \frac{349}{5,485} \cdot 100 = 6.4 \text{ percent}$$

$$\text{RC:} \quad \frac{419}{5,455} \cdot 100 = 7.7 \text{ percent}$$

For deaths due to cerebrovascular disease, which are far fewer
in number, we would prefer to use a referent that leads to values
with a number to the left of the decimal, such as 1,000. Ignoring
the minimal number of persons lost to follow up or deceased from
other causes, the risks, again over 5 years, are:

$$\text{SC:} \quad \frac{29}{5,485} \cdot 1,000 = 5.3 \text{ per thousand}$$

$$\text{RC:} \quad \frac{52}{5,455} \cdot 1,000 = 9.5 \text{ per thousand}$$

Because neither the difference in overall mortality nor that in the
risk of death from cerebrovascular disease are likely to be due to
chance, it is fair to conclude that the treatment had a protective
effect in reducing the risk of death in this population.

If we wish to estimate mortality *rates* in these data, we need
an estimate not of the number of persons who entered the study
cohorts but of the average population at risk during the 5-year
period. This could be estimated for each year and summed over
the period, but a simplifying assumption can be made that deaths
and losses to follow up were evenly distributed over the period.
The assumption may in fact be incorrect, but because of the small
numbers of deaths and losses the estimates are not seriously
affected in this instance. In other situations, however, the estimate of average population must be made more carefully. With
the assumption, the average populations can be estimated as
the entering populations minus half the deaths and losses, or

5,299 and 5,227 in the SC and RC groups, respectively. These numbers can be multiplied by five to give the number of person-years of observation. Estimates of the mean annual mortality rates are:

$$\text{SC:}\quad \frac{349}{5{,}299 \cdot 5} \cdot 100 = 1.3 \text{ percent}$$

$$\text{RC:}\quad \frac{419}{5{,}227 \cdot 5} \cdot 100 = 1.6 \text{ percent}$$

Mortality rates from cerebrovascular disease are 1.1 and 2.0 per thousand per year in the two groups.

Ratios and Other Proportional Measures

Certain other measures, although loosely called rates, are actually ratios. A common form of ratio expresses the number of affected persons relative to the number unaffected in the same population, not to the total number (affected plus unaffected) of persons. For example, in the United States it is common to express the number of fetal deaths relative to the number of livebirths. This is the *fetal death ratio* and should be distinguished from the *fetal death rate* (actually itself a proportion), which would have in its denominator the sum of fetal deaths and livebirths.

Numbers of cases of a disease are sometimes expressed relative to the total number of cases of all diseases, rather than to the population. For example, the number of deaths ascribed to a particular disease may be expressed as a proportion of all deaths. A common term for this measure is the *proportional mortality ratio*. Similarly, in clinical studies the "incidence" of a disease is sometimes reported as the number of cases of the disease as a proportion of all patients seen at the same institution. Such proportions do not express the risk of the population contracting or dying from the disease; comparison of such ratios between areas or between population subgroups may suggest that a difference exists that is worth investigating. Yet, until true rates can be computed against a population base, it will not be known whether the difference relates to differences in the sizes of the numerators or the denominators of the compared ratios.

For example, Berman noted that 91 percent of cancers seen in Bantu laborers in Witwatersrand gold mines were primary cancers of the liver.[26] In this instance, all cancers, rather than all other diseases, were used as the denominator of the proportion. Because the liver generally contributes only about one percent of cancers, it was inferred that the Bantus suffered an extraordinarily high rate of primary liver cancer. However, Gilliam esti-

Table 4-1. Mortality Rates from Cancer in Bantu Mine Workers and African Americans

	Mortality rate*	
Cancer site	Bantu	African Americans
Liver cancer	12.7	3.0
Other sites	1.3	61.5
All cancer	14.0	64.5

Adapted from Gilliam AG. A note on evidence relating to the incidence of primary liver cancer among the Bantu. J Natl Cancer Inst 1954;15 : 195–199.
* Rates are annual mortality rates per 100,000 population and are not age standardized.

mated population rates on the basis of the data given by Berman.[145] The results, shown in Table 4-1, indicated that the Bantus did indeed have higher rates of liver cancer than, for example, African Americans, but an even greater discrepancy existed with respect to the other cancers that, with the liver cancers, made up the denominators of the proportions. Thus the difference between the proportions, using all cancers as denominators, greatly overstated the excess frequency of liver cancer in the Bantu and did not reveal the marked difference between these two populations in cancers of other sites.

A similar situation exists when the frequency of a disease is expressed in relation to the frequency of some other disease. For example, there are many comparisons between populations of the ratio of cases of cancer of the body of the uterus to cases of cancer of the cervix. Such comparisons may suggest that a difference exists between two populations, but they do not reveal which of the two diseases is more or less common in one population than the other.

Multiple Incidence Events

When expressed as a rate of all events (rather than first such events), incidence (unlike prevalence) does not necessarily refer to a fraction of the population. The numerator may be made up of the number of attacks, rather than of individuals, because in some illnesses, such as acute alcoholic delirium or the common cold, some individuals may experience more than one episode during a period of observation. In such a circumstance the rate describes the rate of episodes of illness in the population rather than the rate of individuals becoming ill. It is preferable, for epidemiological purposes, to reduce the numerator to individuals so that the probability of an individual having one or more attacks during the period might be estimated. Further subdivision into the risk of having one, two, three, and so forth, attacks during the period are useful in identifying and describing groups of individuals who have a higher frequency of episodes.

In addition, although attacked only once during the period of observation, some individuals may be experiencing a recurrence of an illness, such as reactive depression, of which their initial attack occurred prior to the current observation period. Under this condition an incidence rate is a measure of the risk of individuals having an episode during the period of observation, whereas it would usually be more helpful for the understanding of causal mechanisms to identify those individuals having their initial episode of illness during the period. Separate incidence rates could then be presented for instances of first attacks, later episodes, and all episodes.

The denominators of incidence rates may also be limited to specific components of a population. For example, if the denominators of incidence rates contain persons who are not at risk of contracting the disease, important epidemiological differences between rates may be obscured. Thus, for those infectious diseases in which an attack confers permanent immunity, the majority of a population may not be at risk during the study period because of prior encounter with the disease (or vaccination). For this reason, the denominator in a secondary attack proportion usually excludes previously affected persons when the disease is one for which immunity follows a first attack. An analogous situation may exist in common chronic or relapsing diseases of long duration where the denominator may contain an appreciable proportion of persons who are either currently ill with the disease or have had it in the past and are therefore not at risk of having an initial attack. Ideally, an incidence rate would have its population base confined to those persons who have not had and do not currently have the disease under study. This is a refinement that has not been commonly practiced and that in fact may usually be ignored without serious error unless the proportion of such persons in the population is large and potentially variable. An example of a situation in which it would be unwise to ignore this principle is cancer of the endometrium. Because between 30 and approximately 50 percent of women over 50 years of age in the United States in the last 30 years have had a hysterectomy,[317,577] rates of endometrial cancer among women in this country cannot meaningfully be compared with those in countries where the hysterectomy rate is much lower.

Crude, Specific, and Standardized Rates

Crude Rates

The term *crude* refers to rates that are based on cases occurring in the total observed population, disregarding any demographic subgroups of the population. Crude rates in two populations may differ simply because the demographic structures of the populations differ, not because of any real difference in disease rates. The most common example is with respect to age. Age is so strongly associated with risk of almost all diseases that two populations that have different age distributions will almost invariably differ in their disease experience, even if their age-specific rates are the same. Similarly, there are many diseases for which one would not wish to compare crude rates in two populations that differed in the proportions of males and females.

Specific Rates

Specific refers to rates that are limited to individuals having the characteristics specified. Thus gender-specific rates provide separate estimates of rates for males and females in the population. Rates that are specific for age and gender are more likely to reflect true difference in disease risk between populations, but of course they do not guarantee that other demographic forces, such as ethnicity and socioeconomic status, are not also playing roles.

Standardized Rates

Specific rates eliminate the role of the characteristics specified in the rates if sufficiently fine categories are used. If the frequency of the disease varies by both age and gender, however, comparison of specific rates might involve the estimation of 20 or more rates for each population (at least 10 age groups in each gender). The populations may not be large enough or the disease common enough for such rates to be reliable. *Standardized* rates are then used. A number of statistical techniques are available for comparison of overall rates after making allowance for demographic differences. The most simple of these is called *standardization* or *adjustment*. The various techniques are described in statistics textbooks and are not discussed at length here. Fleiss[128] treats the subject fully. An early description that is still one of the best is that of Linder and Grove.[290] There is, however, one issue that comes up repeatedly in epidemiological writings that should be mentioned—the difference between *direct* and *indirect* standardization.

To illustrate, suppose that we are attempting to standardize only for age. In direct standardization, a *standard population* with a known age distribution is selected. The selection of this population is arbitrary; it may be constructed by selecting one of the compared populations or a combination of populations, or by arbitrary selection (e.g., assuming equal numbers in each 5-year age group). In the United States, it is common to use the national population of one of the decennial census years. For international comparisons, three standard populations modified from earlier proposals—the so-called African, World and European populations—were suggested by Doll, Payne, and Waterhouse[100] for use in presentation of cancer incidence data. The proposed World population has become widely used, although the heavy weighting of young age groups in this standard reduces the precision of standardized estimates for diseases in which rates increase rapidly with age.[100] Broad acceptance of a common standard population may have no advantage to any individual comparison, but it greatly facilitates comparison of new with previously published data or comparison between sets of data for which comparison was not originally intended. At a minimum, the distribution of the standard population used should be readily accessible to other investigators.

Age-specific rates (preferably in groups no wider than 5 years) are then computed for each of the populations to be compared. These rates are applied to the number of persons in the corresponding age group in the standard population, and the results are summed to obtain the total number of cases that would have occurred in the standard population had it experienced the same age-specific rates as the study population. This sum is divided by the total number of persons in the standard population and given an appropriate base to become the standardized rate in the study population. A directly standardized rate can be compared with any other rate standardized to the same standard population.

Direct standardization is preferable to indirect standardization, but its use is limited by the very feature that makes a standardized rate desirable in the first place—there are frequently inadequate numbers to compute age-specific rates in the study population(s). Indirect standardization is, therefore, often used, and in one form or another is probably more common than the direct procedure. Instead of a standard population, a set of age-specific *standard rates* is selected. These are commonly the national rates for the country or area in which the study was undertaken, but they may not necessarily be so; again, the selection is arbitrary, but rates approximating those in the populations of which the rates are to be standardized are desirable. The standard set of rates is applied to the number of persons in each age stratum in the population of interest and the results summed to estimate the number of cases that would have occurred in the population of interest if it had had the same rates as those in the population from which the standard rates were derived. The ratio of the resulting overall rate in the study population to that in the standard is a measure of the effect of the study population's age distribution on the disease rate for all ages combined. The crude observed rate in the population of interest is then multiplied by this ratio to derive an indirectly standardized rate. This indirectly standardized rate can be compared with the overall rate in the population from which the standard rates were derived. Two indirectly standardized rates, however, cannot strictly be compared with each other, even if the same standard set of rates has been used, because the weights in the indirectly standardized rates are determined by the age distribution of the population whose rates are being standardized, which may differ between compared populations.[602] The only valid comparison of an indirectly standardized rate is with the population from which the standardized rates were derived.

Standardized mortality ratios (SMRs), and *standardized incidence ratios* (SIRs) are forms of indirectly standardized ratios. The numerators are the total numbers of observed cases and the denominators are expected numbers calculated as shown earlier. Traditionally, the results of this ratio have been multiplied by 100; an SMR of 100 implies that the study population had the same risk of disease as the standard population after correction for differences in age and any other variables that are specified in the standard rates. Recently, it has become more common not to apply the 100 factor but to simply present the ratio itself. In this form, the null SMR of 100 would be expressed as 1.0. Miettinen has pointed out that SMRs share the problem of indirectly standardized rates—that of not being directly comparable themselves.[354] Thus, one often sees SMRs of different exposure levels compared to examine an exposure–response relationship. Although the procedure is theoretically incorrect, as Miettinen points out, it is continued. This is probably because of an intuitive dislike for using the wildly fluctuating age-specific rates that might occur in a small series and are necessary for direct standardization. It may also be because of the belief that only in the more extreme instances will the indirect estimates be seriously out of line—a belief, however, that can only be confirmed by comparing directly standardized rates.

Specification of Time

We have noted that time must be specified for calculation of both incidence rates and prevalence proportions—in one instance a time period, in the other a point in time. Thus far calendar time has been implied, but there are several ways of specifying time.

Calendar Time

A period of time may be defined as the period between two calendar dates, and a point in time may be defined as a particular date. These are probably the most common ways of defining time for incidence rates and prevalence proportions.

Age

A second way to specify time is in terms of chronological age. This is frequently used with birth as the starting point. For example, the infant mortality rate is the number of deaths in the first year of life per 1,000 babies born in a particular year. Not all the infants have both birth and death in that year, but this is important only when wide year-to-year fluctuations in fertility are occurring. The period of observation may be a single year or a longer period. Pyloric stenosis of infants is a disease essentially limited to the first 3 months of life; therefore, a measure based on those 3 months could be referred to as a risk. It would not increase with longer observation.

Another example of the use of age to specify time is to say that at the age of 10 years 20 percent of the population are tuberculin positive. Clearly, however, these persons may not all reach age 10 at the same calendar time.

Other Methods of Specifying Time

Without direct reference to either age or calendar time, the occurrence of some life event may be the point at which observations begin. For example, one can calculate the prevalence of certain serologic findings at the time of premarital blood examination, at the time of entrance to school or military service, or incidence of illnesses occurring within a certain period after childbirth. Although age may be highly correlated with some of these life events, it is not the defining characteristic.

Case fatality ratios and disease complication frequencies are also of this nature, with the period of observation beginning with the onset (or diagnosis) of the disease. There may, of course, be specification of the calendar time or the age of the individual if these are relevant, but they are not the variables that define the point or period of observation.

Interrelation of Measures

Incidence and Prevalence

Because incidence is derived by dividing person by person-time, the physical dimension of incidence is $(time)^{-1}$. Indeed, it has been shown that in a population with steady rates and no competing risks, incidence equals the average time until the occurrence of the disease.[368] Thus, situations that impart immediate death are associated with a hazard that approaches infinity. In a steady state, the inverse of mortality from all causes, which is about 10 per 1,000 person-years and has no conceivable competition, is the *mean* life expectancy at birth (about 100 years). Similarly, the inverse of the termination rate per person-days (whether by recovery or death) among a group of patients equals the average duration of their disease in days.

It has also been shown that in a steady state situation, the prevalence odds of a disease (i.e., the ratio of prevalence expressed as a proportion to its complementary quantity) equals the product of the incidence of the disease and its average duration (until recovery or death).[135,358,368,576]

$$\frac{P}{1-P} = I \cdot D$$

where P is the prevalence, I the incidence, and D the duration.

When prevalence is low (say less than 10 percent or 0.1), then

$$P \sim I \cdot D$$

Clearly, given two of the variables in this equation, the third can be calculated. Duration of disease is measured from the same point in time in its natural history (e.g., the date of diagnosis) as is used to define its time of incidence. Likewise, prevalence includes only cases existent at or subsequent to that point.

A change in prevalence from one time to another may be the result of changes in (1) incidence, (2) duration, or (3) both incidence and duration. For example, improvements in therapy that delay death but do not produce recovery may give rise to an apparently paradoxical increase in prevalence of the disease. In addition, decreases in prevalence may result not only from a decrease in incidence but also from a shortening of the duration of illness, through either earlier death or more rapid recovery.

At times, attempts have been made to utilize this relationship to estimate the duration of a disease process when the duration could not be measured directly because discovery of the condition led to interference with the natural course of events. For example, if a program to screen for cervical cancer is to be efficient it is desirable to know how long precancerous or presymptomatic stages of the disease exist before they convert to more serious and perhaps irreversible lesions. However, when one of these conditions is diagnosed, the lesion is therapeutically removed, destroyed, or at least disturbed, and the natural history of the disease is thereby changed. Theoretically, estimates of the incidence and prevalence of the various stages of the disease would permit estimates of their durations from this relationship. Prevalence can be estimated from the frequency of the lesions among women presenting for screening for the first time, and incidence can be derived from women who present for screening subsequent to a negative test. Some useful work of this nature has been done, but it has been limited essentially to cancer of the cervix and its precursor lesions, and even for this disease there is some uncertainty about the accuracy of the estimates derived.[109,369] This uncertainty stems from the manifest violation of the assumption that the disease should be in a steady state over time and uncertainty over whether apparently incident cases are indeed incident cases or result from earlier false negative screenings.[387] Furthermore, for purposes of planning (e.g., of the desirable interval between screenings), information is needed not only on the *average* duration of the lesions but also on the distribution of the durations of individual lesions in the population to be screened; and this cannot be obtained from the formula.

More important than the use of this relationship in its strict algebraic form is to understand that prevalent cases (and prevalence proportions) have duration of illness as an important component, whereas incident cases and incidence rates do not. This fact has several implications.

First, one cannot meaningfully compare incidence and prevalence rates. A classic disregard of this principle created a dispute over the role of exogenous estrogens in the causation of endometrial cancer. It has been shown by many investigators that women who take estrogens for the relief of menopausal symptoms have an increased risk of endometrial cancer. One proffered explanation of this association was that women who take estrogens tend to have bleeding from the uterus as a side effect. They may as a consequence undergo more frequent medical examinations, and therefore be more frequently found to have endometrial cancer, which otherwise would have remained latent. That is to say, there is allegedly a "detection bias" that leads to more frequent diagnosis in exposed women. For this explanation to be accepted it must be shown that there is a large reservoir of undetected uterine cancer in women who show no symptoms or at least have not had symptoms investigated. To evaluate this possibility, Horwitz et al. assembled data on the frequency of postmortem diagnosis of uterine cancer in two large teaching hospitals among women over 45 years of age who had an intact uterus and had not previously been diagnosed as having uterine cancer.[217] The proportions of uterine cancer first diagnosed at necropsy were 22 and 31 per 10,000 autopsies, respectively, in the two hospitals. The authors compared these figures with annual rates of 4.7 and 5.5 per 10,000 from reports to a local tumor registry of endometrial cancer in roughly corresponding time periods and concluded that "the rate of detection at necropsy is about four to six times greater than the rate of detection during life,"[217] and therefore there is opportunity for the existence of a substantial detection bias. Of course, the frequency of cancers detected at necropsy is a prevalence proportion, and the cancer registry data yielded annual incidence rates—they simply cannot be compared. Using appropriate methods of computing life-time cumulative incidence rates (risks) and comparing these with the number of undiagnosed uterine cancers found at necropsy, Merletti and Cole[346] estimated that the proportion of endometrial cancer that was not diagnosed during life was closer to 10–20 percent than to the 56 percent estimate of Horwitz et al. Although the issue is more complex than has been indicated in this outline, the basic principle to be learned is that it is necessary to understand the dimensions of any estimates of disease frequency that are to be compared.

The second implication is that in the context of case-control and cohort studies, to be discussed later, it is important to interpret data relating to incident cases separately from those relating to prevalent cases. For example, in case-control studies it is not uncommon, in order to increase the number of cases available for study, to include cases who are still alive at the beginning of the study but whose disease was diagnosed several years before. These are prevalent cases, and it must be recognized that associations found among them may be related not to their risk of acquiring the disease but to their probability of surviving it and, if it is required that the patient have the disease at the time of the study, to the duration of the disease.

Third, important distinctions between incident and prevalent cases are to be made in the context of evaluating the efficacy of screening for the early detection of diseases, particularly diseases of fairly long but variable duration. The efficacy of screening is often defended by the argument that patients with diseases detected at screening tend to have less advanced disease and to survive longer following diagnosis than patients whose disease was detected in the ordinary course of practice. Two obvious reasons for such an observation are now well recognized. One is sometimes referred to as *lead-time bias*. It relates to the fact that if, because of screening, a patient's disease is diagnosed earlier than it would normally have been then the interval between the time of diagnosis and death will be longer in the screened than in the unscreened patient, even if the early detection did not alter the natural history of the disease or affect the time of death in any way. This will be reflected not only in a longer duration of the interval between diagnosis and death but in time-dependent survival ratios and all other measures of survival following diagnosis. If the early detection does not result in more effective treatment that changes the prognosis, the patient "gains" only the additional period of knowing that he or she has the disease. Hutchison and Shapiro reported an early recognition of this bias and an attempt to estimate its size in the context of a randomized trial of screening for breast cancer.[227]

The other reason to expect that survival will be longer for cases diagnosed by screening, regardless of any beneficial effect of the screening, is often referred to as *length bias*. This stems from the relationship between incidence and prevalence. Cases detected by screening are prevalent cases; those diagnosed in the normal course of events are incident cases. Because less aggressive forms of the same disease are likely to develop slowly and therefore exist for a longer time in the preclinical stages, the proportion of nonaggressive forms will be higher in a prevalence sample (screening) than in the usual incidence-based clinical detection. In an extreme situation, for example, a very slowly growing cancer might never become apparent during the patient's lifetime but will still be detected by screening. Therefore, the better survival of the cases detected by screening cannot automatically be attributed to their early detection. These issues and their technical backgrounds are covered extensively by Cole and Morrison[69] and more recently by Morrison.[368,369]

Incidence and Mortality

A second relationship between measures of disease frequency is between incidence and mortality rates. It may be expressed as follows: M varies as the product of I and F, where M is the mortality rate, I is the incidence rate, and F is the case fatality ratio

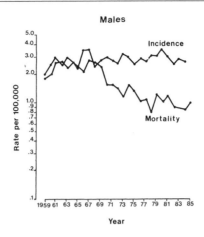

Figure 4-1. Annual incidence and mortality rates from Hodgkin's disease in males in Scotland, 1959–1985. Rates are per 100,000 population and are age standardized. (Source: Boyle P et al. Improving prognosis of Hodgkin's disease in Scotland. Eur J Cancer Clin Oncol 1988;24 : 229–234.)

the proportion of affected individuals who die of the disease). With the same assumptions as to stability of these measures over time, the relationship would be such that *M approximates I · F.* Thus for a stable disease with a case fatality ratio of 0.5, the mortality rate would be about half the incidence rate. This relationship can yield a general idea of the case fatality ratio for a disease given incidence and mortality rates in the population, but the necessary assumptions are seldom fulfilled with sufficient strictness to be confident about the accuracy of such estimates.

An illustration of this relationship is shown in Figure 4-1. Incidence and mortality rates for Hodgkin's disease in Scottish males are shown for the period 1959 to 1985.[38] Until approximately 1970, Hodgkin's disease was regarded as a uniformly fatal disease; this is reflected in the similarity of incidence and mortality rates. In the early 1970s, clinical series of "cures" of Hodgkin's disease began to be reported, particularly among young adults, and, as shown, the curves of incidence and mortality began to diverge. The divergence appeared to level off in the 1980s with an incidence about three times that of the mortality, which suggests that about two-thirds of cases were in fact being cured or at least not dying of the disease.

Comparison of incidence and mortality rate in this way is more than an indirect, and somewhat inaccurate, way of estimating a case fatality ratio, which can usually be measured directly. It provides additional information. Thus, given that directly measured case fatality ratios for Hodgkin's disease in the 1960s were close to 100 percent and in the 1980s approximately 40 percent, could we be sure that the change represented an increasing cure rate? The answer is no. This is because the possibility could not be ruled out that there had been a change in the criteria for diagnosis leading to the inclusion in clinical series of patients with different or milder forms of the disease who would have survived regardless of treatment. However, the fact that incidence rates have remained essentially unchanged argues against that possibility, because if additional milder cases had been diagnosed then the "true" disease must have decreased by almost exactly the same amount. The more parsimonious explanation is that diagnostic criteria have remained unchanged and cases are indeed being cured.

Selection of Measures

A number of measures of disease frequency have been described. The utility of one rather than another depends on the problem being addressed. It may be particularly useful to recapitulate some of the features of incidence rates and prevalence proportions.

Incidence

Attempts to elucidate causal factors focus on explaining the occurrence of illness. The measure most descriptive of occurrence is the incidence rate. Causal factors necessarily operate prior to the onset of disease, and the closer in time that the stage of disease at which incidence is measured comes to the actual time of onset, the more directly the operation of causal factors will influence the measure. For these reasons, incidence measured as early in the disease as practicable is the measure of frequency most useful for studies of causal factors.

Because of their ready availability, death rates are sometimes used as surrogates of incidence. Routine registration of deaths, together with specification of cause of death, enables death rates to be derived for many diseases and among many populations for which more direct measures of incidence are not available. Death rates are most useful as surrogates of incidence when the case fatality ratio is high and the interval between onset of illness and death is short.

Prevalence

For epidemiological purposes, prevalence measures are inferior to incidence rates for reasons discussed earlier in this chapter. Yet, when incidence rates are not obtainable, patterns in prevalence proportions may give clues as to possible variations in incidence.

The main value of prevalence data is, as noted earlier, in administrative situations requiring knowledge of how many patients with a given disease exist in the community. Incidence rates are of uncertain value in such situations because for a given incidence diseases of long duration usually impose a greater burden on the community than those of short duration. Here, too, however, knowledge of incidence rates is important when facilities for new cases differ from those required for patients who do not recover within a short period of time.

5 Strategies of Epidemiology

We open this chapter with an apology—the word *strategies* is too bold for what we have to offer. We are mindful, however, that despite the fact that graduates of war colleges often lose battles and less learned soldiers often win them, it is still considered pertinent that generals attend war college, where strategy is presumably of the essence. Strategy is an attempt, with help and evaluation provided by history, to draw guidelines that favor the side that applies them. A guideline may either favor success (e.g., the element of surprise) or decrease the likelihood of failure (e.g., holding soldiers in reserve). Guidelines of both types can be drawn from the history of epidemiology, and we have attempted to describe them in this chapter and in the rest of the text. Yet, no battle is won entirely by appropriate strategy and some are lost despite it. The outcome of each battle alters the knowledge base and the perception of the "best" strategy in a specific situation. In epidemiology, we are at a very early and fluid stage in the development of the knowledge base.

Describing the Distribution of Disease

Study of the distribution of disease in populations is sometimes referred to as *descriptive epidemiology*. As noted in Chapter 1, it serves many purposes other than helping to understand the causes of disease, including administrative, economic, and political purposes. In this text, however, we are concerned primarily with the understanding of disease causation and will limit the discussion to that purpose.

An inquiry into the nature of an unknown entity opens logically with general questions. For example, in a now outworn but still challenging parlor game, an unseen or imagined object must be identified on the basis of answers to 20 questions. Because the object is frequently one of great rarity, such as the mummified foot of an Egyptian pharaoh, the chance of success through unguided guesses is small. Devotees of the game have developed opening questions aimed at rapidly reducing the number of possibilities. The inquiry usually opens with the question, "Is it animal, vegetable, or mineral?" Whether or not a helpful answer is received to this question (in the present example, it is not clear that an appropriate answer could be given), the inquiry proceeds with further general questions as to the object's age, color, consistency, and so forth. After about 10 questions, the inquirer hopes that the number of possibilities compatible with the answers received may be sufficiently reduced to allow specific guesses.

Similarly, epidemiologists have developed their own set of general limiting questions. Because epidemiologists' questions are not so readily answered as those in the parlor game, the value of an answer to a general question must be weighed against the time and expense involved in obtaining it. Because the collection of data is by far the largest component of the cost of answering epidemiological questions, the exploratory phase of epidemiological investigation is heavily influenced by what information is available. The questions most frequently asked are those for which information is already collected, and sometimes collated and published for other purposes, such as birth and death certificates or census records that are collected primarily for political uses.

The variables most commonly examined can be classified as descriptive of time, place, and person. They include the following:

1. Characteristics that describe the *time* in which the persons were affected by the disease: For example, is there any unusual feature of the distribution of cases by year, month, day, or hour of occurrence?
2. Characteristics that describe the *place* of occurrence: For example, are cases equally distributed with respect to country, state, or district within countries, urban-rural residences, or within the affected local community?
3. Characteristics that describe the *persons* affected: For example, what is their age, gender, ethnic group, occupation, education, socioeconomic class, and marital status?

It is evident that the variables listed are not necessarily those most likely to have causal association with the disease being investigated. Thus, an association with a particular place might be due to characteristics of the persons that inhabit that place, and an association with a variable that is descriptive of a person, such as his or her race, might be the result of factors related to the place of residence. The grouping of variables into categories of time, place, and person should be thought of as an initial separation, possibly helpful to the investigator (but perhaps not, as in the parlor game) and useful as a mnemonic to remind the investigator of the things that should be known about the disease under investigation. Examples of the uses of descriptive variables in forming etiological hypotheses are given in later chapters.

A valuable and comprehensive list and description of data resources in the United States, with characterizations of data limitations, that is useful for the objectives of descriptive epidemiology, but not limited to that purpose, has been prepared by the National Center for Health Statistics and appears as an appendix to *Health, United States, 1995.*[380] A detailed account of the statistical methods appropriate to descriptive epidemiology has been published recently by Estève and his colleagues.[119]

Forming Hypotheses

In epidemiology, as in science in general, a new and convincing hypothesis can be one of the most powerful forces influencing the direction of future research, and the success or failure of that research frequently depends on the soundness of the hypothesis. Yet, the thought processes involved in forming hypotheses are not clearly formalized or classified.

In the early stages of the epidemiological investigation of a disease, hypotheses are formed that seek to explain the patterns of its distribution in populations. Four methods of reaching these hypotheses are discussed here: methods of difference, agreement, concomitant variation, and analogy. The first three are patterned after Mill's five canons of inductive reasoning,[361] which consider the definition and proof of causation.

Difference

If the frequency of a disease is markedly different under two separate circumstances, and some factor can be identified in one circumstance that is absent in the other, this factor, or its absence, may be a cause of the disease.

The difficulty with this method of forming epidemiological hypotheses is usually not one of being unable to identify a factor that is present in one circumstance and not in the other (or relatively so), but rather of the multiplicity of hypotheses that are often suggested on the basis of the difference in disease frequency. For example, literally dozens of possibilities may be suggested to explain differences in disease frequency between males and females, or between the United States and India, or between middle age and elderly persons. For this reason any one descriptive observation, even though revealing a striking characteristic of the disease, is usually not sufficient for the establishment of a sound hypothesis. For example, the predominance of males among patients with gout is more striking than in any other non–sex-organ specific disease; however, it has not resulted in any practically useful hypothesis about the causes of the disease. Usually it takes the concordance of ideas from at least two descriptive observations to make an attractive hypothesis. For example, the correlation of cigarette smoking and lung cancer risk, both by gender and over time, led to a much more powerful hypothesis than either alone would have supported.

Agreement

If a factor is common to a number of different circumstances that are associated with the presence of the disease, this factor may be a cause of the disease. For example, cervical cancer is associated with multiple sexual partners and low socioeconomic status. A common factor may be a virus transmitted through venereal contact. Similarly, seromarkers of hepatitis B virus are found with increased prevalence among both homosexuals and prostitutes, which suggests sexual transmission of this virus.[397]

Concomitant Variation

The method of concomitant variation merges imperceptibly into the two previously described methods because in many situations it is not a matter of a factor being present or absent but of its being present in a greater or lesser degree. The method involves the search for a factor whose frequency or strength varies with the frequency of the disease. It involves a quantitative rather than dichotomous approach. Well-known examples are the many attempts to relate the various dietary constituents to the risk of coronary artery disease in different areas of the world.[254] Another example is the comparison of the fluoride concentration in drinking water in various communities with the prevalence of dental caries in children.[88]

Analogy

The distribution of a disease may be sufficiently similar to that of some other disease that has been more completely and successfully investigated as to suggest that certain causes may be common to both. This method uses the process of deductive reasoning, whereby epidemiological principles already established are applied to other situations. Thus, we tend to associate diseases occurring in certain parts of the world during the summer months with vector transmission.

Even though there are no general laws or principles applicable to the process, this method may be of service. For example, the observation that the geographic distribution of Burkitt's lymphoma in Africa is similar to that of malaria and yellow fever led to the hypothesis that, as with these diseases, an insect vector may be involved in the etiology of this type of lymphoma.[206] Likewise, the similarity of the geographic distribution and certain other epidemiological features of multiple sclerosis to those of paralytic poliomyelitis led Poskanzer et al to suggest that the clinical illness of multiple sclerosis might also be an unusual manifestation of a widespread infection usually acquired at an early age.[421]

The method of analogy, although useful, can also be treacherous; major errors have been made as the result of false analogies. Thus, because genetically determined diseases tend to run in families, there has been a temptation to assume that all familial concentration of disease is evidence of genetic determination. This view is now known to be false; many nutritional and other environmental determinants of disease also run in families. In a different context, John Snow, who, having demonstrated the feces-to-drinking-water transmission of cholera, observed that plague and yellow fever shared the association of cholera with crowding, lack of personal cleanliness, and a tendency to attack towns located on rivers, was led to the mistaken idea that plague and yellow fever were transmitted in the same way as cholera.[508] More recently, the reluctance to accept diseases that are not obviously transmitted directly or indirectly from person to person with some rapidity as having microbiological origin no doubt delayed the recognition of the role of viruses in a number of human cancers and neurological disorders.

Hypotheses that Arise from Data

Specific hypotheses come to attention not from any rational consideration of the distribution of disease and its possible determinants but from serendipitous examination of data collected with some other purpose or no particular purpose. For example, although there are possible biological mechanisms to link alcohol consumption with increased risk of breast cancer, there is nothing in the descriptive epidemiology or biology of the disease that would make one seek such an association. Yet, in the early 1980s reports began to appear associating alcohol consumption with the risk of breast cancer. A combined analysis ("meta-analysis") in 1988 of all the data published on the topic found strong evidence for the existence of an association, as well as a relationship between the amount of alcohol consumed and the level of risk.[296] By 1994, the number of reports on the subject had more than doubled, and a second meta-analysis confirmed the existence of the association and of an exposure-response relationship, although the slope of the relationship was quite modest—daily consumption of one, two, or three alcoholic drinks was associated with increased risks of 11, 24, and 38 percent, respectively, compared to the risk for nondrinkers.[295] Data from the largest case control study of breast cancer to date confirmed this association in independent data.[297] Although mechanisms have been suggested, none of them has been established as the explanation of this association.

Use of alcoholic beverages is the topic of another serendipitous discovery first noted in the mid-1970s. Because it had been accepted for many years by a large proportion of the population that alcohol consumption could be harmful to health, the idea that moderate consumption of alcohol might be protective against coronary artery disease and its consequent heart attacks was not readily accepted by the general public or the growing body of neoprohibitionists in the Western world. Nevertheless, around 1980 there were reports that regular consumers of alcohol in moderate amounts (generally considered between one and three drinks per day) had lower risks of nonfatal and fatal heart attacks (by between 25 and 40 percent) than did nondrinkers.[331] A thorough review of the literature in 1986 supported the existence of such an association,[366] which in fact is compatible with ecological evidence.[279] The association was thought of as U-shaped because at higher levels of consumption (generally five or more drinks per day) the problems of cardiomyopathy, hypertension, and cardiac dysrhythmias begin to appear. There were attempts to show that the lower rate of cardiac disease among moderate drinkers than among nondrinkers was a "myth"[6] because of individuals in the nondrinkers category who were already at high risk because of previous problems with heart disease, alcohol, or both.[489] However, it has been shown in subsequent prospective studies that such explanations are not compatible with the data. Moreover, if the association is U-shaped, the U has a very broad base. In one study females who drank up to 25g of ethanol (2½ drinks) per day had slightly more than half the risk of nondrinkers,[510] and in males the risks remained low for consumptions of up to six or more drinks per day.[32,258] Since these observations, a great deal has been learned about the effect of alcohol on fractions of blood lipoproteins that appear to be protective against coronary artery disease;[142] however, these biochemical associations with alcohol consumption played no role in developing the hypothesis that moderate alcohol use may be protective against coronary disease.

Knowledge of the previously unsuspected toxic potential of many specific chemical and physical substances was also obtained during routine surveillance in occupational medicine.[363] It is also part of clinical routine to take a history from patients as to current and past use of medications, and whether or not such use seems related to the current symptoms. This practice has been adopted by epidemiologists, resulting in the discovery of numerous previously unsuspected associations. For example, aspirin was discovered to lower both recurrence risk and risk of first attack of coronary artery occlusion. This protective effect of aspirin was recently confirmed in a large randomized trial of American physicians.[516] Similarly, accumulated data indicate that use of postmenopausal estrogens by women substantially reduce their risk of coronary heart disease, although biological mechanisms might have predicted associations in either direction.[512]

No doubt, as the number and size of human populations studied increases, and statistics and computers enable more efficient analyses, the number of associations between specific diseases and past experiences discovered by serendipity or pure chance will increase.

Considerations in the Formation of Hypotheses

Although any combination of the methods and variables described may lead to a useful hypothesis, it may be helpful to consider situations that have been particularly productive in the past.

1. New hypotheses are commonly formed by relating observations from several different fields. In the area of disease causation, epidemiological findings are most profitably viewed in the light of clinical, pathological, and laboratory observations. Thus, Snow interpreted the epidemiological characteristics of cholera in the light of the clinical and pathological observations that the intestine was the obvious focus of the disease. In Vienna in 1847, an obstetrician, Ignaz Semmelweis, was attempting to explain the high incidence of puerperal fever in women who delivered by medical students compared to those who delivered by midwives. The clinical observation that certain features of the disease (fever, venous engorgement) were evidenced by a colleague who died of sepsis following a cut he received during an autopsy led Semmelweis to suspect that medical students' attendance at autopsies might be the characteristic that made them more dangerous than midwives to women in labor.[488]

2. The stronger a statistical association, the more likely it is to suggest a causal hypothesis. Strength does not refer to the level of statistical significance, but to the degree to which a disease that is entirely absent in one circumstance and invariably present in another is approached—a situation measured, as is discussed later, by the *relative risk*. The fact that this situation is more nearly the case for the association between smoking and lung cancer than for that between smoking and coronary heart disease led to a much more rapid acceptance of the former association as causal; although, as it turned out, attention should have turned with equal rapidity to the latter. Associations of low strength, however significant statistically, are rarely immediately productive of hypotheses.

3. Observations of change in frequency of a disease over time have been very productive. This is particularly true of changes that have occurred over relatively short periods of time. For example, the rapidity of the rise of an epidemic of unusual congenital malformations in the years 1959 to 1961 called immediate attention to the fact that some new factor must be operative. This led to the rapid identification of thalidomide as the cause.[280] Yet, even changes taking place over several decades can be productive of hypotheses if the changes are striking, as with lung cancer,[94] or if they follow unusual patterns, as did the epidemics of chronic nephritis in Queensland[205] and of Parkinson's disease in the United States.[422]

4. An isolated or unusual case should receive particular attention in the formation of hypotheses. Such cases, for example, in persons living in communities otherwise free of the disease, have been of great value in the study of infectious diseases and figure prominently in the investigations of Snow on cholera,[508] Budd on typhoid fever,[48] and Panum on measles.[396] In this connection, Bradford Hill drew attention to what he referred to as "the curious case of the Hampstead widow" encountered by John Snow in his investigation of the Broad Street outbreak of cholera in London in 1854. In Snow's words:

In the "Weekly Return of Births and Deaths" of September 9th, the following death is recorded as occurring in the Hampstead district: "At

West End, on 2nd September, the widow of a percussion-cap maker, aged 59 years, diarrhoea two hours, cholera epidemica sixteen hours." I was informed by this lady's son that she had not been in the neighbourhood of Broad Street for many months. A cart went from Broad Street to West End every day, and it was the custom to take a large bottle of water from the pump in Broad Street, as she preferred it. The water was taken on Thursday, 31st August, and she drank of it in the evening, and also on Friday. She was seized with cholera on the evening of the latter day, and died Saturday, as the above quotation from the register shows. A niece, who was on a visit to this lady, also drank of the water; she returned to her residence, in a high and healthy part of Islington, was attacked with cholera, and died also. There was no cholera at the time either at West End or in the neighbourhood where the niece died.[508]

5. Observations that appear to be in conflict or to create a paradox are particularly worthy of consideration. For example, the fact that nurses and attendants in asylums did not develop pellagra, in spite of their close contact with the inmates who did, led Goldberger to favor hypotheses relating the disease to diet rather than to infectious agents.[151]

Selection of Hypotheses for Evaluation

Almost any set of observations will be compatible with more than one hypothesis. From all the possibilities it is necessary to select a few that seem particularly worthy of further investigation or at least to establish priorities for order of investigation. The process of evaluating one hypothesis against another usually proceeds concurrently with the formulation of the hypotheses. The following considerations may be kept in mind.

First, the value of a hypothesis is inversely related to the number of acceptable alternatives. The number of these alternatives in turn depends on a variety of circumstances, as follows.

1. The greater the number of separate associations that can be explained by the hypothesis, the fewer the number of acceptable alternatives. Whereas an association involving only one variable may lead to the development of several hypotheses, an association with two independent variables will narrow the field considerably. For example, several hypotheses could explain the high incidence of leukemia in radiologists,[338] but relatively few would explain both this observation and the high leukemia rate in patients given x-ray therapy for ankylosing spondylitis.[83] When yet a third observation is added—the increased rate of leukemia in survivors of the atomic bombings of Hiroshima and Nagasaki[426]—

the possibilities are reduced even further. So far as we know, exposure to ionizing radiation at levels substantially greater than average is the only factor common to these three disparate groups.

2. The more closely two variables found to be associated with a disease are associated, the less their independent value is in the formation of a hypothesis. For example, racial or ethnic minorities are frequently among the least privileged members of a society; the fact that a disease shows association with one such minority group and also with some measure of low socio-economic status, such as income, does not give us two independent bearings on the same disease. In contrast, the fact that three early known risk groups for AIDS—male homosexuals, hemophiliacs, and transfused infants—had little in common other than the opportunity for exposure to the blood and other body fluids of other persons gave strong impetus to the search for a microbiological agent present and transmissible in such fluids—a search that was successfully concluded in 1983.

3. Association with certain variables, for example, specific occupations or religions, may be more stimulative of hypotheses than those with other variables, such as gender and age, because the unique environmental circumstances associated with the former may be fewer than those associated with the latter.

The second consideration in evaluating a hypothesis is that it is useful to make a deliberate search for specific demographic information that may be relevant, particularly that which might appear to refute or at least contradict the hypothesis. For example, if a genetic predisposition to cancer of the stomach is hypothesized on the basis of the high frequency of the disease in Japan, one would predict that stomach cancer would be more common in all peoples of Japanese ancestry, regardless of current environment. In fact, Americans of Japanese ancestry have stomach cancer rates quite similar to those of Americans of European ancestry, and the genetic explanation of the high rates in Japan must be discarded.[189] Similarly, the low rate of cervical cancer in Jewish women suggested for many years that circumcision of the sexual partner might be protective against this disease. Abou-Daoud therefore compared cervical cancer rates among religious groups in Lebanon, where the Moslem men are circumcised and the Christians are not.[3] The fact that there was no apparent difference in cervical cancer rates between the two groups weakened the circumcision hypothesis.

Third, a hypothesis need not explain all existing observations. Inconsistencies may be due to several factors, including:

1. Multiple independent causes of a single manifestational disease: Causes other than the one defined in the hypothesis may be responsible for observations that do not fit. For example, the occurrence of lung cancer in persons who have never smoked is clear evidence that there are constellations of causes of this disease that do not include smoking tobacco.

2. Crudity of the disease classification: The disease "entity" under investigation, for example, epilepsy or lung cancer, may in fact comprise several different entities that could even be distinguished manifestationally if the proper evaluations were performed. Etiological differences between the subentities may produce inconsistencies with a hypothesis that is valid for only one of them. In fact, if the hypothesis is otherwise supported, the inconsistencies may provide the stimulus for separating the associated subentity from the others.

Stating a Hypothesis

Ideally an epidemiologic hypothesis should specify the following:

1. The characteristics of the persons to whom the hypothesis applies
2. The cause being considered—usually an environmental exposure
3. The expected effect—the disease
4. The exposure–response relationship—the amount of the cause needed to lead to a stated risk of the effect
5. The time–response relationship—the time period that will elapse between exposure to the cause and the appearance of the effect.

A well-developed hypothesis describes each of these elements with a high degree of specificity. For example, current knowledge might allow us to formulate the hypothesis that among adults without any previous exposure to the disease or its vaccine, the ingestion of a million viable typhoid bacilli will result in an attack rate of typhoid fever of 50 percent within a period of 30 days. In practice, the components of an epidemiological hypothesis are usually less well specified and may indeed be no more than implied. The hypothesis that dirty water causes diarrhea lacks specificity in the two components that are stated (cause and effect) and implies the concepts that the population involved is human and that the time–response relationship is within a reasonable observation period. Even though unstated, these last components must be made explicit if the hypothesis is to be susceptible to test.

Although a relatively unspecific hypothesis may have some utility, as does linking dirty water to diarrhea, its usefulness would be enhanced by increasing the specificity of any one of its five components. The added specificity may not lead immediately to a more practical preventive program, but it may provide the basis for further investigation that does.

Testing Hypotheses

Some epidemiological aspects of testing hypotheses by direct experiment in humans are discussed later, but let us assume for the moment that the hypothesis under consideration cannot be tested by direct experiment, as is true of the majority of situations in epidemiological investigation.

Ecological Testing

As noted previously, in descriptive epidemiology the unit of observation is a population or subgroup of a population defined in terms of some common characteristic, usually place, time, or person. The disease rates of groups with specific characteristics are compared with those not having the characteristics. In sociology, such studies are referred to as *ecological studies*, and that term has been adopted for similar studies in epidemiology. As noted in the previous section, ecological studies provide one of the sources of information that may lead to the development of causal hypotheses. After the development of a hypothesis a careful search should be made for descriptive data that did not enter into the development of the hypothesis initially but that may be relevant. For example, the hypothesis linking cigarette smoking to lung cancer derived from observation of differences in lung cancer rates by gender and over time; subsequently the hypothesis was evaluated by examining lung cancer incidence in groups whose religion discouraged smoking. The fact that Mormons[118,300] and Seventh Day Adventists,[130] whose religions share this feature, have low lung cancer rates supported the hypothesis. Ecological studies can therefore help in the formation, development, and, to some extent, assessment of hypotheses.

Ecological to Individual Correlation

Whether an association is causal or not, it becomes more meaningful if it can be demonstrated that it exists for individuals as well as in an ecological context; for example, not only do populations that demonstrate frequent cigarette smoking have high lung cancer rates, but *individuals* who smoke also have increased lung cancer risk. This step from ecological to individual correlations is often thought of as the dividing line between descriptive and *analytic* epidemiology. Although the distinction works to some extent, it is not sharp. Thus, smokers comprise a population, just as do males, and the correlation between smokers and lung cancer could have been considered ecologic had vital statistics cross-tabulated lung cancer and smoking as well as lung cancer and gender. Similarly, the observation that nickel workers had an elevated risk for cancer of the nasal sinuses[230] could have been considered either ecologic or analytic, depending on how the data on the association were generated. In fact, one practical distinction between descriptive and analytic studies is that descriptive studies are based on the study and analysis of routinely collected data, whereas analytic studies require the ad hoc collection of information. The terms descriptive and analytic are also sometimes used to distinguish the hypothesis forming from the hypothesis testing stages of epidemiology, and there is considerable, although not total, overlap of studies classified on this basis with those classified by either of the other distinctions stated earlier. It is usually evident from the context in which sense the terms are being used, and there is little to be gained by being purist about the definition.

Case-Control and Cohort Studies

Suppose that a study is planned to test the hypothesis that a particular drug taken during pregnancy causes congenital malformation in the offspring. With respect to the two sets of events— exposure to the drug and the occurrence of malformation—every individual mother–child pair belongs to one of the categories in Table 5-1. The cells in each category are indicated by the letters *a*, *b*, *c*, and *d*. The question posed is whether the proportion malformed is higher in the offspring of mothers who took the drug than in the offspring of those who did not. In other words, is the number of infants in cell *a* higher than would be expected if the two events were unrelated? The method by which the expected number of individuals in cell *a* is obtained distinguishes two basic types of study—cohort studies and case-control studies. This basic distinction between the two types of study was pointed out

Table 5-1. Distribution of Individuals with Respect to Presence or Absence of Two Characteristics

	Malformation in offspring		
Drug use during pregnancy	Present	Absent	Total
Exposed	a	b	$a + b$
Not exposed	c	d	$c + d$
Total	$a + c$	$b + d$	$a + b + c + d$

by White and Bailar in 1953,[588] although recent methodological work has highlighted the unifying elements.[358,576]

Cohort Studies

In cohort studies, using the example in Table 5-1, the investigators select a study population consisting of some pregnant women who took the drug and others who did not. They then observe the groups over time to determine how many exposed and how many nonexposed infants developed malformation. They can then compare the proportion of malformed infants in the exposed group, $a/(a + b)$, with the proportion of malformed infants in the nonexposed group, $c/(c + d)$. Note that this method permits a direct comparison of rates and risks.

This kind of study has also been called a *follow-up* study because exposed and nonexposed persons are followed over time to determine the proportions that become affected. The term is, in our view, insufficiently unique. It is shared not only by clinical studies in which persons already ill are followed to determine the outcome of their illnesses, but also by many kinds of programs in public health that are not in fact research but practical application programs, such as the follow up of patients with a known infectious disease. Furthermore, the *process* of a cohort study may not, as we shall see, involve actual follow up at all; it may involve simply the merging of two or more computer files. For these reasons the term *cohort study* is preferred.

Case-Control Studies

Another sampling approach is to select a study population consisting of some infants who were malformed (cases) and some who were not (controls). The investigator must then determine the frequency with which the mothers in both groups took the drug. The frequency of exposure of cases, $a/(a + c)$, is compared with the frequency of exposure of controls, $b/(b + d)$, the latter being considered a sample of the source population. Even though in a study of this type the study groups are selected from affected $(a + c)$ and unaffected $(b + d)$ individuals, they usually represent unknown proportions of the respective populations; therefore, rates or risks of disease cannot be computed directly in such studies. There are methods by which such risks can be estimated, but they depend on information other than that collected in the case-control study (see Chapter 10). An exception to this generalization occurs when a well-defined population is the source of both cases and controls, and the sampling ratios are explicitly defined.

Choice of Study Design

More detailed descriptions and examples of cohort and case-control studies and their many variations are given in Chapters 9 and 10; however, it may be useful here to note the special features that influence the choice of one or the other type for study of a particular relationship. Cohort studies have some methodological advantages, but they are economical only when the disease under investigation is relatively frequent. For uncommon diseases, very large cohorts are required to obtain reliable estimates of disease rates and risks, and the case control approach is usually preferable. This problem may be overcome if the information can be collected from records assembled over a long period of time or from a large population—usually from computer storage—and there is a computerized mechanism for identifying cases among them. Yet, if new information has to be collected this may not be true. The methodological advantages of the cohort approach are that it takes the intuitively proper sequence, from cause to effect; it more frequently permits direct estimates of rates and risks; and it is less susceptible to selection and information bias.

Perhaps the principal limitation of the case-control study is that information on the supposed cause must be retained—either in memories of persons, in biomarkers (e.g., serological markers or DNA adducts), or in written documents—until after the person can be identified as having the disease. The Health Interview Survey of the US National Center for Health Statistics has provided a good deal of information about the reliability, or lack of it, of people's recall of medical and other events. For example, in a large survey of a random sample of the US noninstitutional population, 30 percent of visits to physicians were not recalled in interviews between 1 and 2 weeks after the visit and more than 30 percent of hospitalizations of less than 5 days that had occurred 41–52 weeks prior were not reported.[51] However, Willett and his colleagues have studied the repeatability and validity of dietary information elicited through specialized food consumption frequency questionnaires and found it reasonably satisfactory, at least when the study subjects were nurses or other health professionals.[440,595] Written documentation is often lacking for variables of epidemiological interest, and information drawn from memory must be carefully evaluated for possible bias (so called *information bias*) relating to the development of the disease in one group (the cases) and not in the other (the controls).[472,581]

In contrast, a case-control study is usually more powerful, in the statistical sense, and less costly than a cohort study in terms of both time and resources. For example, an increased risk of lung cancer among women who did not smoke but who were married to smokers was reported almost simultaneously from two studies. The two estimates of the size of the risk were very similar. One study was a concurrent cohort study that involved interviews with more than 142,000 women.[211] The other was a case-control study involving only 214 interviews.[539] Case-control studies are frequently undertaken as a first step to determine whether or not an association exists or to select between several hypotheses that could explain the observed distribution of the disease. Cohort studies may then be undertaken to gain added confidence in the existence of the relationship and to measure more accurately its characteristics. For example, approximately 15 case-control studies of the relationship between lung cancer and smoking had been published before the publication of the first cohort study in 1954.[94]

Other Terminology

Historical and Concurrent Studies

An important element of the cost of a cohort study is the waiting time that elapses between the selection of exposed and nonexposed cohorts and the development of the disease. In a typical *concurrent* study, such as the Framingham Heart Study of the US Public Health Service,[86] even when a relatively common disease, such as coronary heart disease, is under investigation, many years elapse between the selection of the study cohorts and the appearance of sufficient cases for the computation of reliable disease rates and risks among exposed and nonexposed cohort members.

The cost of such a study can be substantially reduced if the cause and effect under investigation are such that they can both be ascertained *historically* from existing records. For example, in 1960 Beebe assembled from US Army records a cohort of men who were hospitalized for mustard gas poisoning in 1918. Two comparison cohorts were also assembled from military records of the same vintage.[19] Mortality of the cohorts between 1919 and 1955 was ascertained from Veterans Administration records, with a significant excess of deaths due to lung cancer being found in the cohort exposed to mustard gas. Because both the exposure and the effects occurred prior to the time the investigation began, the waiting period required in a concurrent study was eliminated. Such studies combine the economy of the case-control study with the advantages of the cohort study in providing direct estimates of risk and reducing the danger of information and selection bias.

Prospective and Retrospective Studies

The terms *prospective* and *retrospective* have also been used to describe these two forms of cohort study, and we have encouraged such use. The terms *concurrent* and *historical* were suggested by Lilienfeld[286] and seem preferable, not because they are more descriptive but because they avoid the confusion engendered in the epidemiological literature by the terms prospective and retrospective. In a terminology that is now more or less defunct (courtesy of White and Bailar[588]) they were once used to designate what are now called cohort and case-control studies, but they have been used in a variety of other senses. We suggest that they be used in epidemiology only in the sense in which they are used in everyday language, that is, pertaining to things in the future and in the past, respectively. In fact, it seems that confusion would be lessened if the words prospective and retrospective were phased out in describing epidemiological studies and the alternatives suggested by Lilienfeld adopted instead.

Cross-Sectional and Longitudinal Studies

Epidemiological studies can also be characterized by whether the ascertainments of cause and effect relate to two different points or to a single point in the life of an individual. In a *longitudinal* study, the observations relate to two different points in the life of the individual study members, even if both items of information are ascertained at the same point in the life of the investigator. Most cohort and case-control studies are longitudinal in nature. In a *cross-sectional* study, however, measurements of cause and effect (or of the two components of the hypothesis if a causal relationship is not suspected), relate to the same point in the study members' lives. Although the cross-sectional study is easier and more economical than the longitudinal study, it is limited to studies of causes that are long-standing characteristics of the individual, so that his or her status at the time the disease was manifested has a high probability of reflecting the status at the time the disease originated. For example, a cross-sectional study would be a reasonable way of investigating the relationship between histocompatibility antigens and disease. A longitudinal study would be required, however, to investigate the relationship between neonatal jaundice and mental development. In practice, the distinction between cross-sectional and longitudinal studies is not clear. For example, cigarette consumption is a variable that tends to remain a long-standing characteristic of an individual, and the relationship between lung cancer risk and prior cigarette smoking is so strong that it would probably be detected by asking lung cancer patients about their current smoking habits. The relationship would, however, be less strong than that between lung cancer and smoking habits 20 years previously. There is a considerable range of stability of individual characteristics over time.

Cross-sectional studies are frequently made on total population samples. For example, the US National Health Survey has reported a number of studies in which correlations between possible causal factors (e.g., current occupation, parity, blood chemistry) and disease (e.g., hearing deficiency, diabetes mellitus, hypertension) have been based on observations made at a single examination of a random sample of the US population. It should be borne in mind that such studies describe the patterns of disease prevalence, not incidence, and that these will be affected by factors influencing disease duration as well as incidence (see Chapter 4). Studies of genetic markers and disease, however, exemplify cross-sectional studies that may use the case-control method of subject selection, and in these instances may be based on incident rather than prevalent cases of disease.

The categorizations and terminology just described are presented for the purpose of describing some of the techniques and problems associated with particular aspects of study design. Although many studies may be described as "typical" examples of a case-control study or a historical cohort study, for example, there are also studies that defy such classification. For example, there are studies that have been designed as cohort studies but analyzed as case-control studies;[394] such studies are sometimes referred to as case-control studies "nested" in a cohort study. A recent example is the analysis of contraceptive histories among cases (and noncases) of cervical dysplasia identified during a concurrent cohort study.[386] There are also case-control studies that are population based and do permit rather direct estimates of disease rates in exposed and nonexposed groups.[364] It would be unfortunate if epidemiologic methodology were to lose flexibility and become constrained within these or any other definitions of "typical" kinds of study.

Refutation in Epidemiology

In 1975, Carol Buck introduced the logic of the late Karl Popper to epidemiologists.[47] Others have compared in detail, and in general favorably, the essence of Popper's philosophy with what they see as current practice in epidemiology.[275,304] Popper's principal point is that science advances by drawing deductions from postulated hypotheses and, by showing the deductions to be false, refuting the hypothesis.[418-420] In what has become almost a self-caricature, Popper uses the hypothesis that "All swans are white" as an example of a hypothesis that can never be confirmed, no matter how many white swans are observed, but that can be refuted by the appearance of a single nonwhite swan. The concept of testing hypotheses by examining the consequences of what can be deduced from them is not new to epidemiologists and other scientists; however, in emphasizing the need to define hypotheses in terms that are refutable, Popper has made an unwitting contribution to the discipline. What is less broadly accepted is the centrality that Popper assigns to this particular process. Several readers have challenged his position that anything other than refutation, and particularly the processes of verification and induction, may not be science at all.[304,520] Susser writes: "The second aspect of my disagreement [with Popper] is in the matter of induction: to rule out induction as well as verification is to rule out much of the rational (and nonrational) procedure of daily science, and to deprive the scientist of his small arms if not of his biggest guns. Certainly epidemiologists are in the habit of generating hypotheses by induction from the arrays of descriptive data and existing knowledge with which their studies are bound to begin."[521]

We should keep in mind that science is by definition a body of knowledge, not a method or even a group of methods by which that knowledge has been obtained. If we are to separate science from nonscience the argument should therefore be around whether or not the facts are science (i.e., known to be true), not whether the methods used to ascertain them were scientific. In any discipline, the range of methods used to assemble the existing database is extremely broad and constantly changing. A focus on what is probably the single most incisive way of testing hypotheses should not discourage the use of other methods.

Others have trouble not only with what Popper leaves out, but with whether his exclusive demand for falsification can be met within the framework of epidemiology. Karhausen[246] points out that *existential* statements, such as "There is at least one black swan," can only be verified and not falsified, but many interpret Popper as regarding existential statements as "outside of the domain of science."[402] Furthermore, a good deal of epidemiology (as science) has little to do with the testing or refutation of hypotheses,[403] but is concerned with describing what has been called the "Furniture of the Earth."[515]

We have included a brief review of this debate so that readers will at least be aware of it and to provide some references for those interested in pursuing the arguments in more detail. There are other informative papers, in addition to the ones we have quoted, in the group of essays assembled by Rothman.[468]

6 Time

I look under the lids of Time

Others have shared Thoreau's curiosity about time, but none so avidly as epidemiologists. As the quotation implies, Time has several lids to look under; a few of them are described in reference to epidemiology in this chapter.

Rapid changes in the frequency of a disease may occur within days, hours, or less. In such circumstances the existence of an epidemic is obvious, and, sometimes, although by no means always, its causes are easy to determine. Yet, major epidemics often develop slowly over periods of years or decades; their growth may be so insidious that even the fact that a temporal epidemic exists may not be known to the affected population. The elucidation of the causes of such epidemics is likely to involve the linkage of events and illnesses widely separated in time and perhaps also in place.

Also evident are changes in disease frequency associated with the natural cycles of the year, the lunar month, and the day, as well as with the cycles of the calendar. These vary in the utility of the information that their study yields.

The incidence of many diseases (e.g., scarlet fever, cholera, suicide, peptic ulcer, and coronary heart disease) shows characteristics of several kinds of temporal trends—broad ups or downs spanning decades or centuries, with transient periods of epidemicity affecting particular populations (or sometimes the entire globe) superimposed for brief periods. For the purpose of understanding and, therefore, being able to influence, temporal changes in such diseases, it is useful to think of the determinants of the long-term trends separately from those of the acute episodes because they may not be the same. Similarly, the important determinants of acute or chronic episodes, even of what is clinically the same disease, may differ from episode to episode so that what is learned from one may not be applicable to another. For example, even if it were true, as is suspected, that the high rates of mortality from childhood infections in the industrial nations of the nineteenth century were attributable in large part to inadequate nutrition, the information would be of little help to a health officer faced with an outbreak of streptococcal infection today.

Short-Term Changes

Sharp increases in disease frequency that occur within hours, days, or weeks are often the result of almost simultaneous exposure of a group of people to a single source of contamination—a *point source*. The term is a useful one, although it cannot be precisely defined. For example, are episodes of intense air pollution, such as that which affected London in 1952,[362] or sources of chemical contamination that have been long standing, or an HIV carrier who happens to be a world traveler, point sources? Any answer is arbitrary and the term has meaning only in context.

One of the classic and probably best known point source epidemics was the epidemic of cholera in the Golden Square area of London in 1854, described by John Snow, whose work was referred to in Chapter 1.[508] The rise and fall of this epidemic, shown in Figure 6-1, suggest that a short transient exposure was involved.

The downward slope of the epidemic shown in Figure 6-1 is less steep than the upward slope, as is typical, because the distribution of incubation or latency periods (the period between internalization of an agent and the appearance of clinical illness) tends, in both infectious and noninfectious disease, to be positively skewed. In this instance the downward slope is relatively smooth. Sometimes in infectious diseases the downward slope of the epidemic is interrupted by waves of *secondary* cases occurring at intervals corresponding to the average incubation period of the disease and attributable to persons infected by the primary cases arising from the point source. Such curves are typically seen in disease spread by personal contact, particularly when the setting is a closed or partially closed community.

Specification of Time

As we described in Chapter 5 in the context of measures of disease frequency, a point in time or the beginning of a period of time may not always be defined in terms of a calendar date. It may be specified in terms of age or the occurrence of some event that happens at different ages and different calendar times to different individuals.

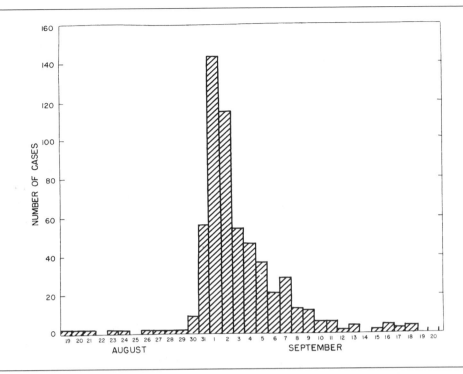

Figure 6-1. The outbreak of cholera in the Golden Square area of London, August and September, 1854. (From Snow J. *On the Mode of Communication of Cholera* [2nd ed.]. London: Churchill, 1855. Reproduced in Snow J. *Snow on Cholera.* New York: Commonwealth Fund, 1936. Reprinted New York: Hafner, 1965.)

For example, Aycock and Luther obtained histories of tonsillectomy from patients with poliomyelitis.[17] Among 36 cases of poliomyelitis that occurred within 12 months of tonsillectomy, there were 16 in which the poliomyelitis occurred within one month of the operation. All 16 of these had onset within 7 to 18 days of tonsillectomy, a period compatible with the known incubation period of poliomyelitis. Even though no data were available to determine how many children selected at random might have given a history of tonsillectomy within 7 to 18 days, the marked clustering suggested a causal relationship between the two events.

Similarly, the marked clustering in onset of episodes of psychotic depression within a few days or weeks of childbirth suggests a relationship between the two, even though the general frequency of episodes of psychotic depression in women of childbearing age is not known.[527]

A method to assess the role of potential causes of acute onset disease events occurring over the time span of the lives of the same individuals (in the absence of external controls) has been developed by Maclure in what he has termed the *case-crossover* design.[305] For a series of individuals, the occurrence of an acute disease event (e.g., acute myocardial infarction) in the person-time following a short transient exposure (e.g., heavy physical activity) is compared with the event-density experience of the same individuals when an exposure did not occur. Statistical methodology is proposed to derive rate ratios associated with specified periods of time after exposure, and the empirical latency following exposure is identified by maximization of the rate ratio. The technique would seem to be of value particularly in the context of assessing the risk of triggering exposures, when assump-

Figure 6-2. Distributions according to week of onset and according to interval between yellow fever vaccination and onset of jaundice, for 5,917 cases of jaundice in US military units in California, 1942. (From Sawyer WA, et al. Jaundice in army personnel in the Western Region of the United States and its relation to vaccination against yellow fever. *Am J Hyg* 1944;39 : 337–430.)

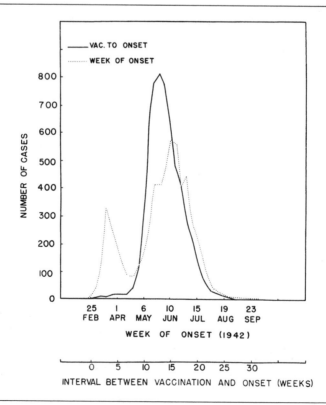

tions can reasonably be made about the likely duration of effect of the exposure and when comparison subjects cannot be sampled.

Measurement of the mean and variance of the interval between an event and its apparent effect is another technique that has been used. In an investigation of the possible relationship between vaccination for yellow fever and possible hepatitis among troops bound for Asia during World War II, it was not possible to compare vaccinated with unvaccinated persons because nearly all the military personnel involved had been vaccinated. Investigation of the time relationships, however, showed that the interval between vaccination and onset of jaundice was less variable than the calendar date of onset of the disease. The standard deviation for the date of onset for 5,917 cases in California, around their mean of June 1, was 5.7 weeks, whereas the standard deviation of the interval between vaccination and onset of jaundice, around a mean of 14.6 weeks, was only 3.5 weeks, supporting a link between these two events (Figure 6-2).[478] A statistical procedure for testing the significance of the difference between correlated variances is given by Snedecor and Cochran.[506]

Secular Changes

Secular changes are those that occur over long periods of time. In epidemiology the term usually implies changes in disease frequency encompassing several decades. Examination of secular changes has been a powerful tool that helped identify the cause of the twentieth century's epidemic of lung cancer[35] (see Figure 6-3) and that challenges solution of such questions as why deaths from atherosclerotic heart disease have been declining so consistently in many countries during the last two decades and those from stomach cancer for an even longer period. However, the study of secular trends is fraught with more than the usual number of problems associated with observational studies in free-living populations.

Until the middle of the twentieth century, the study of secular trends was practically limited to the study of causes of death obtained from death certificates. For diseases that had a high case fatality rate and countries that had a good death reporting system, death certificates served well.

Notification of certain infectious diseases has also been in existence for many decades and has functioned to pick up short-term changes that may warn of the approach of epidemics. Yet, infectious diseases (apart from the major quarantinable diseases, and at times even those) have been greatly underreported, and in a manner that varies from time to time and place to place. Reports based on infectious disease notifications, whether voluntary or under legal authority, have, therefore, not been good sources of information on long-term trends, with some exceptions.

Starting from approximately the 1940s to the 1970s, there have been excellent data on incidence as well as mortality from cancer derived from a hundred or more registries throughout the world. Congenital defects constitute another group of disease for which registry data have been established for some time, although usually in limited geographic areas. The detection of short-term, sharp increases in particular defects, indicating the presence of a new teratogen in the environment, provides the usual stimulus for these registries; they have not been useful for the study of long-term trends. Changes in a variety of biochemical and other physiological parameters in the United States—and to a much lesser extent some disease states—can be monitored subsequent to the inauguration of the US National Health Survey in 1957.

Before concluding that a change in disease frequency over time, particularly over a long period of time, can be linked to changes in the environment to which the observed population has been exposed, it is first necessary to exclude possible alternative explanations. Some common reasons for apparent secular changes in disease frequency include the following:

1. Changes in the completeness of the source of data: At least in the industrialized world, death registration has been reasonably complete for at least 50 years, but it is a common phenomenon to see incidence rates rising for several years after the start of a new registry, the introduction of a new diagnostic technique, or publicity attending the use of such a technique. Also to be considered is the completeness of the information on the certificate if the event is indeed registered. For example, in 1917 the percentage of US death certificates listing more than one pathological condition as an underlying or contributing cause of death was 35 percent; in 1979 it was 73 percent.[231] It is possible that some of this increase reflected the fact that the population dying in 1979 was older than that dying in 1917 and in fact had more pathological conditions present at the time of death. Yet, it may also be that physicians and other certifiers had become more aware of the value of a complete picture of the circumstances leading to the death, and that factors that were in fact present in the earlier deaths had simply not been recorded because a single diagnosis provided a seemingly adequate explanation of the death.

2. Changes in diagnostic ability of physicians and others contributing relevant data: Such changes may reflect real changes in the profession's ability to diagnose because of experience or better technology, or they may simply reflect the fact that many diagnoses come and go in medical circulation without much scientific justification.

3. Changes of practice in data classification: Most striking in this regard are some of the changes introduced by modifications in numerical coding of diseases following the revisions of the World Health Organization's International Classification of Diseases. These were referred to in Chapter 3.

4. Demographic changes in the population in which the trend is being observed: In the societies for which secular data are available, the tendency has been for the age distribution to shift to the right (become older) during long periods of observation. This results in an increase in rates for the great majority of diseases, other than those of infancy and childhood. Provided the age distribution of the population during the period is known, this is readily adjusted for, as discussed in Chapter 4. The problem may not, however, be limited to age. Changes in the distribution by ethnic background, socioeconomic status, education, marital status, residential living patterns, and other factors may also produce changes in disease rates. Sometimes these problems can be dealt with analytically in the same way as age, but there are two difficulties. First, the investigator may recognize the possibilities of such factors influencing the data but may not have the information necessary to adjust for them. Second, the investigator may not recognize the occurrence of changes in some potentially important demographic variable.

5. Concomitant changes in environmental circumstances other than those that the investigator postulates to be the explanation of the observed changes in disease frequency: Such changes have been the source of much ridicule of the concomitant variable ecological method (e.g., the correlation between sales of nylon stockings and the frequency of lung cancer), and most investigators are sufficiently cautious to hedge their hypotheses appropriately. Nevertheless, the possibility of being deceived by some unknown variable remains. The increase over the last two decades in both the incidence of perforated ulcer in the older population, particularly women,[63] and the use of nonsteroidal anti-inflammatory drugs for the treatment of arthritis is a recent example of a temporal correlation that should probably be considered as causal. However, it cannot be so interpreted with certainty.[237]

6. Depending on the nature of the events that are being assembled by the registry or data source, apparent changes in incidence or mortality may reflect a change in the natural history of the disease other than that in which the investigator is interested. Thus a decline in incidence rates does not immediately translate into a decline in mortality; there may be a large group of prevalent cases whose death is still pending. The relationship between incidence, prevalence, and mortality rates was discussed in Chapter 4. Beyond those relationships, an improvement or deterioration in the prognosis of a disease over time (whether due to unknown biological factors or to changes in therapy) may, by bringing the disease more or less often to medical attention, produce a change in reported incidence rates.

The components of secular change that are most difficult to deal with are those relating to the effect of changes in clinical concepts, diagnosis, and terminology because such changes evolve gradually, and, although it is frequently possible to be confident that they have occurred, it is rarely possible to quantify their impact. Some approaches that have been attempted are as follows:

1. Comparison of trends for the disease under investigation with those for other diseases judged equally susceptible to changes in diagnostic ability: For example, Figure 6-3 makes it clear that, although lung cancer is by no means the only cancer site that showed an increase or decrease at some point in this time period, the data leave little doubt that something happened for lung cancer that did not happen for cancers of other internal sites. If it was of a diagnostic nature, it betrays a past ignorance that was remarkably localized from an anatomic point of view. Reasoning of this type can only be suggestive because such an anatomically localized oversight is not inconceivable and because it is usually not possible to find two disorders in which improvement in diagnostic procedures advanced at an equal rate. Such evidence must of course be evaluated in light of what occurred in the practice of medicine during the relevant time frame.

2. Comparison of the frequency with which a disorder is present at autopsies performed at different points in the observation period: This procedure will be more satisfactory the less fatal the disease under investigation, or in other words, the greater the probability that the autopsied patients died of some other cause. In a nonfatal disease, the number of patients in whom the disease is found at autopsy is a measure of the prevalence of the disease at the age at which the patients died. The number can be related

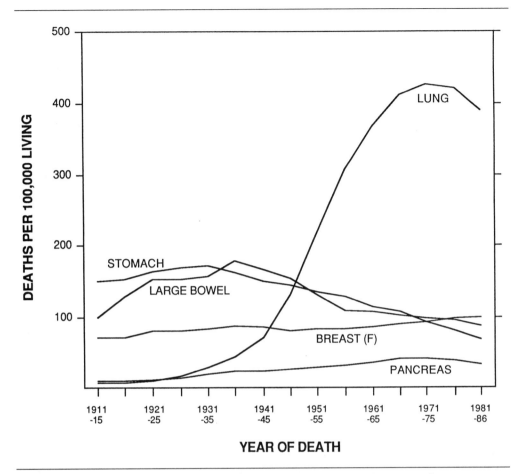

Figure 6-3. Age-adjusted annual mortality rates from selected causes of cancer in males, aged 50–74, Scotland, 1911–1986. (From MacFarlane GJ, Boyle P. Scottish Mortality Data, 1911–1985. Mimeographed. Personal communication, 1987.)

to the number of autopsies at that age to derive age-specific prevalence proportions.

3. Examination of the extent to which the apparent trend might result from secular changes in the proportion of cases ascribed to other diagnoses, with assessment of the reasonableness of the assumptions necessary to account for the observed trend: This method was followed by Gilliam who examined the effect on the trend in lung cancer death rates if various proportions of patients who died of the disease in earlier years had been erroneously certified as dying from other respiratory diseases.[146] Because the number of deaths attributed to other respiratory diseases was much larger than the number attributed to lung cancer, particularly in the earlier years of the twentieth century, a small proportion of them would have made a substantial addition to the number of deaths attributed to lung cancer and markedly reduced the secular trend in lung cancer rates. However, the proportion of misdiagnosed cases necessary to eliminate the trend entirely was so large that the assumptions did not seem reasonable when viewed in conjunction with available data from autopsies.[146]

There are also a number of general arguments that can be applied to the assessment of the epidemiological significance of an apparent secular trend. Thus, trends that are markedly different for certain age, gender, or ethnic groups living in the same community are less likely to be artifacts than those that are evident in all such subgroups. Also it may be illuminating to ask (e.g., in the case of lung cancer) whether diagnostic ability became more sophisticated between 1950 and 1970 at the same rate as it did during earlier years when such diagnostic aids as X ray and bronchoscopy were being introduced.

Secular changes such as those seen in this century for lung cancer are unusual in the chronic diseases, although a decline of almost comparable slope has been seen for cancer of the stomach in Europe and North America and appears to be beginning in Japan. Frequently, after all the considerations have been judged, the question of whether or not a secular trend really exists may remain in doubt. It is important to keep in mind that, whatever the role that a secular trend played in suggesting a hypothesis, the ultimate validity of the hypothesis must rest on evidence other than the secular trend. The latter merely suggested the desirability of assembling that evidence. It was an early tactic of the tobacco companies to distract attention from the real evidence linking cigarette smoking and lung cancer by focusing on the much more easily attacked data on the secular trend.

Generational (Cohort) Secular Time Trends

In Chapter 5 we used the term *cohort study* to describe the observation over time of one or more groups of people (cohorts) for whom information on certain variables potentially productive, or at least predictive, of disease were available. A special type of cohort is one formed of persons born within a specified period of time (e.g., a 1-year or a 5-year period). It has been observed that time trends in chronic diseases may be to some extent characteristic of such *birth cohorts*; that is, they follow a pattern of disease frequency that is in part predicted by their year of birth independently of the cohort's age or of the time in which it is observed. When the birth cohort does not predict the frequency of disease, the patterns observed are characteristic of the time of observation and the individuals' ages at the time, regardless of when the individuals were born. Sometimes several types of pattern can be seen in the same data set.

The distinction between these patterns is important in two contexts: when interpreting the shape of a graph illustrating changes in disease frequency with age and when seeking explanation for or predicting changes in disease frequency over time. The issue was first noted by Andvord in 1930;[9] it was brought to wider attention by Frost in 1939[138] and, in the context of noninfectious disease, by Dorn and Cutler in 1959.[104] The earlier authors noted that the relationship of tuberculosis mortality to age was much more consistent if the age curves were drawn for individual birth cohorts than if cross-sectional data were illustrated at particular points in time. The consistency of the age pattern for birth cohorts was intellectually satisfying because it also indicated that, to some degree, the tuberculosis mortality of a generation was established early in its life—a fact consistent with knowledge of the biology of the disease. Lancaster provided an even more dramatic example in showing how the peak of age-specific prevalence of deaf-mute persons in New South Wales advanced 10 years in each successive 10-year census—a function of the fact that the birth cohort born in 1899 was exposed in utero to a severe epidemic of rubella.[274] The relevance of cohort patterns to the study of time trends was emphasized by Case in 1956.[52]

Consider the data illustrated in Figure 6-4.[36,53] They suggest that the time trend in mortality due to lung cancer has been different in different age groups. In the oldest age groups (70 and older), rates increased throughout the period of observation, whereas in the younger age groups rates were more or less stationary or declining since the late 1950s. Immediately intriguing about this pattern is that the levelling off began earlier in time the younger the age group that was observed. This is shown in Figure 6-5 by realigning the curves so that a vertical line joins the rates exhibited by persons belonging to the same birth cohort. The trends are now consistent over all age groups. Cohorts of persons born until approximately 1900–1905 experienced increasing rates (in all age groups), but cohorts born thereafter experienced stationary or declining rates in all age groups. It is not necessary therefore to seek an explanation for the trends in time-related experience that varied differentially across age groups. It is true, of course, that the latter cannot be excluded,

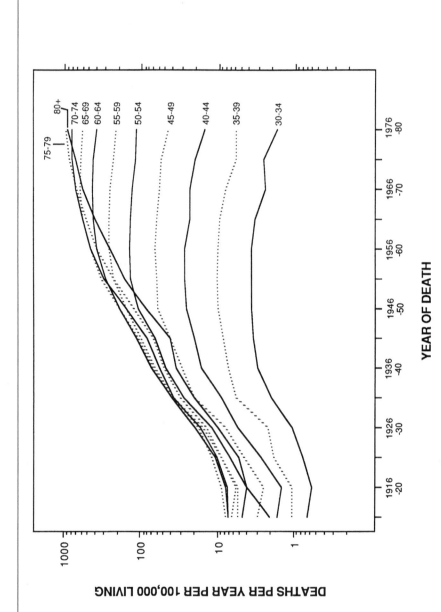

Figure 6-4. Age-specific annual death rates from cancer of the lung and pleura in males, England and Wales, 1911–1980. (Data for 1911–1970 from Case RAM, et al. *Serial Mortality Tables. Neoplastic Diseases, Volume 1. England and Wales, 1911–1970.* Mimeographed. London: Division of Epidemiology, Institute for Cancer Research, 1976. Data for 1971–1980 from Boyle P. Personal communication, 1987.)

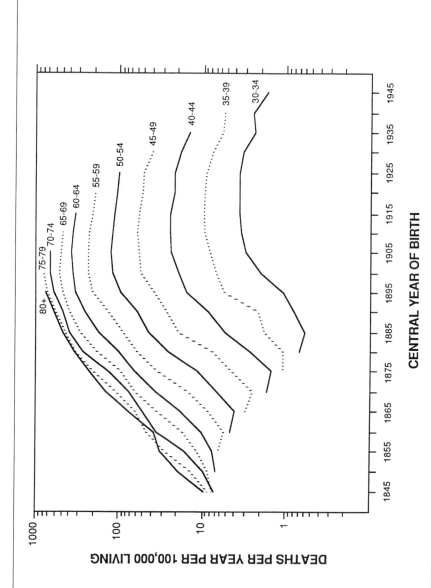

Figure 6-5. Data from Figure 6-4 rearranged to show age-specific rates for birth cohorts born between 1846 and 1906. (Data for 1911–1970 from Case RAM, et al. *Serial Mortality Tables. Neoplastic Diseases, Volume 1. England and Wales. 1911–1970.* Mimeographed. London: Division of Epidemiology, Institute for Cancer Research, 1976. Data for 1971–1980 from Boyle P. Personal communication, 1987.)

but the more parsimonious hypothesis is that the change that induced the decline was one that affected successive generations and remained with them throughout life.

Initially, the "analysis" of birth cohort trends was visual, dependent on bringing into consistency an inflection in either the age trend or the time trend. Initiated by important work by Stevens et al,[518] Holford,[214] and Breslow and Day,[43] the 1980s brought mathematical modeling (Poisson regression) to the problem, and we are no longer dependent on the presence of an inflection to distinguish birth cohort from period effects. Tarone and Chu give a good review of the mathematical developments following those papers.[526] They show that the procedures can be used nonparametrically, and they apply their nonparametric formulation to the study of recent trends in breast cancer mortality. Breast cancer appears to be an example of a disease in which both cohort and period (cross-sectional) effects are at work.

Boyle and Robertson analyzed Scottish mortality data for lung and laryngeal cancer for 1960–1979.[37] For lung cancer, the trends appeared to be predominantly dependent on cohort effects that were stronger among men than women in the older cohorts, but stronger in women than men in the younger cohorts. The observation would be compatible with the observed increase in consumption of cigarettes among young women. The authors suggested that a small cross-sectional effect in both sexes could be attributable to the increased coverage of cancer registration in Scotland since 1960. Because the data are for mortality, any increase in treatment efficacy, if it had occurred, might also have contributed to the cross-sectional component of the trends. Mathematical models of cohort effects are obviously more efficient if data are available for individuals rather than for groups.

With techniques for birth cohort analysis well formulated, there needs to be more work devoted to the identification of explanations for cohort effects when they are observed and to the perhaps more difficult task of testing the hypotheses suggested.

Cyclic Changes

Many of the world's major diseases have ebbed and flowed over the centuries, as with the seventeenth century's plague, the nineteenth century's cholera, and the twentieth (and certainly twenty-first) century's lung cancer. Sometimes such long-lasting outbreaks are referred to as "cycles;" however, in epidemiology the word has a more limited meaning. It indicates repetitive cycling

predictable to some extent in terms of an external measure of time, such as the season of the year. The variation is most frequently evaluated simply by plotting the occurrence of cases against the season or month. Use of a reference population and calculation of rates are usually unnecessary, unless periodic changes in the size of the population are likely, as might be expected in a vacation resort or military camp. However, for accuracy, account must be taken of the fact that different months have different numbers of days and therefore different periods of risk. Thus, for Figure 6-6, numbers of suicides were computed on a daily basis, and the average number for each day was expressed as a percentage of the overall daily mean. The data for each month represent the average for the month. Visual inspection is usually sufficient to detect any meaningful relationships (the trend shown in Figure 6-6 is

Figure 6-6. Corrected monthly suicides expressed as percentages above or below the overall daily mean. United States, 1972–1978. (Corrected for number of days in each month.) (From MacMahon K. Short-term fluctuations in the frequency of suicide, United States, 1972–1978. *Am J Epidemiol* 1983;117 : 744–750.)

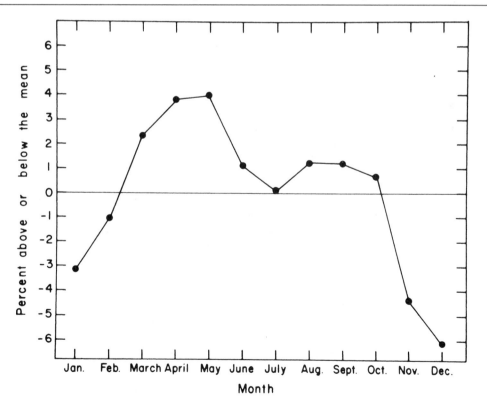

typical for what has been reported for suicide), otherwise statistical tests can be conducted.

The disadvantage of statistical tests based on modeling is their complexity. An efficient test, based on the parameters of a sine curve, which computes both the strength and the statistical significance of a seasonal association was developed by Edwards.[113] The efficiency of the test depends on an underlying model of a condition with a single high and a single low period of risk. Conditions with more than one seasonal peak, as in Figure 6-6, cannot be analyzed by this technique.

The greatest utility stemming from the study of cyclic variations in disease frequency has to date come in the context of seasonal variation; a great many biological phenomena vary with the seasons, including the life cycles of plants and insects, many of which influence strongly the occurrence of human disease. Investigations have ranged from the study of pollens involved in hay fever to the search for insect vectors with relevant seasonal patterns of reproduction or feeding. For example, in the United States, diseases contracted from ticks, such as Rocky Mountain Spotted Fever and Lyme disease, show marked concentrations in the spring and early summer, corresponding to the feeding activity of adult ticks. The mosquito-borne encephalitides, however, are concentrated in the late summer and early fall.

Seasonal variation in occupational or recreational activities may also account for variation in exposure to sources of infection. Thus, the marked concentration of human leptospirosis during the summer months is accounted for by increased exposure to infected waters in the course of bathing and fishing. Increased crowding during cold weather leads to conditions conducive to the spread of airborne infections.

Seasonal variations in the acute infectious diseases of childhood pose some of the major unsolved mysteries of infectious disease epidemiology. In spite of the consistent occurrence and magnitude of these variations, they remain largely unexplained. There appear to be no seasonal variations in the secondary attack rates of measles, chicken pox, or mumps once an infection is introduced into a household,[497] suggesting that seasonal factors relate more to opportunities for infection than to variation in characteristics of the virus or potential host. Seasonal circumstances that are entirely man-made may play a part. Thus, Friedman et al. showed rises in serum cholesterol of accountants corresponding to critical dates in the tax calendar.[137] If this is a real phenomenon, it is unlikely to be limited to accountants.

There are cyclic trends other than seasonal, which may have both biological and sociological determinants. Variation in the

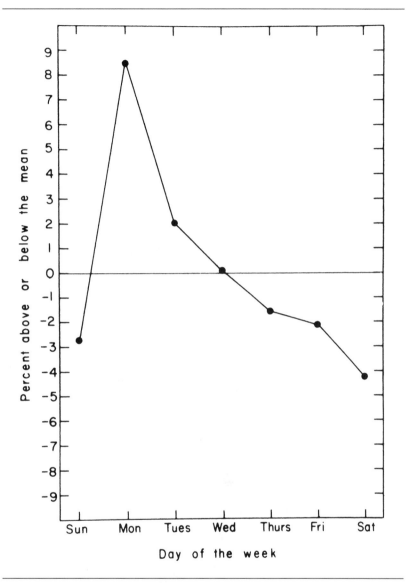

Figure 6-7. Suicides by day of the week, expressed as percentages above or below the average daily mean. United States, 1972–1978. (From MacMahon K. Short-term fluctuations in the frequency of suicide, United States, 1972–1978. *Am J Epidemiol* 1983;117 : 744–750.)

frequency of suicide by day of the week, as shown in Figure 6-7, has a pattern for which most of us think they can feel some understanding in sociological terms. Variation by day of the week and time of day in birth (particularly by Caesarean section) or death undoubtedly have both medical and social determinants.

Diurnal variation in the frequency of myocardial infarction is of great interest. Onset of infarction, whether assessed by onset of pain or by elevation in certain serum enzymes, is more frequent in the morning hours than during the night.[372] At the peak of the cycle (9 A.M.), the frequency of infarction is three times as great as at the ebb (11 P.M.). Willich et al. took account of the time of wakening of the patients and found that the morning increase occurred during the first 3 hours after wakening (Figure 6-8).[599,600] A similar pattern has been reported for sudden cardiac deaths occurring out of the hospital.[372] Stroke, also frequently the result of arterial occlusion, shows a similar morning peak.[327,548] There are concomitant cycles in platelet aggregation potential and other relevant physiological changes that may suggest mechanisms underlying the cycle,[374,534] and that an external factor is at least partly responsible is suggested by the fact that the cyclic pattern is not seen for infarctions that occur on Saturday or Sunday.[373] As noted earlier (Chapter 5), joint action of two variables,

Figure 6-8. Time of sudden cardiac death in relation to hours after awakening. (From Willich SN et al. Increased onset of sudden cardiac death in the first three hours after awakening. *Am J Cardiol* 1992;70 : 65–68.)

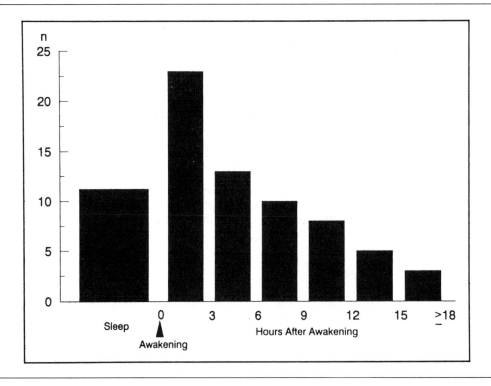

in this instance diurnal and weekly cycles, should present a powerful opportunity for hypothesis development. Cohen and Muller offer a recent review of the possible triggers and mechanisms involved.[64]

7 Place

Place, like time, presents many facets to epidemiologists. In Chapter 1, we gave recognition to Hippocrates for his understanding of the importance of variation in disease manifestations from place to place. Early knowledge of the geographic distribution of disease was entirely qualitative and derived from sporadically published observations of medical practitioners and other observers. Hirsch's three volume *Handbook of Geographical and Historical Pathology*, translated into English in 1883, is an enormous accumulation of such observations and represents the full flowering of anecdotal epidemiology.[212]

As with many of the associations described in the previous and subsequent chapters, current quantitative knowledge of this topic is based on data collected and published routinely in the course of registration of vital events (birth and death), surveillance of special diseases, medical care reports, and special surveys.

International Comparisons

Data relating to causes of death and notifications of specific infectious diseases are collected and published by the World Health Organization and, in the case of cancer, by the International Agency for Research on Cancer. Although the published data are restricted to countries in which reporting is believed to be adequate, differences in accuracy and completeness of diagnosis and reporting often pose serious difficulties. Nevertheless, the large differences that have been shown, and even those that are less striking, should not be ignored simply because of this uncertainty. They may at least merit special studies to test their validity.

For some diseases, for example, the major infectious diseases, the fact that they are epidemic in some areas and virtually absent in others is immediately obvious from review of published reports. The international differences seen for most noninfectious diseases are generally smaller; however, these differences may be even more important from an investigative point of view because most of them concern diseases of unknown etiology, and in many instances the international differences are the most striking feature of their descriptive epidemiology. Japan, for example, has relatively low rates of death from coronary heart disease, but it has very high rates of hypertension and cerebrovascular accidents; Germany, Iceland, and Japan have unusually high death rates from stomach cancer, although the rates in Japan appear to be declining; the United States has very high rates of coronary artery disease, as well as a number of specific cancers. Perhaps the main value of routine international data is to provide a basis for the broad classification of countries into those with probably high, probably average, and probably low rates of particular diseases. The data are too fragile to support finer classifications at the present time.

Cross-National Surveys

International differences in disease rates observed in crude data may be further investigated in special surveys, one purpose of which may be simply to ascertain whether an unusual frequency of disease suggested in routine data is real or the result of diagnostic or reporting differences. Ideally, this question could be answered by conducting surveys using identical protocols in the countries where differences in disease frequencies are suspected. More commonly, however, the issue is approached by surveys that seek to determine whether diagnostic or reporting practices differ sufficiently that they *could* explain the differences observed. For example, routine statistics from mental hospitals have consistently shown that, although overall hospitalization rates for mental illness are similar in the United States and the United Kingdom, the distributions of patients by diagnosis are very different.[266] A US-UK Diagnostic Project was established to compare diagnostic practices in the two countries. In one large hospital in New York, 61 percent of the patients had been diagnosed as schizophrenic, whereas in a comparable London hospital only 34 percent of patients were given this diagnosis. Yet, it was found that when standardized interviews were used to collect clinical information the distributions of diagnoses of the same patients in the two hospitals were very similar.[73] Apparently the diagnostic criteria for schizophrenia were much broader in the United States than in the United Kingdom,[550] and this provided an adequate explanation of the differences found in routine statistics.

Special surveys may also be done to determine whether differences in disease patterns can be explained by differences in environmental exposures. Commonly, what is measured is some marker of exposure rather than the exposure itself (e.g., serum cholesterol as a marker of dietary intake of saturated fat or biomarkers of past exposure to a virus). In theory, the samples that are being surveyed should be random samples of the populations in which the disease frequencies have been measured, but this ideal is rarely achieved. In practice the international differences in rates are often so great that broad excursions from the assumption of representativeness of the sample subjects can be tolerated. Sometimes, measures of disease may be incorporated along with measures of exposure and, indeed, on occasion it is unclear which role a particular variable is playing. Hypertension, for example, is a disease in its own right, but it is also a predictor of stroke and other cardiovascular conditions. A classic example of this kind of survey is that of Keys and his associates in the 1960s.[255] Using standardized forms and procedures and centralized analyses of the output of such portable commodities as electrocardiograms and sera, males 40–59 years old in nine communities in seven countries with widely different rates of death from coronary heart disease were examined and then resurveyed 5 years later. The study focused attention on serum cholesterol levels of individuals and percentage of calories derived from saturated fatty acids in the diets of population groups as predictors of fatal and nonfatal myocardial infarction.

Variation Within Countries

Except in instances of very acute and localized epidemics, the study of variation in disease rates within countries generally is limited to comparisons defined by existing administrative boundaries, such as states or counties, because even if the cases of disease can be distributed without respect to administrative boundaries, population data having sufficient specificity of age, gender, and other variables will generally not be available. Differences in diagnostic and reporting practices are usually less troublesome when comparing administrative areas within countries than in international comparisons, but they cannot be ignored.

Disease Mapping

Whether intranational or international patterns are being sought, it is often desirable to display the results descriptively in the form of a map. The technology for disease mapping has received considerable attention recently in the context of cancer. In 1974, the National Cancer Institute produced a monograph of age-adjusted mortality rates for 35 forms of cancer in the 3,056 counties of the 48 contiguous states of the United States for the period 1950–1969,[335] followed by maps derived from these data for the white[336] and nonwhite[337] populations. For the less common cancers, contiguous counties were grouped into "State Economic Areas" (SEA) to reduce the random fluctuation to which the number of cancer cases in the smaller counties was susceptible. A similar atlas of mortality from diseases other than cancer was also produced,[334] and the cancer data for whites were updated to cover the period 1950–1980.[412] In the latter report, the 506 SEAs, rather than the 3,056 counties, were used exclusively, thus increasing the stability of the rates. These maps identified a number of geographic patterns that were not evident in comparison of state data and generated hypotheses that were subsequently tested in analytic studies.[134] For example, the first maps indicated concentrations of high mortality from respiratory cancer in males along the South Atlantic seaboard and the Gulf of Mexico, which led to suspicion about the role of the large shipyards located in those areas that were very active during World War II. Case-control studies in some of the areas showed elevated lung cancer risk associated with shipyard employment even after adjustment for demographic variables and other known risk factors, such as cigarette smoking and other occupations. Clusters of mesothelioma in the non–shipyard-employed wives of shipyard employees and in other residents of the areas,[525] as well as in the employees themselves, leave little doubt as to the role of asbestos exposure in and emanating from the shipyards in the high mesothelioma and lung cancer rates in these geographic areas.

In the last few years, a number of other countries have produced maps of the distribution of cancer within their borders. Among them are several European countries, the European Union,[498] Japan, and, perhaps most notably, China, where extraordinary variations in the frequencies of major cancer sites are seen.[112,285] Some of the European maps are based on incidence registration, rather than mortality, which has obvious advantages when understanding etiology is the objective of the exercise.[253,428]

These maps are no longer produced by multicolored crayons on the mimeographed outlines of maps of the country with its administrative subdivisions; they are computer generated and produced in vibrant colors. Yet, the basic decisions that confronted the original mapmakers still exist. These decisions are given more formal attention and are described in some detail by Kemp et al.[253] They include the following:

1. Administrative units: Selecting the level of administrative subdivision to be used involves a difficult trade-off. Clearly, the unit has to be one for which both disease occurrence and population numbers and characteristics are available. Beyond that, on the one hand the smaller the units used the more accurately the boundaries of an area of high or low disease frequency can be defined. On the other hand, the smaller the units used the less stable the individual rates will be, and in the resulting picture the real patterns may be obscured by random variation. The size of the population of a unit, the frequency of the disease under investigation, and the general environmental similarity of the contiguous units are relevant factors. Most often the choice is made empirically. Thus, comparisons of the 1987 and 1974 US cancer maps suggest that, for this group of diseases, the use of SEAs shows geographic patterns more clearly and without the distraction introduced by the random variation in data for individual counties.

2. Random variation: The simplest way of preparing a disease map is to fill in the area of each administrative unit according to some color code identifying a range of rates and ignore the unavoidable random variation that occurs around the estimate. The difficulty with this approach, as noted previously, is that the administrative units usually vary in size and, therefore, in the stability of their rate estimates. An apparent focus of disease may be nothing more than a chance elevation in an area with a small population. Furthermore, there is often an inverse association between an administrative unit's population and its geographic acreage (and, therefore, the proportion of the map that it occupies), so that a sparsely settled desert may, by chance, give an impressive appearance of high or low disease frequency.

The US investigators approached this problem by combining in a single scale the level of the rate and its stability. Thus, in the 1987 report,[412] SEAs are colored red if their rate is significantly higher than the overall US rate *and* in the top 10 percent of all SEA rates, orange if they are not in the highest decile but are significantly higher than the US average, purple if they are in the highest decile but not significantly different from the US average, and blue if they are significantly lower than the US rate. SEAs that are not significantly different from the US rate and are not in the highest decile are left unshaded. Although this procedure is helpful, it is still the case that a small SEA needs a greater rate increase to be colored red (because it is less likely to differ significantly from the US average for a given rate increase). The difficulty is lessened by the fact that the creation of the SEAs has produced areas that are less variable in population size than are counties. Although one may wonder what is going on in the unshaded part of these maps, the technique is good for picking out "hot spots," such as the high rates of increase of respiratory cancer in white females in California, the Northwest, New York State, and Florida seen between 1950 and 1980. Still, the combination of the levels of the rates and their statistical precision in a single scale lacks the virtue of simplicity. The reader may have to spend more time than he or she is willing to become familiar with the particular codes before understanding what any particular map is trying to communicate.

In the cancer maps for Scotland,[253] the geographic units were the 53 local authority districts and three island areas. The authors of these maps chose to display the rates for all units, regardless of statistical precision, together with a measure ("D") of the likelihood that the overall geographic variation differs from that of a random distribution. This measure, described by Kemp et al.,[253] is based on the probability that closely ranked units (high or low) will be contiguous by chance alone. Therefore, it is sensitive to large-scale regional patterns (e.g., north-south gradients), but it does not evaluate the significance of deviations in individual units. A nonsignificant value of D does not preclude the occurrence of substantially elevated rates in individual areas, particularly if they are not contiguous.

An interesting method of "smoothing" has been used by Pukkala, Gustavsson, and Teppo to overcome the problem of erratic rates in small administrative areas.[428] The basic units, in which age-adjusted rates were calculated, were the 461 municipalities of Finland. An apparently solid color map was computer-generated from a large number of separate dots. The color of each dot was determined by the weighted average of the incidence rates in the municipalities whose centers were within 200 kilometers of the dot. The weights were inversely associated with the distance between the dot and the center of each municipality and directly proportional to the sizes of the populations of the municipalities influencing the dot. The method effectively smooths the random variation seen in municipalities with small populations; however, as with the method used in the Scottish maps, it tends to obscure elevated rates in individual municipalities if they are not shared by other areas in the same region.

3. Selection of ranges: The ranges of rates that are to be illustrated may be selected in terms of actual rates that are thought to be meaningfully different given what is known about the occurrence of the disease, or in terms of grouped percentiles of the distribution of the actual observed values. The use of grouped percentiles relieves the investigator of the need to define meaningful ranges, but it may conceal differences between diseases in the range of their geographic variation.

Urban-Rural Comparisons

Despite the accumulation of many data on urban-rural differences in disease rates in the United States and elsewhere, they are not very helpful in the development of etiologic hypotheses, although air pollution has frequently been invoked to explain the higher incidence of respiratory and, perhaps, cardiovascular disease in the cities.[93,554] Furthermore, urban-rural distinctions in disease rates, to our knowledge, have not been employed effectively in the planning or administration of health services. Considering prevailing demographic and technologic trends, it seems unlikely that urban-rural disease differences will become more useful in the future than they have been in the past.

Local Clustering of Disease

The preparation of maps showing the distribution of cases of disease within a local community is a long-established epidemiological practice. The classic example is John Snow's plotting of the epidemic of cholera in the Golden Square area of London in 1854 (see also Figure 6-1). By plotting the cases on a map of the local area, Snow was able to center attention on a particular public water pump in Broad Street and to show that the cases declined in number as soon as it became easier for the residents to travel to another source of water. Painstaking investigation of the apparent exceptions to this generalization strengthened the hypothesis that it was the water from the Broad Street pump that was responsible for this epidemic.

There remains a strong interest in investigating what appear to be "clusters" of disease for at least two reasons:

1. The occurrence of geographic clustering may suggest a role for an infectious agent.
2. Geographic clustering may suggest the existence of local environmental contamination, particularly when the cluster-

ing occurs in the locality of some suspected source of pollution, such as a waste dump or an industrial plant.

In some circumstances, disease clustering is very obvious (e.g., the aftermath of a massive environmental contamination or the passage of a familiar infectious disease), and the existence of the clustering, and often even its cause, require little subtlety of investigation. What is more difficult is the search for clusters of diseases that are not known to be of infectious origin and in which clustering, if it occurs at all, is at a very low level, that is, it involves only a minority of cases of the disease. The question of whether or not a disease tends to cluster has a significance beyond those cases of the disease that do appear to come in clusters because it may have implications to the etiology of those cases that do not. This low-level clustering is the particular focus of this section.

The issue arises in a number of ways and the research approaches vary accordingly. Broadly, there are three situations.

1. No clustering has been observed in the population to be studied, and the question of whether or not it is occurring is being approached a priori. It does not matter how the question arises—by the observation of clustering in some other population, suspicions based on the biology of the disease, the existence in the population of potential sources of local contamination, or simply as part of routine disease surveillance. The premise is that the disease distribution in the population in which the study is to be conducted in unknown.

2. The second situation is similar to the first in that nothing is known about the distribution of the disease in the population, but there is a specific hypothesis to be investigated; for example, a leukemia risk is related to proximity to a nuclear power plant, or the occurrence of respiratory symptoms is related to proximity to one or more sources of environmental contamination.

3. In the third situation, a disease cluster has already been observed and the problem for the investigator is to determine whether it is a "real" cluster (i.e., whether it is more than one might expect by chance alone) and whether an explanation can be found for it.

In all three situations, a number of decisions have to be made about what has come to be known as the "boundary problem"— the setting of the temporal and spatial boundaries within which the cluster or clusters are believed to exist.[29,467,574] First is the issue of geographic boundaries. These may be set in terms of the units used for separating the population geographically for political and administrative purposes (electoral wards, towns, counties, etc.), preferably a division for which population data are available for each unit. A secondary decision has to do with the size of the unit to be used. The previous discussion relating to the trade-offs involved in selecting unit size is relevant.

Yet, geography is not the only boundary that must be defined. Others include the dimension of time, the age and gender of the cases (and noncases) to be included, and the specification of the disease or diseases to be investigated (e.g., cases of or deaths from one or more types of leukemia or subtypes, and whether possibly related diseases, such as solid hematologic malignancies, should be included).

Beyond all these decisions is the principle that the boundaries must be established in all their dimensions prior to analysis (or even glimpses of) the data. If the data that exist in the population are allowed in any way, conscious or unconscious on the part of the investigator, to influence the selection of boundaries, all statistical tests applied to the results will be misleading. The issues are considered further in each of the three situations previously outlined.

There Is No Prior Hypothesis

When there is no prior hypothesis the boundary problem is relatively simple. In this situation the use of existing administrative boundaries is most common, but the size of the administrative units to be used remains to be decided. As with all other aspects of the boundary problem, this must be specified in the absence of information on the data. Because in the particular context discussed here the concern is for clusters of a small number of cases, smaller units are generally preferred, but they must be large enough to encompass clusters if clustering is in fact occurring. The other aspects of boundary specification outlined previously must also be accommodated. Some measure or measures of frequency of the disease of interest will then be computed for each of the areas defined by the boundaries. The investigator can then hope for statistically unequivocal evidence of whether or not clustering is occurring in the study population (at least within the constraints of the boundaries set up for the particular study). This could be a χ^2 or other suitable test for heterogeneity among subdivisions of the area *taken as a whole*. No groupings of divisions arrived at after the data are inspected can be subjected to valid statistical testing because the multiple possibilities for grouping change the interpretation of the P value resulting from any single statistical test. Thus, even if one of the divisions is found to have an elevated disease rate that is associated with a P value that may be formally significant (e.g., <0.05), when compared to the rate for the study area as a whole, the difference between this elevated rate and the average rate cannot necessarily be considered significant if this division was not specified in advance of the test. An early illustration comes from the study of Glass, Hill, and Miller of children under 15 years of age dying of leukemia or other malignancies in the county of Los Angeles from 1960 to 1964.[149] There was striking uniformity in the mortality rate from all malignancies combined and from leukemia over the 32 regions into which the county was divided, each of which was composed of about 40 census tracts. However, by visually inspecting the distribution of the cases and drawing tight boundaries of the populations around apparent groups of leukemia cases, the authors were able to create nine leukemia clusters comparable to clusters reported in the literature that were attracting great attention at the time. In all nine artificial clusters the rate of leukemia was greater than in the county as a whole, with a high level of statistical significance. The procedure is illustrated for three of the "clusters" in Figure 7-1. This figure also shows several other groupings around which "clusters" might well have been created artificially in this situation.

The intense public interest in clustering, real or perceived, has stimulated ad hoc conferences[58,234] and the formulation of guidelines for investigating clusters.[57] Among the statistical tests that have been proposed to assess spatial clustering,[333] there are some that do not depend explicitly on the setting of boundaries; these appear to be particularly appropriate in some circumstances. Thus, Cuzick and Edwards have proposed a case-control approach based on selecting controls from the population at risk (the "study base" discussed in Chapter 9) and computing distances from the combined sample (cases and controls) among the locations that characterize the subjects.[81] Testing is based on the number of other cases among the nearest neighbors of each case. This approach does not depend on the variation of population density and allows for control of confounding variables. As originally proposed, Cuzick and Edwards's test required knowledge of the exact location of the subjects, but a modification of the test, suitable for a situation in which only approximate locations are known, is now available.[233]

There Is a Prior Hypothesis

The problem of boundary definition becomes more complex and perhaps more critical with a prior hypothesis. The premise remains that the boundaries of the cluster or clusters are set before

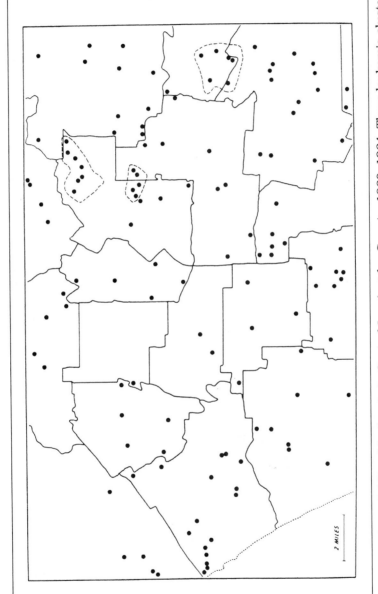

Figure 7-1. Deaths from childhood leukemia in Central Los Angeles County, 1960–1964. Three leukemia clusters constructed by selection of cases within arbitrary boundaries are shown. (From Glass AG, Hill JA, Miller RW. Significance of leukemia clusters. *J Pediatr* 1968;73 : 101–107.)

the distribution of disease in the test population is known. Sometimes a broad population within which clusters are known to have occurred is used for hypothesis testing. For example, there were hypothesis-testing studies of clustering of cancer or subtypes of it in geographic proximity to nuclear power plants in Britain,[71,72,201] France,[209] and the United States[232] following reports of clusters in these countries. Such known clusters may be excluded from the hypothesis-testing study, but one must guard against the possibility that all the clusters in the population are known and that their exclusion leaves only the segment of the data that does not exhibit clustering. The latter is an unlikely, but not unimaginable, possibility.

The setting of boundaries in a hypothesis-testing study involves all the variables that go into the definition of clusters. The specific parameters chosen will depend on the nature of the exposure and disease and of the relation that is hypothesized between them. Geographically, there must be a definition of what constitutes "proximity to" the source of the supposed exposure. Usually, this is defined in terms of a radius. However, because to define the population resident within such a radius is a problem of enormous magnitude, this method usually reduces to the populations of administrative areas whose "centroid" (center of gravity) or some specified proportion of the population lies within the circle. By further dividing such areas into those that have 0.0–9.9, 10.0–65.9, or 66.0+ percent of their populations within a 10-mile radius of a nuclear installation, Cook-Mozaffari et al. introduced a gradient in probability of exposure, crudely comparable to a gradient commonly used to evaluate exposure–response relationships.[72] The temporal boundary must also be defined in terms of time since the beginning and ending of the postulated exposure. If no temporal boundary is specified, the study will test only the hypothesis that at some unspecified time during the period of observation clustering occurred. Any post hoc observation that clustering was limited to a specific period following the opening or closing of the exposure source can be considered only as a hypothesis to be tested in other data. The fact that each of the putative clusters around nuclear facilities in Britain had its own peculiar characteristics since the opening of the facility is one of the features that argues for lack of biological coherence to these clusters.[308]

Once the boundaries of the exposed cluster or clusters are defined, decisions regarding appropriate comparison areas must be made. The first such decision must be whether it is feasible to use the whole of the population (e.g., the country). This requires the existence of appropriate data (e.g., cancer mortality or incidence) for the whole population. If feasible, this is usually the preferable alternative because the selection of supposedly more appropriate comparison subgroups always raises the possibility of unknown procedural or demographic bias.

For example, in one of the earlier studies of cancer occurrence in the vicinity of nuclear installations in England and Wales, cancer registrations and deaths were assigned to Local Authority Areas (LAAs) having more than one-third of their populations living within 10 miles of one of the 15 nuclear installations in the United Kingdom. A comparison LAA with the same urban-rural status and population size as its comparison was selected for each "installation LAA" from the same standard region. Where there was a choice within the region, an area with "comparable social class structure" was selected.[71] In this study there did seem to be a problem with the selection of the comparison LAAs. For example, in persons under 25 years of age with lymphoid leukemia, the SMR (relative to the expected based on regional rates) for the nuclear installation LAAs was 1.13, not significantly different from unity, but in the comparison areas there were 56.1 deaths expected but only 22 observed, giving an SMR of 0.39. Similar differences, although not so striking, were seen for several other cancers. It seems likely that unrecognized biases existed in the selection of the comparison LAAs in this study.[131] Because of this problem, in a later study of the same LAA data, rates were compared with those of the rest of the country, making allowance for social and demographic differences by regression modeling in the analysis of the data.[72] By no means all studies of this type using comparison areas have encountered this problem,[232] but it does seem desirable to gain whatever information can be obtained about the broader population from which exposed and comparison groups are selected to evaluate the possibility of unrecognized biases in either group. Studies that have more than one comparison group for each exposed group may have an advantage over those in which there is only one such group.

Once again, the investigator has only one chance of performing an unequivocally valid statistical test of the guiding hypothesis—that is, of a comparison of the exposed and comparison groups overall, as defined by the a priori boundaries in relation to the hypothesized outcome or outcomes. Differences that are seen for subgroups within the a priori boundaries, even if reaching levels of formal significance when analyzed separately, must be regarded only as hypotheses to be tested in other data.

A Cluster Is Observed

The great majority of disease clusters come to attention not as the result of systematic investigation but because a group of cases in a community are perceived by someone—often a relative of one of the cases—to represent a higher number than one would expect in that community. This is frequently because some kind of social link or demographic commonality is seen between some of the cases. An early and dramatic apparent cluster of childhood leukemia was seen in the town of Niles, Illinois, population approximately 18,000, in which eight cases of leukemia occurred in the 3 years prior to the summer of 1960. Of interest was the fact that seven of the eight cases were of Roman Catholic religion and attended the same parochial school. This cluster was investigated extensively by the Centers for Disease Control (CDC) over a period of many months but no explanation was uncovered.[202]

A major difficulty in the investigation of apparent clusters is that there are no predetermined boundaries (the cases in fact determine the boundaries of the cluster); therefore, it is impossible, except in unusual situations, to determine whether the number of cases is in excess of the number that might be attributable to chance. An egregious example of the distribution of cases being allowed to define the boundaries of the cluster is that of childhood leukemia cases in the village of Seascale in Cumbria in the United Kingdom, which for a period of several years was considered by many to be linked in some unidentified way to Britain's first and largest nuclear reprocessing plant at Sellafield, three kilometers to the northwest. In 1983, a team from Yorkshire Television (YTV) went to Sellafield to study the employees. The reporters became aware of the occurrence of childhood cancer in the village of Seascale. After an investigation of which the methods were described by a subsequent government panel as "unconventional,"[30] seven young people in the village of Seascale who had contracted leukemia between 1950 and 1983 were identified. There are plenty of reasons to consider Seascale in the context of Sellafield, along with dozens of other villages in Cumbria, but it was the occurrence of the cases in Seascale that defined the geographic boundary of the cluster. The occurrence of the disease in children defined the age boundary of the cluster. The time span studied also expanded and contracted in the more systematic studies that followed that of YTV. One hypothesis suggested by limited data put responsibility on genetic mutations in the germ cell lines of fathers employed at Sellafield. After enormous expenditures of scientific, legal, and financial resources, this hypothesis was found to be false.[95,575] The cause or causes of the Seascale cluster, if they are indeed beyond the possibility of chance superimposed on post hoc gerrymandering of boundaries, remain unknown.

Indeed, except those involving infectious diseases with known etiologic agents, very few investigations of clusters observed post hoc have been productive.[22,467] Between 1961 and 1982, the US

Centers for Disease Control investigated 85 clusters of leukemia cases. Forty-one of these clusters involved leukemia alone, and 44 involved leukemia with other lymphomas or other cancers. Some of these clusters, including the Niles cluster, were investigated in great detail. No "clear-cut etiologic relations" were established for any of these clusters.[49] Nevertheless, mysterious clusters, real or apparent, will continue to attract inquisitive epidemiologists[58] and their investigation will occasionally be worthwhile. For example, a recently reported investigation of a cluster of cases of mesothelioma in an Indian pueblo in New Mexico led to identification of a previously unknown source of exposure to asbestos—the manufacture of Indian jewelry and the whitening of leather leggings and moccasins used during ceremonial dances.[107] Investigation of several other obvious place diseases, however, including the so-called Balkan Endemic Nephropathy, which was seen in specific areas of the Balkans for more than a century and whose cause still remains uncertain,[55] have not been so productive.

Clustering by Time and Place

The previous section of this chapter discussed clusters of disease that occur by place and remain characteristic of that place over substantial periods of time. In Chapter 6 we discussed episodes of disease that cluster in time. Now the discussion focuses on a third form of clustering—that which is a function of both place and time. The distinction is somewhat arbitrary because time and place are almost always interdependent, if only because our observations are limited with respect to both variables. In addition, we can never demonstrate unequivocally that the time or place cluster we observe does not have a dimension of the other variable. Nevertheless, it is a useful distinction within the constraints of our observation possibilities. In fact, local clustering of disease in time and place can occur without apparent evidence of variation in the overall distributions in either of the two variables alone. Consider, for example, an epidemic that progresses regularly from one side of a large country to the other, affecting the same proportion of the population of each area as it proceeds. At any point in time, the disease will show marked aggregation within a few districts, and any single district will exhibit a marked time variation as the disease passes through it. However, if rates for the country as a whole are examined over a time span corresponding to that of the epidemic, it would appear that all areas of the country were equally affected and that an equal fraction of cases occurred in each time interval. Although this exact circumstance seems unlikely, it is nevertheless the case that the interaction of time and place may be more important than is revealed by an examination of the effect of either variable alone. Furthermore, the levels of time-place clustering may not be identified by examination of either variable alone.

Time-place interaction is, of course, characteristic of acute contagious diseases, usually being so obvious that no special methods are required to detect it.[150] Problems arise when the individual clusters are small and not sharply located in time and when the circumstances in which they occur are not readily replicable. The principal issue in investigating time-place clustering is that the "boundary" problem referred to previously affects both variables and is consequently difficult to address in a priori-defined, biologically plausible terms.

A number of approaches have been suggested and succinctly reviewed by Smith.[500] A method that is free of the need to define arbitrary time and space boundaries and does not require a control group is based on the "all possible pairs" approach. The device of computing the temporal and geographic distances between all possible pairs in a study series was used by Pinkel, Dowd, and Bross[415] and by Knox in 1963,[261] but was further developed by Knox in 1964. In a series of n cases, there will be $n(n - 1)/2$ possible pairs. The distribution of the time intervals between all these possible pairs will depend on the incidence of cases in the study population and on any change in incidence that may have occurred during the study period. Similarly, the distribution of geographic distances between cases can be interpreted as indicating any tendency to localization of the disease that could have been attributed to, say, localization of the population or purely geographic clustering of the disease. Cross-tabulation of all the possible pairs by time intervals and geographic distances will reveal whether those pairs that are close together in time also tend to be close together geographically. Illustrative data are shown in Table 7-1. The residences of the mothers of 723 cases of neural tube defect (primarily anencephaly and/or spina bifida) in Providence, Rhode Island, were located on a map, and the map coordinates of each residence were recorded. The cases were also identified by the first day of the mothers' last menstrual periods as markers of the dates of conception. The days were numbered consecutively from the beginning to the end of the study period. The 723 cases yielded 261,003 possible pairs. For each pair, both the time interval and the geographic distance were calculated. The time interval was calculated by subtracting the number assigned to the earlier date of conception from the later, and the geographic distance was calculated by the application of

Table 7-1. Distribution of all Possible Pairs of Cases of Neural Tube Defects in Providence, Rhode Island, 1936–1965, by Observed and Expected Geographic and Temporal Distance Between the Members of Each Pair

Distance (km)	Observed or expected	No. of pairs in each time interval (days)							Total pairs
		0–14	15–29	30–59	60–89	90–179	180–364	365–12087	
<0.25	Observed	5	6	5	6	16	42	774	854
	Expected	2.9	2.9	5.5	5.2	15.9	33.2	788.5	854.0
0.25–0.49	Observed	7	8	13	12	41	98	1872	2051
	Expected	6.9	6.9	13.1	12.6	38.1	79.7	1893.8	2051.0
0.50–0.99	Observed	23	26	43	42	96	244	5881	6355
	Expected	21.5	21.3	40.6	38.9	118.0	246.9	5867.8	6355.0
1.00–1.99	Observed	69	79	140	132	403	831	19593	21247
	Expected	71.8	71.1	135.8	130.2	394.7	825.5	19618.0	21247.0
2.00–4.99	Observed	248	261	528	497	1557	3203	75135	81429
	Expected	275.2	272.4	520.4	498.9	1512.5	3163.8	75185.9	81429.0
5.00+	Observed	530	493	939	910	2735	5723	137737	149067
	Expected	503.7	498.6	952.7	913.2	2768.8	5791.8	137638.1	149067.0
Total pairs	Observed	882	873	1668	1599	4848	10141	240992	261003
	Expected	882.0	873.0	1668.0	1599.0	4848.0	10141.0	240992.0	261003.0

Source: Trichopoulos D, et al. A study of time-place clustering in anencephaly and spina bifida. *Am J Epidemiol* 1971:94 : 26–30.

Pythagoras' theorem to map coordinates. The distribution of the 261,003 possible pairs is shown as the observed frequencies in Table 7-1. For example, there were five pairs in which the members were separated by less than 0.25 kilometers and less than 15 days. The expected values are based on the assumption that the distribution of pairs by time interval is independent of that by geographic distance, and they are computed from the marginal distributions.[538] Thus, the value 2.9 expected cases within 0.25 kilometers and less than 15 days is derived from $(882/261,003) \cdot 854$.

A simple descriptive comparison of the observed and expected values in such a table, particularly focusing on the left upper corner, may be of value. There may be insufficient evidence of clustering by simple inspection to warrant further consideration of the issue, or, conceivably, the table may yield evidence of clustering of such a degree that statistical tests of significance are not needed to convince the investigator that it is real. If the clustering is not intense, as in the current example, it may suggest the geographic and temporal distances to use in a subsequent study to test a specific hypothesis. Because there was no such hypothesis in the study, the individual cells cannot be grouped to form a cluster that might be subjected to statistical tests. However, in Table 7-1, there is an excess of observed pairs in the two cells characterized by intervals of less than 30 days and distances of less than 0.25 kilometers that might be worth testing as an a priori hypothesis in a subsequent study.

One statistical problem is derived from the lack of independence of the individual measurements, with each point being represented $(n - 1)$ times. Knox pointed out that if attention is restricted to the pairs occupying the cells bordered by such small time and distance boundaries, the number of pairs they contain will be small and their members will likely be independent. The observed values can then be compared with a Poisson distribution of which the mean and variance is the observed number of cases.[263] In Table 7-1, comparison of 11 (or more) observed with 5.8 expected in the two cells with less than 0.25 kilometers and 30 days gives $P \sim 0.03$ (one-tail test); however, as noted, this was not a prior hypothesis. David and Barton subsequently calculated the exact mean and variance of Knox's criterion and showed the appropriateness of the Poisson model in most situations.[84] Mantel described the procedures for computing variances by an exact permutational method in circumstances in which the appropriateness of the Poisson model may be in doubt,[324] and Pike and Bull provided an algorithm.[414]

In simulation experiments, Chen, Mantel, and Klingberg compared several of the available tests for time-place clustering and found none particularly sensitive, although the Knox method was somewhat more sensitive over the range of examples used.[60] Not many positive results of the Knox test can be cited, although Mangoud et al. successfully detected time-place clustering in Hodgkin's disease by this method.[321] The sparsity of positive results may not be a function of the limitations of the method so much as of the rarity of this kind of clustering outside of highly contagious diseases.

8 Person

Chapter 5 listed some of the characteristics of persons that have been identified as risk factors for disease. Information on several of these factors, such as age, gender, race, and income, is collected routinely by medical and social agencies for their own purposes, and the data are readily available in tabular form. For many of these variables, their association with disease risk is striking. Some of the relationships have been influential in the development of etiological hypotheses, but knowledge of them has been even more important in clarifying disease relationships with other variables that otherwise might be misleading because they were confounded. This is particularly true for the age variable.

Age

Age as a Confounding Variable

In most diseases the variation in frequency that occurs with age is greater than that with any other variable. Although knowledge of the form of the relationship between age and a disease occasionally has been of assistance in formulating hypotheses of causation, much more important is that a disease's relationship with age is often so strong that associations with other variables may be misleading unless the overwhelming importance of age is taken into account. An illustration is given in Table 8-1. Age-adjusted mortality rates for whites in the United States are only about 65 percent of those for blacks, in both males and females. Yet, the crude (unadjusted) rates in the two racial groups are not very different for males, whereas among females they are actually higher for whites than for blacks. The National Center for Health

Table 8-1. Total (All Causes) Average Annual Mortality Rates per 100,000 for the Black and White Populations of the United States by Gender, 1989–1991

Gender	Crude rates		Age-adjusted rates (A)		Age-adjusted rates (B)	
	White	Black	White	Black	White	Black
Male	930	1,009	643	1,062	1,055	1,533
Female	848	751	370	582	661	906

Source: National Center for Health Statistics. *Health, United States, 1993.* Hyattsville, MD: Public Health Service, 1994. DHHS Publ. No. (PSH) 94-1232.
The age-adjusted rates (A) are those given in the source monograph and used as the standard total US population in 1940. The age-adjusted rates (B) are computed using the total US population in 1991 as the standard.

Statistics (NCHS) in adjusting these rates used the US population in 1940 as a standard population,[379] which accounts for the dramatic differences between the crude and adjusted rates for whites. It is generally preferable, although not critical, that the standard population used is close in age distribution to the age distribution of the populations of which the rates are being standardized. The 1940 population was probably used here by NCHS to maintain long-term historical continuity. When the 1991 population is used as the standard, the two sets of adjusted rates are strikingly different, but the relationship between the racial groups remains unaffected.

Technical Influences on Age Curves

In the context of age, it is particularly relevant to note the differences between trends noted in *numbers* of cases and population-based *rates*. Clinicians and others dealing with patients frequently make their impressions of the shape of age associations from the age distributions of the patients they see, which overlooks the fact that the shape of such a distribution is determined not only by the likelihood of the disease occurring but by the number of living persons in whom it can occur. Currently in the United States, the latter declines steadily after the mid-thirties. This point was discussed in Chapter 4, but it is important to note here that the distinction is perhaps more frequently ignored for age than for any other variable.

There are a number of sources of error that vary with age and may affect the shape of observed age-risk curves. For example, accuracy of diagnosis varies with age, a fact that is particularly likely to affect the newborn and the oldest age groups and that is probably more significant in the context of mortality than of incidence data. There is, for example, often less concern to establish an exact cause of death in a person of 80 years of age than in one of 40 years. This tends to reduce age-specific rates in the oldest age groups for diseases of difficult diagnosis and to increase rates in the same age groups for "wastebasket" diagnoses, such as "senility." In addition, base population data may be less accurate in the older age groups, which leads to further distortions. In the United States, this lack of accuracy applies particularly to the rural and nonwhite populations. Although probably not a problem in the United States, failure to report very early deaths may lead to underestimates of infant death rates in many parts of the world.

The shape of an age-risk curve will also depend on whether it is based on rates of incidence, prevalence, or mortality, and on the stage of the disease at which incidence or prevalence is measured. For example, Figure 8-1 shows that in New Zealand in the mid-1980s rates of reported cervical cancer increased regularly between the ages of 20 and 39 (the only age range for which cervical dysplasia information was available), but both prevalence and incidence of cervical dysplasia (an acknowledged precursor of invasive lesions) declined with age. The figure also indicates that for a condition lasting more than 1 year prevalence will be higher than annual incidence, which is expected from the relationships of the various measures (discussed in Chapter 4). The contrast may be reduced in cervical dysplasia by the spontaneous reversal of dysplasias in some individuals.

The issue of causal factors that appear to be characteristic of generations or birth cohorts was discussed in Chapter 6 in the context of their effect on time trends. Such factors also must be considered in interpreting age patterns. Indeed, as we noted in that chapter, it was in the context of interpreting age curves for tuberculosis that the concept of cohort effects first came to attention. The role of cohort factors on the age association for malignant disease was first noted by Dorn and Cutler with respect to lung cancer.[103] As shown in Figure 8-2, while cross-sectional age curves (i.e., curves drawn by linking the rates in each age group at a given time) declined in the older age groups, cohort age curves (i.e., drawn by linking the rates in each age group at the calendar time in which that generation attained that particular age) continued to increase throughout the life span. Successive cohorts in the observation period had increasingly higher lung cancer rates, but the later-born cohorts were not represented in the older age groups, accounting for the lower rates in the older age groups. As

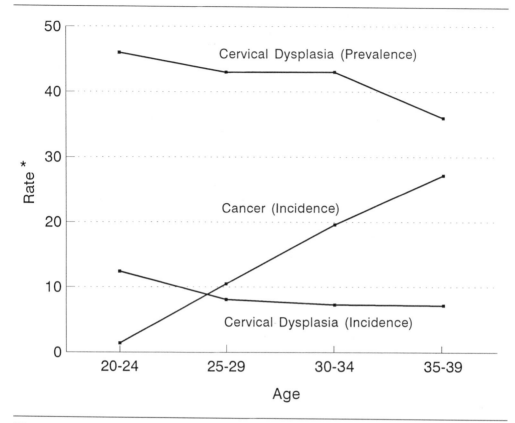

Figure 8-1. Prevalence and incidence of cervical dysplasia and incidence of cervical cancer in New Zealand in the mid-1980s. (Prevalence is per thousand population. Incidence of dysplasia is per 1,000 person-years; incidence of cervical cancer is per 100,000 person-years.) (Sources for cervical dysplasia data: New Zealand Contraception and Health Study Group. The prevalence of abnormal cervical cytology in a group of New Zealand women using contraception: a preliminary report. *NZ Med J* 1989;102 : 369–371; and New Zealand Contraception and Health Study Group. An attempt to estimate the incidence of cervical dysplasia in a group of New Zealand women using contraception. *Epidemiology* 1995;6 : 121–126. Source for cervical cancer data: Parkin DM et al. *Cancer Incidence in Five Continents. Volume VI.* Lyon: International Agency for Research on Cancer, 1992. IARC Scientific Publications No. 120. The two sources are not comparable in several ways, but these are unlikely to affect the overall shape of the age trends.)

noted in Chapter 6, such patterns are now known to be common in other cancers and in other noninfectious diseases. They must be considered when interpreting patterns of association between age and disease rates.

Interpretation of Age Associations

Figure 8-3 shows mortality rates by age for four gender and race groups in the United States in 1992. Overall age curves such as

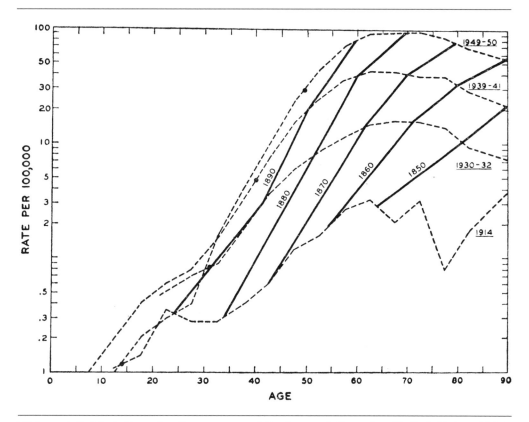

Figure 8-2. Mortality rates from cancer of the lung; white males, United States, 1914 to 1950. Solid lines are birth-cohort curves, broken lines are cross-sectional or current age curves as of the dates of the successive surveys. (Adapted from Dorn HF, Cutler SJ. *Morbidity from Cancer in the United States. Part 1. Variations in Incidence by Age, Sex, Race, Marital Status, and Geographic Region.* Washington DC: US Government Printing Office, 1955. Public Health Monograph No. 29. Public Health Service Publication No. 418.)

these are of great importance from a demographic point of view, but their usefulness in epidemiological terms is rather limited. They do draw attention to the high mortality in the first year of life, which actually occurs mostly in the earliest days of life, and to the uninterrupted increase in mortality with age after the first decade of life.

Early Mortality

The latter half of the nineteenth and the first half of the twentieth centuries saw major progress in the partial understanding and control of the diseases responsible for the peak of mortality in early life. In most developed areas of the world, infant mortality rates by 1950 were only about 10 percent of what they had been at the beginning of the century. In the United States Death Registration Area, between 1900 and 1940 the expectation of life at birth increased by about 15 years in both genders.[556] However,

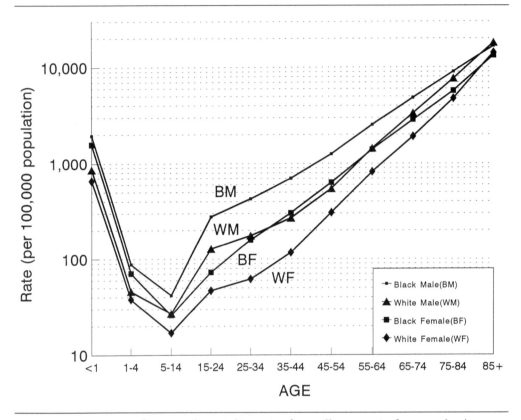

Figure 8-3. Age-specific annual mortality rates from all causes in four gender/race groups, United States, 1992. (Rates are per 100,000 population. Note that the first two points are not drawn to scale on the age axis, so as to distinguish the four lines.) (Source: National Center for Health Statistics. *Health, United States, 1993.* Hyattsville MD: Public Health Service, 1994. DHHS Pub. No. (PHS) 94-1232.)

this was a function almost entirely of the decline in deaths at very early ages, which carries considerable weight in computing the expectation for the whole population. Expectation of life for persons who reach age 45 has changed substantially less. Epidemiological observations played a considerable part in bringing about the decline in early deaths by pointing to the strong link of childhood diseases with poverty, malnutrition, and overcrowding. These observations were an important adjunct to the revolutionary advances in microbiology.

The Diseases of Aging
In addition to continuing progress in controlling diseases of early life, the second half of the twentieth century has provided evidence that the rising age curve in later life may also be at least in part modifiable. Observations in humans and other species support

the view that the duration of life is indeed finite, but its upper limit may be greater than we have been led to believe. There are two direct pieces of evidence to this effect: one is the potential for the control of lung cancer and an even larger number of deaths due to other diseases attributable to cigarette smoking, and the other is the steady decline in mortality from ischemic heart disease that has occurred in the last two decades for reasons that are not clearly understood but are probably multiple. Additional evidence, which a tobacco company executive might characterize as "only statistical," comes from recent life expectancy data. White females 65 years old in the United States in 1990 had a life expectancy almost 50 percent higher than did women of the same age in 1940. The expectation of additional life for white females 65 years old is currently approximately 19 years more than in 1940.[556,559] White males and blacks have also shown increases in life expectation, but not of such magnitude. Again, epidemiological observations have played crucial roles in bringing about these changes, although not specifically by the study of age patterns.

The major features of the overall age-mortality curves that we have discussed represent the summation of the age associations for a multitude of diseases that may lead to death and that, by and large, have individual patterns of association with age (Figure 8-4). Within the broad disease categories shown in Figure 8-4, specific diseases show marked differences in age associations. For example, within the hundred or so diseases that make up the category of malignant neoplasms, there are several distinguishable age patterns. Age patterns in mortality are, of course, determined not only by the factors that influence the likelihood of occurrence of those diseases, but also by those that affect the probability that they will lead to death and those that determine the length of the average interval between occurrence of the disease and death. Most, if not all, the factors known to be associated with either risk of disease or mortality also vary with age. Generalizations are, however, difficult.

Irregularities in Age Curves

Sometimes irregularities in overall age curves, such as those shown in Figure 8-3, may indicate age groups in need of further investigation. The figure shows a deviation upward in the otherwise almost log-linear trend from 5–14 years to 85+ years, affecting males 15–24 years old and to a lesser extent the two following age groups. The deviation is seen to some degree in white females only in the 15–24 age group, and minimally, or not at all, among black females. Further investigation reveals that these deviations, which appear trivial in the log-linear trend for deaths from all

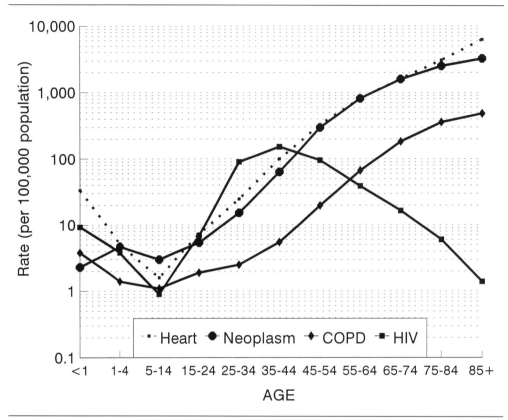

Figure 8-4. Age-specific annual rates of death from diseases of the heart, malignant neoplasms, chronic obstructive pulmonary disease (COPD), and infection with human imunodeficiency virus (HIV) in black males, United States, 1991. (Rates are per 100,000 population. Note that the first two points are not drawn to scale on the age axis, so as to distinguish the four lines.) (Source: National Center For Health Statistics. *Health, United States, 1993.* Hyattsville MD: Public Health Service, 1994. DHHS Pub. No. (PHS) 94-1232.)

causes, stem from two rather substantial and remarkable epidemics—one of deaths in motor vehicle crashes (Figure 8-5) and one of deaths from firearm injuries (Figure 8-6). The automobile deaths are more common in whites, particularly in the youngest age group affected (15–24 years) and particularly in males, which is perhaps a function of differences in the group members' access to motor vehicles. The firearm deaths, however, are strikingly more common in blacks, particularly males (note the different vertical scales in Figures 8-5 and 8-6). In the age group 15–24, 60 percent of the deaths of black males in 1992 were due to firearm injuries and another 12 percent to motor vehicle crashes. Among white males in the same age group, only 27 percent of all

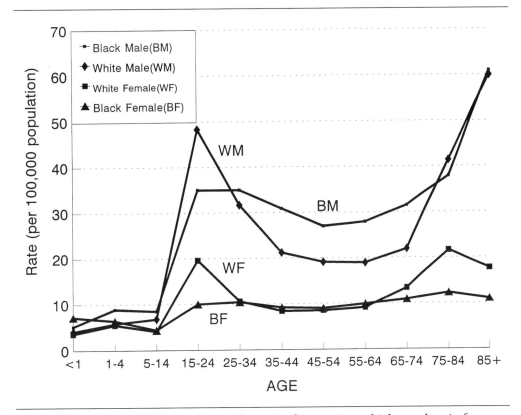

Figure 8-5. Age-specific annual mortality rates from motor vehicle crashes in four gender/race groups, United States, 1991. (Rates are per 100,000 population. Note that the first two points are not drawn to scale on the age axis, so as to distinguish the four lines.) (Source: National Center For Health Statistics. *Health, United States, 1993.* Hyattsville MD: Public Health Service, 1994. DHHS Pub. No. (PHS) 94-1232.)

deaths were due to firearm injuries, but 35 percent were due to motor vehicle crashes.[380]

These data, although perhaps doing no more than quantitating phenomena that may readily be discerned from the daily news media, illustrate that the process of interpreting an age curve for total mortality or morbidity involves two steps. These are determining what disease or diseases contribute to different segments of the age curve and understanding the age patterns for the individual diseases.

Bimodality

The occurrence of two separate peaks in the age-incidence curve of a disease is always of interest. Even when the disease entity under examination has been defined in terms of causal, rather

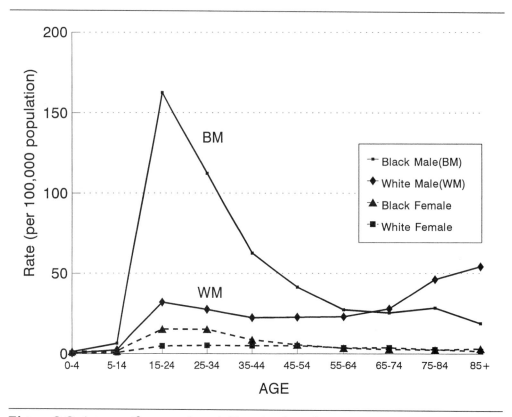

Figure 8-6. Age-specific annual mortality rates from firearm injuries in four gender/race groups, United States, 1991. (Rates are per 100,000 population. Note that the first point is not drawn to scale on the age axis.) (Source: National Center For Health Statistics. *Health, United States, 1993.* Hyattsville MD: Public Health Service, 1994. DHHS Pub. No. (PHS) 94-1232.)

than manifestational, characteristics (see Chapter 3), bimodality suggests the existence of causal differences other than those on which the classification of the disease is based. For example, age curves for tuberculosis are bimodal, showing one mode in the 0–4 age group and a second in the 20–29 age group. Tuberculosis is defined in terms of exposure to the tubercle bacillus, so that both these modes affect the same "disease." The existence of the two modes, however, suggests that two distinct sets of other component causes must be taken into account to explain the age distribution.

Another example of bimodality in a disease defined in causal terms was seen in Figure 8-5 with regard to deaths in motor vehicle crashes. Although the motor vehicle is a common factor in the deaths of young adults and the elderly, it is likely that there

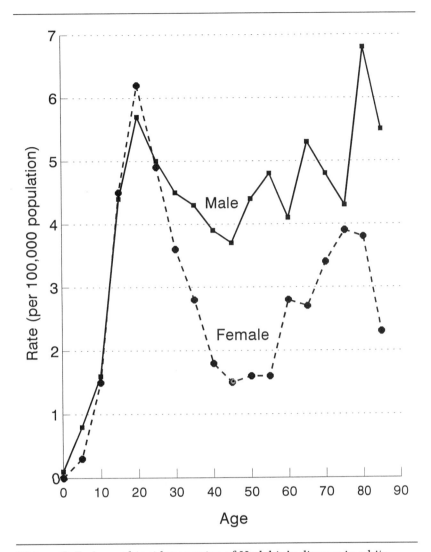

Figure 8-7. Annual incidence rates of Hodgkin's disease in white Americans in 10 US cancer registries, 1983–1987, by age and gender. (Rates are per 100,000 population.) (Source: Parkin DM et al. *Cancer Incidence in Five Continents. Volume VI.* Lyon: International Agency for Research on Cancer, 1992. IARC Scientific Publications No. 120. Data are from the Surveillance, Epidemiology and End Results Program of the National Cancer Institute.)

are substantial differences in the other components of the causal web in these two age groups.

When two modes are seen for a disease entity that has been defined manifestationally, for example, tumors of the testis[186] and Hodgkin's disease (Figure 8-7),[399] the need to investigate separately the etiology of the disease as it occurs in the two modes becomes more compelling. The need becomes even stronger when the histology of "the disease" differs between cases occurring in the two modes of the age distribution. That this is the situation for tumors of the testis is well known clinically; it has also been shown for Hodgkin's disease.[383] Accumulating evidence calls for a role of the Epstein-Barr virus in a substantial number of cases of Hodgkin's disease,[371] but it remains unclear whether this role differs between cases in the two age modes.[121] The possibility that these are two meaningfully separate entities is strengthened by the notable difference in gender distribution of the disease in the two age modes—a difference that existed when the bimodality was first noted in the 1950s.[307]

Gender

The Gender Ratio

As with other descriptive variables, associations between gender and a disease are most convincingly demonstrated by comparing disease *rates* between males and females. At times, deviations of the percentage of males from 50 percent of the total cases (commonly referred to as the *sex ratio*) are interpreted as evidence of a gender difference in disease rates, based on the assumption that the percentage of males in the population from which the cases are derived is about 50. This assumption is frequently unjustified. For example, in the US population aged 75 or more in 1991, the percentage of males was 35, not 50. The gender (sex) ratio *at birth*—generally varying between 50.5 and 52 percent—is a biological phenomenon that has attracted much interest from epidemiologists and other scientists. It varies with race, birth order, and over time in ways that are often predictable but of which the mechanisms are not understood. It is of course a prevalence ratio and both a function of the ratio of males to females that existed at the time of conception and the differential mortality of the two genders during intrauterine life. It has been thought that knowledge of the factors related to this variable might give leads as to the nature of factors affecting mortality during intrauterine life, but studies to date have not been informative in this respect.

Gender Differences in Mortality

As noted previously, more males are born alive than females—a ratio that is generally about 106:100. Except in areas where obstetrical care is poor, death rates are higher for males than for females at all ages, as was shown in Figure 8-3. Although this has been true in the United States throughout the twentieth century, the contrast has become more marked over time. Thus, in the US Registration states of 1900 the age-adjusted mortality rates for males and females were 16.2 and 15.0 per thousand, respectively,[290] and the life expectations were 46.3 and 48.3 years at birth and 11.5 and 12.2 years at age 65, respectively.[379] In 1992, provisional age-adjusted all-causes mortality rates for males and females were 6.6 and 3.8 per thousand, respectively, and the life expectations for the two genders were 72.3 and 79.0 at birth and 15.5 and 19.1 at age 65.[379] In contrast to the distinct separation of the gender-specific mortality rates seen for 1992 in Figure 8-3, in 1900 the curves by age for the two genders virtually overlapped. As a result of these mortality differentials, in most populations males and females have different distributions by age, the mean age of females commonly being higher than that of males. Therefore, small differences in gender-specific rates must be viewed with caution until the possible effect of age differences has been evaluated. For example, several of the causes of death listed in Table 8-2 in which the ratio of male to female rates is close to 1.0 (including hypertensive heart disease, cerebrovascular disease, and diabetes mellitus) actually show higher crude mortality rates for females than for males, but, as seen in the table, when the rates are age standardized they are higher for males than for females.

Explanations for the increasing discrepancy between the mortality of males and females in the twentieth century are not hard to find. They include, overwhelmingly, the much earlier onset of heavy cigarette smoking in males (beginning in the first quarter of the century); the later epidemics of deaths due to firearms and motor vehicle crashes (both affecting males primarily); and, most recently, the epidemic of AIDS, which up to this point has affected males predominantly. However, the higher overall mortality of males is the result of serious disadvantages in most of the common causes of death (Table 8-2). These rate ratios are not dissimilar to those published for 1955 and 1967,[314,316] except for respiratory cancer, in which the earlier male to female rate ratios were around 6 : 1; they have now dropped to 2.2 : 1. This, however, is more the result of bad news for women than of good news for men. Rates of respiratory cancer for men have declined slightly in the last decade, but the change in the ratio reflects primarily the increase over recent years in the corresponding rates for women.

Table 8-2. Annual Age-Adjusted Death Rates from Leading Causes of Death, United States, White Population, 1990

Cause of death	Male (M)	Female (F)	Ratio M/F
Ischemic heart disease	145.3	68.6	2.1
Hypertension (± heart or renal disease)	6.2	4.6	1.3
Cerebrovascular disease	27.7	23.8	1.2
Malignant neoplasms*	160.3	111.2	1.4
Of respiratory system	59.0	26.5	2.2
Of digestive organs	37.0	22.0	1.7
Leukemia	6.5	3.9	1.7
Chronic obstructive lung disease	27.4	15.2	1.8
Diabetes mellitus	11.3	9.5	1.2
HIV† infection‡	16.7	1.3	12.8
Motor vehicle crashes	26.3	11.0	2.4
Homicide and legal intervention	8.9	2.8	3.2
Suicide	20.1	4.8	4.2
Firearm injuries‡	20.7	3.7	5.6

Source: National Center for Health Statistics. *Vital Statistics of the United States, 1990. Volume II: Mortality. Part A.* Hyattsville, MD: National Center for Health Statistics, 1994. DHHS Publ. No. (PHS) 94-1100.
All rates are per 100,000 and are standardized to the total US population in 1940.
* Tumors of organs functionally limited to one gender are not shown separately, but are included in this total category.
† Human immunodeficiency virus
‡ Source: National Center for Health Statistics. *Health, United States, 1993.* Hyattsville, MD: Public Health Service, 1994. DHHS Publ. No. (PHS) 94-1232. (Data are for 1991.)
Note that rates that are not standardized to the same population cannot be meaningfully compared.

Gender Differences in Morbidity

The ratios of male to female incidence rates for individual diseases cover a wide range of values. Women have higher morbidity rates than men for many chronic diseases. In some instances the differences are striking, for example, thyrotoxicosis, diabetes mellitus, cholecystitis and biliary calculi, obesity, arthritis, and psychoneuroses. In contrast, other diseases are predominantly diseases of males when examined in morbidity data. These include ischemic heart disease, malignant and nonmalignant respiratory disease, peptic ulcer, inguinal hernia, gout, and accidents.

Any attempt to evaluate whether the excess mortality for males overall is reflected in overall excess morbidity is immediately encountered by the hurdle that we have no *measure* of overall morbidity—the distinction between healthy or unhealthy lacks the clarity of that between living or dead. Health is a scaled, rather than dichotomous, variable, and it can be and has been defined in innumerable ways. In fact, many measures that are used as indices of health status are not measures of health at all but of utilization of health services (e.g., visits to health care providers, hospital admissions).

It is paradoxical, however, when viewed in the light of the findings in mortality data, that many summary indices show more frequent reporting of ill health and greater use of medical resources by women than by men, particularly among adults and the elderly. This paradox was pointed out by John Graunt 350 years ago when he wrote:

> there were fourteen men to thirteen women (christened) and . . . they die in the same proportion. . . . Yet I have heard physicians say that they have two women patients to one man. . . . Now it should follow from this that more women die than men, if the number of burials answered [is] in proportion to the number of sicknesses.[158]

Graunt is not, of course, allowing for the distinction between the *risk* of death (one per person) and the death *rate*, and so he is actually understating the paradox (assuming the accuracy of the estimate made by his physician friends).

Some recent data from the US National Health Survey are given in Table 8-3. The picture is not entirely clear. Men do experience fewer acute conditions and associated bed days than women, and they apparently have fewer physician office visits. The data on physician office contact do not exclude visits associated with pregnancy, delivery, and the puerperium, but even when the data are restricted to ages 45 and higher, women still have a somewhat higher rate of physician contact than men. Yet, when deliveries are excluded, rates of hospitalization and length of stay in the hospital are approximately equal in women and men. These data are not strong. Despite the high level of interviewer training and other technical aspects of the National Health Survey, the findings still depend ultimately on self-report. Furthermore, the age groups used for adjustment are broad, and the use of narrower ranges would presumably reduce most of the rates for women relative to those for men. Although not strongly supporting Graunt's impression that rates of morbidity are higher in women than in men, it is probably fair to say that there is no evidence that women enjoy, with respect to morbidity, the considerable superiority they hold with respect to mortality.

Table 8-3. Selected Measures of Morbidity in Adult Males and Females, United States, 1993

| Measure | Per 100 persons | | Ratio M/F |
	Male	Female	
Acute conditions reported*‡			
Annual incidence	126	169	0.72
Associated bed days	262	387	0.68
Associated work-loss days	267	326	0.82
Prevalence of impairment due to chronic conditions†			
Some activity limitation	29.8	30.2	0.99
Unable to carry on major activity	10.3	8.7	1.18
Bed days due to acute and chronic conditions in previous year†	890	1190	0.74
Physician office contacts per year*	293	421	0.70
Physician office contacts per year†	415	489	0.85
One or more short-stay hospitalizations, previous year*‡	7.2	7.6	0.95
Annual hospital days*‡	73	69	1.05

Source: Data from National Center for Health Statistics. *Current Estimates from the National Health Interview Survey, 1993.* Hyattsville, MD: National Center for Health Statistics, 1994. DHHS Publ. No. (PHS) 95-1518.
Rates are standardized in broad age groups to the estimated total population of males and females in 1993.
* Ages 18 years and up
† Ages 45 years and up
‡ Excludes events of pregnancy, delivery, or the puerperium

Interpretation of Gender Differences

We are not sufficiently bold to offer a list of the differences between men and women, but clearly they are many, and any or all may play a role in the differences in the health experience of the two genders. However, we should note that, as a descriptive epidemiologic variable, gender differences have not played as large a role as might have been expected in the formulation of etiologic hypotheses. A notable exception relates to the gender difference in mortality rates from cancer of the lung, which, triangulated with the marked increase in incidence of the disease during this century, pointed clearly to the possibility of the role of cigarette smoking in the disease. Yet, almost equally strong gender differences in ischemic heart disease have not played any substantial role in understanding the etiology of this disease and, in fact, remain largely unexplained.

Race and Ethnic Group

Race and ethnic group are descriptors that are widely used but inconsistently defined. They may denote categories as broad as the human race or imply narrowly the descendants of a single couple or a small group of common ancestors. The term *ethnic group* is broader and perhaps preferable to *race* in epidemiologic contexts because, while it encompasses racial distinctions, it does not necessarily have implications with respect to ancestry. For epidemiological purposes, any group whose members have lived in proximity and shared customs and values for a length of time sufficient to have acquired common characteristics (e.g., diet), whether by biological or social mechanisms, is of interest. Some such groups, such as Seventh Day Adventists or Mormons, would not usually be thought of as ethnic groups, but others, such as Jews and Hispanics, would. The greater the influence of ancestry in the development of the specific characteristics of the group, the more closely it relates to our concept of an ethnic group. Yet, the dividing line between cultural groups that are considered ethnic and those that are not is indistinct.

For more than a century in the United States, the ethnic distinction that has been foremost in epidemiology (and elsewhere) is one based on "race," particularly between the two racial groups that until the last two decades predominated in this country—the population of primarily European origin (usually referred to as white) and that of predominantly African origin (referred to as black, or African American). In 1940, in an introduction to a review of the findings during the previous 41 years that the Bureau of the Census had compiled and published in annual vital statistics reports, Linder and Grove wrote:

> The classification of mortality and natality data by race is difficult, and the results tend to be ambiguous and incomplete. No practicable and acceptable ethnological classification has been developed for vital statistics, and it would be difficult to obtain the necessary information required for such a classification of mortality statistics. The classification of deaths into white, Negro, Indian, Chinese, Japanese, and "Minor races" is used in the vital statistics reports for the United States. More frequently the shorter classifications of "White," "Negro," and "Other races" or of simply "White" and "All other" are used. None of these classifications are adequate in providing for mixed types or in breaking the large group of "White" into more homogeneous groups. Owing to the lack of precise definition of race and of exact information regarding race on the birth and death certificates, any further attempt to subdivide by race results in a confusion with the concepts of nationality, country of origin of parents or other characteristics.[290]

Fifty years later, this description could stand with little modification as a statement of the position today, despite serious efforts in the intervening years of many demographers, statisticians, and epidemiologists at the Bureau of the Census, the National Center for Health Statistics, and in the individual states. Some recent work toward standardization, at least among US federal agencies, is referenced by Feinleib.[123] The problems are, as we shall see, perhaps intractable. Although considerable progress has been made toward uniformity of definition and measurement overall, not all movement has been in a forward direction. One major state (New Jersey) for a short period in the early 1960s removed the question on race from its birth certificate. Under pressure from the federal government and other jurisdictions, the item was replaced fairly quickly, but the action left an irreparable 2-year gap in national historical trends. The New Jersey action was motivated by politics rather than science, but, to the extent that science was an issue at all, not all scientists regarded it as a step in the wrong direction. In understanding and describing the diversity of the human population, race has an important place in the views of anthropologists and geneticists, but some sociologists have questioned its utility for their purposes.[156,284,365] Furthermore, the relative importance of race and ethnic group among the many descriptors of human diversity, whether for political or epidemiological purposes varies markedly with time and place. In the 1990s it has taken on overwhelming significance in some areas of the world, for example Rwanda and the former Yugoslavia, and with less dire consequences in North America.

As a historical note we might recall that in published statistics it was quite common to provide detail for the white population (which in 1980 comprised 83 percent of the whole) and comparable detail only for all other racial groups combined, which were identified as "nonwhite" or "all other." At one time it was reasonable to suppose that the data for "all other" reflected disease patterns in the black population because that group constituted more than 90 percent of the nonwhite population. Although the supposition was reasonable on a national basis, it was always questionable for certain geographic areas of the country, and the origins of recent immigrants to the country have made it even less sound. At the 1990 census, only 76 percent of the nonwhite population was black, and in the West Region of the United States the black population constituted only 13 percent of the nonwhite population.[560] This trend is recognized by the increasing proportion of federal statistics that provide separate data for blacks, as well as for other major ethnic groups.[379]

In the compilation of statistics on population, illness, and mortality by race, there have been numerous changes in the ways that individuals have been classified. From definitions based on the proportion of recent ancestors (usually grandparents) who were of particular racial background, the move has been to categorize individuals on the basis of the racial group he or she identifies with by self-report, or, in the case of deaths, in the opinions of the next of kin or the funeral director. Most health statistics now collected are on the latter basis. It should be noted, however, that all of the methods used, including those currently in use, are arbitrary and lack underlying conceptual definition.[190] From an epidemiologic perspective, the way in which racial groups are defined is less important than that they be defined similarly in the numerators and denominators of rates in populations in which race-specific rates are being compared. Herein lie some difficulties.

Inconsistencies in Racial Classification

Hahn, Mulinare, and Teutsch used the linked birth/infant death tape prepared by the National Center for Health Statistics to compare the racial classification at birth to the classification reported at death for the same infants.[192] Some results are shown in Table 8-4. The authors conclude that the coding of race and ethnicity of infants at birth and death is "remarkably inconsistent, with substantial impact on the estimation of infant mortality rates." Certainly there is inconsistency, but its remarkable nature is peculiarly limited in its scope. With the possible exception of the 4.1 percent of black infants who were reported as white at death, the data for white and black infants seem no more inconsistent than would be expected from clerical errors in a large body of data. What is remarkable is the high frequency with which infants classified as "other," who are largely Asian or American Indian, were reported as white at the time of death. The source or sources of these discrepancies are not known. Their effect on infant mortality rates is of course to raise the infant mortality rate for whites and to lower those for the racial groups whose members are being classified as white at the time of death. Correction for the errors lowers the rate for whites and raises those for the groups that are being misclassified as white at the time of death. The effect on the infant mortality rate for whites is fairly trivial because these deaths form a very small proportion of the very large population of deaths of white infants, but the effect on the rates for the Asian and American Indian groups is substantial—the "true" rates being considerably higher than those based on recorded race at

homogeneity. The Jewish religion, however, does currently appear to identify groups that are more homogeneous than the population at large with respect to some characteristics (e.g., eastern European ancestry, male circumcision, moderation in use of alcohol, genotype).

Whereas religion may be the classificatory item used to identify population groups, it is clear that explanations for observed differences in disease rates between religious groups may or may not be found in a feature of the religious practice. Specific methods of birth control, circumcision, and abstinence from tobacco are features of, respectively, Catholics, Jews, and Seventh Day Adventists that may be thought of as part of religious practice. Prior to the study of Zinsser on endemic typhus in New York City the disease was thought to be a disease of Jews. Zinsser, however, showed that it was a function of the fact that the majority of the immigrants from Eastern Europe at that particular time were Jewish, and the organisms had been carried in dormant form from their homelands on migration.[613]

A great deal of interest in religious differences has been focused in the field of cancer, most recently in the hope of discovering from the dietary practices of groups such as the Mormons and the Seventh Day Adventists clues about dietary factors related to cancer etiology, as referred to in Chapter 5. Originally, however, this interest was stimulated by the well-known rarity of cancer of the cervix in Jewish women and its possible relationship to the circumcision of Jewish males, a relationship for which there now appears to be only limited support. Nevertheless, an early study of cancer mortality in New York City, while finding few differences in rates between the Catholic and Protestant populations, showed comparatively high rates among Jews for lymphoma and leukemia as well as for cancers of the breast, brain, kidney, pancreas, and large intestine, and low rates for cancers of the tongue, upper respiratory tract, and esophagus, as well as for cancer of the prostate and the uterine cervix.[384] With the exception of the low rates for the alcohol-related cancers of the upper respiratory tract, these differences remain essentially unexplained.

Local Reproductive and Social Units

Small local populations that have maintained some degree of genetic homogeneity through inbreeding and have preserved environmental consistency have been the subjects of intensive anthropological study. Populations of this type have so far not received a great deal of epidemiologic attention, perhaps because of the great variability in rates of disease that could be expected in groups of small size. Nevertheless, the addition of accurate medical data to anthropological studies has produced some interesting findings. The identification of the probable role of cannibalism in the dissemination of kuru in the Fore people of New Guinea,[339] and indeed the entire story of the elucidation of the etiology of this disease, provides a good example of the usefulness of the combination of anthropologic and epidemiologic information. Investigations of certain North American Indian tribes show disease patterns so strikingly different from those of North America in general that closer study seems likely to be informative.[187,503]

Within the populations of Europe and the United States, a few such localized groups have been studied. Most of these studies have been interpreted with particular reference to genetic hypotheses. Religious belief is also sometimes associated with the formation of local groups that maintain various degrees of inbreeding. One of the most long-lasting of such groups are the Hutterites, who have maintained an almost completely isolated genetic and social unit for three centuries. The unique characteristics of this group have been utilized in studies of the frequency and nature of mental disorders among them.[110]

Interpretation of Racial and Ethnic Patterns of Disease

There is probably no cultural or ancestral characteristic of a racial or ethnic group that does not carry its own determinant of the overall health of members of the group. The catalog of racial and ethnic determinants of disease is too broad to be fully described here. We can only list a few of the general categories of disease determinants that should be investigated when an apparently racial or ethnic peculiarity is noted for a specific group.

Mutations in Single Major Genes

A number of important diseases are determined by mutations in single major genes, the inheritance of which has been limited, or essentially limited, to certain groups.[524,531] These include:

Sickle cell anemia: Common in West African blacks and their descendants in the United States and elsewhere.

Cystic fibrosis of the pancreas: High in Europeans and US Caucasian populations.

Tay-Sach's disease: Essentially restricted to Ashkenazi Jews.

Alcohol dehydrogenase deficiency in Japanese and some other Asian populations.

Thalassemia, which occurs mainly in persons of Greek or Italian descent and in other areas around the Mediterranean Sea.

Polygenic Inheritance

There are genetic factors in disease susceptibility other than those determined by single major genes that vary in their frequency distributions between ancestrally defined ethnic groups. They may be responsible for ethnic variation in susceptibility to tuberculosis, diabetes mellitus, hypertension, and many other diseases. Although the influence of such factors is undoubted, the specifics are poorly understood at the present time.

Geography

Ethnic groups are frequently congregated by residence, either over very large areas (e.g., an Indian reservation) or within a few contiguous city blocks. Any feature of that geographic congregation that is associated with disease susceptibility may be reflected in an apparent association of the disease with an ethnic group.

Socioeconomic Status

Associations between ethnic groups and socioeconomic status in a community are common. Since the end of slavery in the United States, in comparison to whites, blacks have been economically deprived. Although there are prominent exceptions today, and the overall differential is progressively decreasing, it is still true that the black population as a whole is economically disadvantaged relative to the white population. This is reflected in trends in infant mortality rates, one of the most sensitive health indicators of economic status, which have fallen dramatically in both groups, but remain more than twice as high in the black as in the white population. Many other apparent ethnic differences may also only be reflecting underlying differences in economic status.

Cultural Practices

Cultural, including religious, practices associated with particular ethnic groups may have influences on disease patterns. Diet in particular is one of the most important of such potential influences, but attitudes toward, and practice of, such things as sexual behavior, exercise, sports, and spiritual life should also be considered.

Migration

The study of disease patterns in migrants overlaps somewhat with the evaluation of ethnic differences because the occurrence of more than one ethnic group in a region is often the result of recent or remote migrations. Studies of recent migrations are of most interest to epidemiologists. In addition, a comparison with rates in the population or populations from which the migrants came strengthens the simple comparison of disease rates among ethnic groups within a region.[400] Studies of migrants, therefore, add the dimension of *change* in disease rates that may accompany a change in environment.

Studies of migrants have been used mainly to evaluate the role that different gene pools may play in accounting for international differences in disease rates. In theory, studies of migrants may also be used to compare disease frequencies in successive generations after migration to evaluate how deeply entrenched in a culture the environmental factors responsible for a particular disease may be. Also, by examining the role of age at migration, the studies may be used to seek hints as to the time in life during which etiologic factors are operating.[256] In practice, however, the logistic difficulties of migrant studies have limited the inferences that can be drawn from them in some of these respects. Comprehensive reviews of studies of migrants, with particular respect to cancer risk, have been published recently by Parkin[398] and Geddes et al.,[144] and many principles and methods are illustrated in the review by Benfante of morbidity from cardiovascular and other diseases among populations of Japanese origin in the Pacific region.[20]

The Role of Genes

In the 1950s, distinctive differences in rates of chronic diseases between nations, particularly in the contrasts between Oriental and Western populations, became apparent. Smith called attention to the difference between observed and expected cancer mortality among Japanese and Chinese in the United States,[501,502] and Segi[483] and Segi and Kurihara[485] produced a series of reports, beginning with data for 1950–1957, comparing cancer mortality around the world by compiling statistics reported to the World Health Organization. Segi et al. went on to show that cancer incidence, as well as mortality, was very different in Myagi Prefecture in Japan than in registration areas in the United States.[484]

These reports did not initially receive the attention they deserved. After all, there were so many differences between Western and Oriental populations, particularly at that time, shortly after World War II, that it was hard to pin down hypotheses that might explain the differences in cancer rates. Furthermore, it was not out of the question that the differences might lie in the different gene pools and, therefore, have no practical implication for manipulation or prevention.

Great credit must be given to William Haenszel of the US National Cancer Institute for not only recognizing the significance of studies of migrants in this situation, but for acting on this recognition. In an extensive series of studies conducted in collaboration with Oriental, European, and American investigators, Haenszel showed that in the case of migrants from various European countries and from Japan to the United States, the migrants, after periods of time that varied for different sites of cancer, came to have rates more similar to those of the host population than of the country from which they migrated. Early findings are shown in Table 8-5. The table illustrates that the effect of migration on disease risk is not the same for all diseases or even for all cancers. The distinctions shown in Table 8-5 for Japanese migrants to America have also been seen in migrants from Europe to the United States,[514] Italy to Canada,[143] Estonia to Sweden,[388] and Poland to France,[552] among others.[340,611]

For several of the diseases listed in the table (e.g., intracranial vascular lesions, cancer of the cervix), the Japanese Americans, even those born in Japan, show rates similar to those of white Americans, and quite different from those of the Japanese in Japan. For some other causes of death, notably cancer of the

Table 8-5. Standardized Mortality Ratios (SMRs)* for Selected Causes of Death in Japan, Among American Residents of Japanese Ancestry, and in White Americans, 1959–1962

Cause of death for males (M) and females (F)	Japan	Japanese Americans		White Americans
		Not US born	US born	
Cancer				
Esophagus (M)	100	132	51	47
Stomach (M)	100	72	38	17
Stomach (F)	100	55	48	18
Intestine (M)	100	374	288	489
Intestine (F)	100	218	209	483
Breast (F)	100	166	136	591
Cervix uteri (F)	100	52	33	48
Intracranial vascular lesions (M)	100	32	24	37
Intracranial vascular lesions (F)	100	40	43	48
Arteriosclerotic heart disease (M)	100	226	165	481
Arteriosclerotic heart disease (F)	100	196	38	348

Adapted from Haenszel W, Kurihara M. Studies of Japanese migrants. I. Mortality from cancer and other diseases among Japanese in the United States. *J Natl Cancer Inst* 1968;40 : 43–68.
* SMRs relative to a death rate of 100 in Japan

stomach and the intestine, rates for Japanese Americans are intermediate between those for Japan and those for white Americans. For one of the conditions listed in Table 8-5—breast cancer—the death rate for Japanese Americans is much closer to that of the Japanese than to that of the white American, even among the American born.

Multigeneration Studies

At the time that these data were assembled, the Japanese Americans who were not American born were mostly born in Japan, and most of those born in the United S ates had parents who were born in Japan. With the passage of time since the major immigrations of Japanese and Chinese populations to the United States around the turn of the century there has been greater opportunity to study the rate of acquisition of American disease patterns over the generations. There is not always consistency in the use of terminology, but we shall refer to the migrants themselves as the "first generation," the American born children of the migrants as the "second generation," and so forth.

The pattern illustrated in Table 8-5 for several diseases in which the first generation already acquires rates approaching those of the host country has been noted for other diseases and in other migrant groups.[611] It has been seen, for example, for several cancers, most consistently for cancers of the lung in most migrant groups and of the colon in migrants from Poland, and in male but not female Chinese migrants. That such a change in disease experience could come about within the lifetime of the migrant population is unequivocal evidence that some feature or features of the environment in the country of origin are responsible for the low or high rates of these particular diseases. It also indicates that these are not features of the environment that migrants take with them unaltered when they migrate. This conclusion does not imply that genetic factors are irrelevant in these diseases, but simply that such factors do not explain the observed international differences in rates for these cancers.

For the group of diseases for which rates in the first and the second generations are intermediate between those in the country of origin and the host country—this is the case for most cancers—the significance of environmental factors is again strongly suggested. That the rates among foreign-born Americans do not come closer to those of the US population might be explained by a long induction period for the disease, long duration of disease prior to death, some retention of the relevant environment, or other mechanisms. Age at migration is a potentially relevant variable, which is addressed later. However, the fact that even those Americans of Japanese ancestry who were born in the United States had rates substantially different from those of white Americans indicates that either the responsible environmental factor is retained for a considerable period in the host country, as dietary customs might be, or that more intrinsic features also play a role.

Such an observation is compatible with the hypothesis that the international difference in rates has a genetic basis. Yet, even if the same observation were made over several generations of the migrant population, the example of circumcision of Jewish male infants is a reminder that some environmental factors remain firmly bound to the home culture several generations after migration. In addition, it should be noted that the observation in Table 8-5 is essentially limited to a single generation born in the host country. If a disease were dependent in part on, for example, diet in childhood, it is not surprising that the first generation of migrants would experience rates more characteristic of the home than of the host country.

In an interesting approach to the multigeneration problem, the case-control approach (see Chapter 10) was used by Ziegler et al. to study the birth places of breast cancer cases, their matched controls, and their parents and grandparents.[611] The cases and controls were of Chinese, Japanese, or Filipino descent, aged 20–55, and living in San Francisco, Los Angeles, or Oahu, Hawaii, between 1983 and 1987. The cases and their ancestors were classified as to whether they were born in the "West" (primarily North America, but including Europe and Australia and New Zealand) or the "East" (primarily Southeast Asia and off-lying islands). Odds ratio estimates among the migrants themselves increased with increasing duration of residence in the West, although they did not reach the levels characteristic of Asian-Americans who were born and lived their entire lives in the West. Interestingly, Asian-American women with one or more grandparents also born in the West actually had rates exceeding those of the white population. This tendency of the rates in the third and, occasionally, second generation migrants to "overshoot" those in the local host population has also been seen in Polish migrants to the United States[514] and Australia[344] and some other groups.[287,381] An explanation of this phenomenon in terms of methodologic issues, including differential ascertainment of cases in the host country and the country of origin, has been offered by Parkin,[398] but it does not seem a satisfactory explanation of the generational pattern noted by Ziegler et al.[611]

Biases in Migrant Studies

A comprehensive account of the potential biases in migrant studies has been assembled by Parkin.[398] They include:

1. Diagnostic, reporting, and coding practices may be different in the country of origin from those in the host country. Such differences would affect particularly comparisons of migrants with rates in the country of origin, but could even affect comparisons within the host country if, because of geographic distribution, socioeconomic status, or other factors, migrants differed from the native born in access to medical facilities or were predominantly seen within different systems of care.

2. Migrants are not representative samples of the populations of their home countries of origin and may be selected in terms of geographic area (important if the disease of interest varies by geography within the country of origin), age, gender, race, socioeconomic, and, perhaps most important, health status. The healthy and physically able are most likely to migrate. These are features that may be strengthened by health-related restrictions or job opportunities in the host country.

3. The stresses of migration may in some circumstances pose disease risks not present, or present to a lesser degree, in either the country of origin or the host country. Such stresses may be of particular significance in the context of studies of mental illness among migrants.

4. Biases may be introduced by inaccuracies in denominator data because the accuracy of numbers and levels of information on such variables as age, gender, and race will vary according to statistical resources available in both the countries of origin and the host country.

Few studies of migrants have eradicated the possibility of bias from any of these sources, and none has dealt with all of them. There is room, therefore, for considerable caution in the interpretation of migrant studies. Nevertheless, the differences noted in many studies are so great that very strong biases would have to be operating to explain them. To be overconcerned about possible biases and ignore the inferences that may be drawn from the observations, even if partially biased, would be a greater error than to accept the observations without concern for potential biases. Where differences are small, greater caution is warranted.

Socioeconomic Status

Socioeconomic status (SES) is one of the most important demographic determinants of disease risk. In the US National Health Survey, restricted activity due to poor health, and in particular average days of bed disability per person, declines markedly with increasing family income (see Table 8-6). The trend is seen at all ages (except for non–bed-disability in children under 5 years), but is particularly striking in the age group 45–64 when activity restriction due to ill health becomes a prominent problem. Although the trend is not seen in these morbidity data for persons under 5 years of age overall, socioeconomic factors are more important in the first year of life than at any other age. They are a very influential factor in infant mortality. Virtually all causes of ill health participate in these trends, which are evident in data on mortality, both before and after the first year, as well as morbidity. Similar trends are seen in all countries for which such data are available.

However, SES is a concept that is not uniformly defined. Indeed, the concept has so many components—income, occupation, living conditions, social prestige—that in practice a single variable that can be defined objectively is often used as a surrogate for the whole, as shown in Table 8-6. Another variable that is frequently used as a measure of SES is occupation. Probably the best known examples of such use are the series of reports produced by the Registrar General for England and Wales (now the Office of Population Censuses and Surveys [OPCS]). Deaths for a number of years surrounding the decennial censuses have been classified in these reports by assessed SES of the decedent's occupation (using the husband's occupation for a married woman), ranging from professional to unskilled and related to the occupational status distribution of the population derived from the corresponding census. Since the beginning of the twentieth century, a decrease in mortality with an increase in SES measured by this classification of occupation has been observed.[434]

When the distribution of an epidemiologic variable in a series that comprises all deaths (or cases) in a population during a certain period is compared with the corresponding distribution from a census of that same population (at a relevant time), there should be no bias due to selection of the study series. However, this does not eliminate information bias resulting from the different sources of information on the variable between the deaths or

Table 8-6. Number of Days of Restricted Activity per Person per Year, by Type of Restriction, Age, and Family Income, United States, 1993

Age	Family income (thousands of dollars)			
	<10	10–19	20–34	35+
ALL TYPES OF RESTRICTION:				
<5	9.9	13.3	10.3	10.7
5–17	14.9	10.5	10.1	8.7
18–24	12.5	10.1	9.5	7.3
25–44	31.2	22.5	13.8	10.8
45–64	65.7	35.8	20.6	12.8
65+	51.1	33.4	30.2	22.2
BED DISABILITY:				
<5	6.0	6.1	4.4	3.9
5–17	5.8	5.0	4.2	3.8
18–24	5.5	4.7	4.5	2.7
25–44	12.7	9.4	5.1	3.6
45–64	32.4	14.8	6.8	4.4
65+	17.9	13.9	11.4	9.1

Source: National Center for Health Statistics. *Current Estimates from the National Health Interview Survey, 1993.* Hyattsville, MD: National Center for Health Statistics, 1994. DHHS Publ. No. (PHS) 95-1518.

cases and the census. Occupation is particularly susceptible to this source of error. For example, a man who worked as a carpenter throughout his life, retired at age 65, and worked part time as a market gardener for 5 years before his death at age 70, might be described as a carpenter, a gardener, or a retiree. The choice would be even broader if he had held several different jobs during the course of his life. The respondent is asked for only one occupation, and the choice may be different at the census, when he responds himself, than on a death certificate, for which another person provides the information. For this reason and others, a number of prospective cohort studies have been undertaken, sometimes also involving periodic medical examinations and laboratory tests, in which the occupation of a decedent or anyone who manifests any health abnormality can be determined from the information obtained at entrance to the study or from information updated as the study proceeds. Outstanding examples of such studies are the two studies of British civil servants (Whitehall I and Whitehall II).[328] The first began in 1967 and was limited to males;[436] the second covered the years 1985–1988 and included 6,900 men and 3,414 women.[332] The measure of SES was the individual's civil service grade title, which corresponded to an annual salary range (in 1987) from £3,061 to £62,100. Other recently initiated studies have not been restricted to employees of a single service, which has potential advantages (e.g., greater range in SES) and potential disadvantages (e.g., greater potential for confounding of SES with access to and use of medical services). For instance, the Scottish Heart Health Study is based on a random sample of 10,359 men and women between 40 and 59 years of age from 22 districts across Scotland.[504] Four measures of social status were used: (1) the OPCS's five classes based on occupation referred to earlier; (2) whether employed in "manual" or "nonmanual" labor; (3) level of education; and (4) "housing tenure," that is, whether the subject owned or rented his residence. For coronary heart disease, which is a major contributor to the high morbidity and mortality in the lower economic classes and which we will discuss further later, the strongest association was found with housing tenure.[551,603]

A much larger longitudinal study linking health outcomes to socioeconomic characteristics of individuals is the (US) National Longitudinal Mortality Study (NLMS), in which more than one million people participating in Current Population Surveys[557] between 1979 and 1985 were interviewed in person or by telephone about numerous socioeconomic variables.[453] There was no attempt at personal follow-up, but a file of 530,000 persons over 25 years of age with known values for relevant variables was linked to the National Death Index[376] for the years 1979–1989.[509] The National Death Index, which is based on specific identifying information such as name, birthdate, and Social Security Number, has been shown in several studies to have a sensitivity of around 98 percent for the identification of a known decedent.[439,513,598] Substantial associations have been found in these data with most measures of socioeconomic status.[509]

It is instructive to examine side by side the Whitehall studies and the NLMS to assess the strengths and limitations of the two longitudinal designs. For the study of a fairly common disease—coronary heart disease—which was the objective of both studies, the Whitehall studies are clearly more informative. But for less common diseases, the much larger data base of the NLMS provides information that the Whitehall studies cannot.

Years of schooling (education) received, or in the case of children, years of education of a parent, also correlates well with the general concept of SES. This measure was selected in the Ontario Heart Study[235] and in many other contexts. Indeed, because years of education are more accurately ascertained than family income and they are more easily classifiable than occupation, they often produce more consistent trends with outcomes known to be associated with SES, such as infant mortality,[310] than any of the other single variable surrogates. Whichever single variable is selected, the interpretation of results must take into consideration features that are peculiar to that particular variable, as well as to SES in general.

For most cities, data for census tracts or other units are available that allow classification according to some measure of SES (e.g., median income of their populations; the percentage of their populations in certain occupational categories; measures of housing standards, such as median rental or degree of crowding). Disease frequencies may be computed and compared for residents of areas classified according to these indices. It is important to note that in this method SES is not known for the individuals concerned but is inferred from their place of residence, thus introducing an "ecologic" element in the ascertainment of exposure (see Chapter 5). The reliability of the method varies greatly from one city to another and may also vary within the same city over time. Although there is no question as to the tendency of the residences of persons of high and low SES to cluster in certain parts of cities, the administrative areas for which data are available may not be small enough to discriminate clearly between exposure clusters. If differential disease rates are demonstrated by this method, then (subject to the usual precautions about confounding and other sources of error) it can probably be assumed that an association with SES exists. Yet, if no association is noted, two explanations must be considered: either no association exists or the classification of areas is not sufficiently discriminating to demonstrate an association that does exist.

Occasionally, an investigator will devise an index combining a number of variables by an arbitrary formula to fit with his or her own concept of social class. The index might be based on a weighted combination of some or all of such items as income, rental, family size, occupation, and residence. The last three, for example, were used by Hollingshead and Redlich to develop an index that has been widely applied in psychiatric epidemiology.[215] In a long-term cohort study of 5,249 Copenhagen males, first examined in 1970–1971, an index combining occupation and education was used to define social class.[203] A scale with particular application to New Zealand has been developed by Elley and Irving,[117] and others[536] could be cited. Whereas such indices have utility within the particular populations to which they are applied, they have the disadvantage of seldom being used in exactly the same form by other investigators or in other countries and, therefore, hindering comparison of findings. Certain variables, whether used alone[499] or as part of an index[536] (e.g., access to an automobile), may be useful in some settings and not in others.

An important contribution was made by Diez-Roux et al., who noted that, in the context of atherosclerosis, within the same community a single marker of social class may not have the same implication for all gender or racial groups.[92] In four communities across the United States, education was a better predictor of atherosclerosis prevalence than occupation or income in whites but not in blacks. As might be expected, occupation was a much stronger predictor in males than in females. These observations will add to the debate about how social class is best measured. A useful account of the meaning of social class and its relevance to illness is given by Susser, Watson, and Hopper.[523]

Interpretation

However much one may wish to eliminate differences in SES within or between societies, such a goal has implications far beyond those of disease prevention and is largely outside the scope of public health. For public health purposes we must endeavor to identify the attributes of social class that are most strongly related to disease risk and that can be altered. Some of these are obvious and, indeed, have already been acted upon, for example, the crowded and unsanitary living conditions that aid the spread of infectious disease and the many known diseases associated with undernutrition. Other mechanisms for social class effects are strongly suspect but effective counteractions are not yet known; for example, it is doubtful that the diet favored by the rich over the last 200 years is the most beneficial in terms of health, but the changes that would improve it from the point of view of health are controversial. As another example, the educational underpinnings of a proclivity to violence, although undoubtedly related to social class, are not understood.

There are other relationships of disease risk to SES of which the mechanisms remain totally mysterious. There is probably no better example of such a mystery than that of coronary heart disease, which is summarized here for illustrative purposes. The complexity of the general issue is well put by Marmot:

> The magnitude of the social class differences vary for different causes of death, presumably as a sign of the effect of specific factors for specific disease. The observation that social class differences apply to most causes of death, however, suggest(s) that factors like early life experience, difference in behaviour, material and psychological conditions act in an unspecific way.[328]

Mention should be made of the social "drift" hypothesis, which postulates that illness, either physical or mental, causes low SES, rather than the reverse (e.g., making affected individuals less competitive in both the educational and employment settings). Undoubtedly this does occur in many cases of chronic or financially devastating illness, but the extent to which it determines the major relationships between social class and disease is unknown. Diez-Roux et al., in the context of coronary heart disease, suggest that such a mechanism could not explain relationships with educational attainment because they are usually complete before clinical signs of disease appear and would not be altered by the occurrence of disease.[92] That might be true in the particular context they were discussing because, at least with regard to their data on whites, education was a better predictor of disease than either income or occupation, and the association with education could not therefore be completely confounded by either of the latter variables. However, it is not true as a generalization because even if the drift is attributable to a downward drift in occupation it would still appear in unadjusted associations between disease and education because of the correlation of occupation and education. Marmot found no evidence for health selection of salary grade in the Whitehall studies,[328] and Goldblatt found no evidence that health-related downward drift accounted for social class differences in mortality in Britain between 1971 and 1981.[153]

An Example: Coronary Heart Disease

The prospective cohort studies described earlier, and many others not mentioned, have consistently shown a strong inverse relationship of SES, however it is measured, to risk of coronary heart disease (CHD). Generally speaking, the rate ratio for the lowest compared to the highest classes is greater than three and sometimes higher. For a disease as common as CHD, this excess risk is of great importance—it accounts for about half of the excess mortality associated with low social class. The relationship is even more remarkable because it is of relatively recent origin.[329] In the 1930–1932 analysis of the Registrar General noted earlier, the mortality from CHD in men in the highest economic class was 3.5 times that of those in the lowest class. By 1950 the differential had fallen to 1.7, although still in the same direction.[435] Rose and Marmot followed this series through the report of 1971 and showed the crossover in the trend occurring between 1951 and 1961.[457] They note that this reversal in the trend with SES has not been seen in women. Women in the lowest classes (as assessed from their husbands' occupations) have had higher mortality than those in the upper classes throughout this period. Rose and Marmot also point to the potential roles of changes in disease diagnosis and classification, as well as changes in the implications of the occupational classes over time, as potential players in this striking reversal of SES trends in males over time. However, it does not seem likely that several generations of physicians before 1950 could have been completely misled as to the social class of the males presenting with coronary disease. Moreover, whatever the state of affairs before 1950, there can be no doubt about the strength of the current inverse relationship between SES and CHD. In fact, a number of the prospective cohort studies mentioned earlier were set up primarily to investigate this relationship. During the last three decades a substantial literature has developed, and an extensive review leaves no question as to the reality of the trend and the fact that it is widespread throughout the developed world.[92] Indeed, there are some indications that the differential is increasing over time in some countries.[252,328,330] In the study of Diez-Roux et al., referred to earlier, it was shown that the relationship is seen in preclinical as well as clinical atherosclerotic disease as evidenced by thickening of the intima of the carotid arteries.[92] It is intriguing that this association first became evident at about the same time that CHD began to decline as a cause of death in many Western nations.

A first question is whether or not the association of social class can be explained by known risk factors for CHD. A major suspect in this respect is, of course, cigarette smoking, which is strongly associated with CHD and has shown a steeper decline in the upper socioeconomic groups than in the lower. In the first Whitehall study (1967–1969, males only), four socioeconomic classes were defined, and the percentages of current smokers in the highest and lowest classes were 29 and 61, respectively.[457] In the second Whitehall study (1985–1988), six social classes were defined. The percentage of male smokers in the lowest grade was 33.6, and the percentages in the two grades that corresponded approximately to the highest grade in the first study were 8.3 and 10.2.[332] (The men in the second study were by design 5–10 years younger than those in the first.) Yet, by multivariate modeling, differences in smoking appeared to account for only about 10 percent of the CHD difference between the highest and the lowest economic class. In fact, adjustment for age, smoking, serum cholesterol level, blood pressure, height, leisure time activities, and glucose tolerance accounted for only 35 percent of the difference in CHD.[457] An extensive analysis of gender, serum cholesterol, apolipoproteins, and hemostatic factors in the second Whitehall study led to the conclusion that the most important known factor mediating the relationship between SES and CHD is probably smoking, and, as we have seen, the relationship with smoking in the Whitehall data is not nearly strong enough to explain the SES effect.[45]

In the Scottish study referred to previously,[603] smoking in males was also the most important mediator of the relationship between SES and CHD, accounting for between 16 and 34 percent of the excess risk in the lower class, depending on the variable used to define the SES. In women, smoking was of little importance, the most important mediator being body mass index, which accounted for between 24 and 58 percent of the excess.

The picture is more complicated in the Copenhagen study because of the different forms in which tobacco is smoked.[203] However, the incidence rate ratio for men in the lowest social class compared to those in the highest, after multivariate adjustment for age, blood pressure, physical activity, body mass index, and alcohol use was 3.6. After adding the form of tobacco used, the amount used, and the presence or absence of inhalation to the multivariate model, the relative risk remained almost unchanged at 3.5. Clearly the bulk of the relationship between SES and CHD remains to be explained.

The purpose of reviewing the substantive question of social class and CHD at some length (although still quite superficially) in a text that deals with principles is that it provides so many illustrations of the types of descriptive relationships that have been found to be useful in epidemiology. There is the paradox that CHD has changed from a disease of the affluent in wealthy countries to a disease of the poor in the same countries. There is the coincidence, which is almost certainly not a coincidence, that the change in relationship of CHD with social class began at around the same time as the overall decline in CHD began in the same countries. There can be few hypotheses that would explain this set of circumstances. Then there is the need to consider latency—in smoking and diet effects, for example—when correlating trends in exposures and disease rates. Lastly, there is the consistency of the observations looked for in the Western world, which makes it virtually certain that there are real forces at work that could be of critical importance to understand.

Occupation

We devote little space to occupation as a personal characteristic relevant to descriptive epidemiology, but not because it is not an important descriptor. Occupation has been so important in the development of knowledge of disease causation, and the relevant

principles and methods are so essential, that we cannot expect
to do justice to them in the space available in this text. The reader
interested in this topic would be well served by consulting one or
more of the several textbooks of occupational epidemiology[59,363] or
occupational medicine[454] that are available, including the classic
Hunter's Diseases of Occupations, now in its 8th edition.[429] Only
the principle ways that occupation has been used in the formulation of hypotheses about causes of disease are outlined here.
There are three distinct approaches through which knowledge of
a person's occupation has been used for this purpose. One use
has been described at some length in the previous section of this
chapter—occupation as a surrogate for socioeconomic status—
and will not be discussed further.

A second, and probably the most obvious, approach is to identify occupations at high risk for specific diseases and search for
the noxious agents or processes to which persons in these occupations are exposed. Probably about half the chemicals and chemical processes known to be carcinogenic to humans have been
identified in this way. They include soot, lead, acrylonitrile, asbestos, aniline derivatives, arsenic, benzene, cadmium, coal tar
fumes, chromates, mineral oils, nickel, radium, radon, vinyl chlo-
ride, and wood dust.[303] The associations of silica and other dusts
with chronic obstructive lung disease were also identified in this
way, as was the association of heavy exposure to carbon disulphide with coronary heart disease.[206a,312] Health problems recognized in occupational groups may have implications for populations quite remote from the occupation in which the problem was
recognized. Lubin et al. have used meta-analysis techniques to
derive from the available data on radon-exposed miners the best
equation describing the relationship between level of exposure
and risk of lung cancer.[298] This equation was then applied to
estimates of indoor (nonoccupational) exposure in housing in the
United States to suggest that 10 percent of all US lung cancer
cases might be due to radon exposure and that reducing radon
in all homes to below the Environmental Protection Agency's recommended action level would reduce lung cancer deaths by 2–4
percent. Essential to this use of occupation are accurate data
on exposure. A comprehensive review of methods for obtaining
exposure information and their strengths and limitations has
been published by Armstrong and colleagues.[14] Although the review is not limited to occupational exposures, the principles delin-
eated are very relevant here, as well as in subsequent chapters.

A third use of occupation is as an index of factors associated
with working conditions, rather than specific exposures associated with the occupation. Perhaps the most frequent use of occu-

pation in this sense is as a surrogate of the amount of physical energy expenditure demanded by the occupation. A classical example of this is provided in the studies of Paffenbarger and his colleagues of longshoremen (stevedores) in San Francisco who were classified as to whether their duties involved heavy, moderate, or light physical activity. Prospectively followed, the death rate from coronary heart disease among those with the heaviest energy expenditure was only 60 percent of those among men with moderate or light physical activity.[392] A potential problem in interpreting this observation is that, although all the men were judged physically healthy at the time of employment, men with symptoms or early evidence of heart disease may have sought transfer to activities with less severe physical demands. This problem was minimized, although not entirely overcome, by classifying men according to the level of their activity 6 months before death. This potential selection problem has to be considered in all inferences about health in relation to working conditions, whether these conditions refer to physical activity, monotony of the work, the individual's level of control over his or her activities, or job satisfaction.[332]

Marital Status

Marital status is a descriptive variable that appears on medical and civil records almost as frequently as age and gender, and of which there have been a number of epidemiologic analyses. Although there are distinct differences in disease rates according to marital status, they have not been particularly rewarding as a source of epidemiologic hypotheses. Generally speaking, for most diseases mortality rates are lowest among married people and highest among the widowed and divorced. The major difficulty in interpreting these differences is in differentiating the hypothesis that some factor associated with marital status is a risk factor for a disease from the hypothesis that marital status depends to some extent on the presence or absence of chronic disease. Thus, persons already in poor health may be less likely to marry and, if widowed, less likely to remarry. The fact that certain causes of death or illness that may be associated with "living dangerously" (e.g., automobile accidents, other accidents, sexually transmitted diseases) are particularly in excess among single males suggests that there are lifestyle differences according to marital status. Yet, this provides no more information than everyday observation and leaves unanswered the question of the directionality of the causal path.

Religion

Religion has been of use in identifying groups with particular dietary or other practices, as mentioned in Chapter 5, but otherwise has not been an informative descriptive variable for epidemiologic purposes. In fact, because most of the relevant exposures can be directly ascertained, and nonconfounding factors that affect the likelihood of these exposures should not be controlled in the analysis[416] (see Chapter 10), there is little reason to collect information on religion except to assess comparability of study samples and populations.

9 Cohort Studies

The incidence *rate* is the essential measure of disease occurrence; therefore, the incidence rate ratio and the incidence rate difference are the fundamental measures of association between a disease and an exposure variable, whether the exposure takes two (unexposed and exposed) or several values. Cumulative incidence or *risk* and the corresponding ratio and difference measures (risk ratio and risk difference) may have utility in some circumstances, but they are meaningful only when the rates involved are low and the period of follow-up is relatively short. When the follow-up period is very long, even low rates can generate high risks, and the risk ratio tends asymptotically to the value of one, thus underestimating the underlying rate ratio (when this is higher than one). Furthermore, competing causes of death can directly affect estimated risks and risk ratios because they operate principally on the numerators of the formulae from which the risk estimators are calculated. By contrast, competing causes do not, *as a rule*, affect rates and rate ratios because they influence both the numerators and the person-time denominators of the rate estimators, usually in a roughly balanced way. Thus, the ravaging of certain African countries by AIDS certainly reduces the number of people who die from malaria and, as a result, the corresponding risk. However, the mortality rate from malaria does not necessarily decline, as AIDS kills with no particular predilection for persons who otherwise would have died from malaria and those who would not have died from malaria.

Every analytic epidemiological study involves some type of sampling, although often the sampling process is not clearly defined. The source population over the study period that is sampled is sometimes called the *study base* or *base population*, whereas the

165

subjects that are actually investigated form the *study group(s)* or the *study population*.[358] There are two defining characteristics of cohort studies: (1) they are exposure based, and (2) they are patently or conceptually longitudinal.

In cohort studies, the samples to be studied are considered with reference to exposure. In some studies, the samples are chosen on the basis of a particular exposure (*special exposure cohorts*). In other cohort studies, population groups offering special resources for follow-up or data linkage are chosen, and the individuals are subsequently allocated according to exposure status (*general population cohorts*). The first approach may be necessary when generally rare exposures need to be studied, whereas the second approach is appropriate when the exposure under consideration is fairly common in general populations (e.g., smoking or major components of diet). In some situations, exposure may refer to a particular event (e.g., eating a contaminated salad or exposure in an industrial accident) or to the time of attainment of a particular state of exposure (e.g., being a smoker for at least 6 months or having been occupationally exposed to asbestos for at least 2 years). In other situations, exposure refers to a state itself, which can be either permanent (e.g., being a veteran of the Gulf War) or reversible (e.g., being a current smoker or living under stress).

In cohort studies, individuals are observed over a period of time to determine the frequency of occurrence of disease among them. The distinction between *retrospective* and *prospective* cohort studies depends on whether or not the cases of disease have occurred in the cohort at the time the study begins. In a retrospective cohort study, all the relevant exposures and health outcomes have already occurred when the study is initiated. In a prospective cohort study, the relevant causes may or may not have occurred at the time the study begins, but the cases of disease have not yet occurred, and, following selection of the study cohort, the investigator must wait for the disease to appear in the cohort members. The distinction between retrospective and prospective cohort studies is important, not because of any conceptual differences or differences in interpretability of findings, but because of relevance to some practical issues, mostly the ability to control confounding.

Types of Cohort

There are two types of cohorts and, accordingly, cohort studies: (1) closed or fixed cohorts, and (2) open or dynamic cohorts.[358,576]

Closed Cohorts

Closed cohorts consist of a fixed group of persons who are followed from a certain point in time until a defined endpoint. The starting point of observation may be the exposure defining event, or a point in time related to it, and a comparable point in the nonexposed comparison group. The endpoint is the occurrence of the disease that is suspected of being related to the exposure, death from another cause, loss to follow up, or a defined common endpoint in time, whichever comes first. Preferably, study participants should be followed for the same length of time, except for differences related to the disease under investigation. Examples of closed cohorts are a group of persons who consumed a particular food suspected to be contaminated, workers near the site of an industrial accident, or children exposed to thalidomide in utero. Although the follow up and analysis in closed cohort studies bear some resemblance to those of randomized trials, there are some important differences. First, because in a cohort study the exposure is not assigned at random (or in any other way intentionally administered by the investigator for research objectives), potentially harmful (as well as beneficial) exposures can be studied without ethical objection. However, because of the lack of randomization, confounding by unsuspected or poorly measured factors can rarely be quantified and controlled with complete confidence, whether harmful or beneficial effects are being evaluated.

A second issue that distinguishes clinical follow-up studies from etiologically focused closed cohort investigations is that in clinical studies the frequency of occurrence of many relevant outcomes (e.g., recovery or postoperative complications) is fairly high, whereas the incidence of even common diseases in a generally healthy population is usually low. In the latter situation, longer follow up is therefore required, and this implies aging of the study subjects over the course of the study. Because age is associated with many diseases, a long follow-up may imply changing of exposure status for other risk factors for the disease. In addition, differences between the exposed and unexposed study subjects due to loss to follow-up may also arise. For these reasons, closed cohort designs are commonly utilized in short-term, high-frequency outcome situations, such as food poisoning or other acute outbreaks. There are certainly closed cohorts that are not short-term and that are not directed to high-frequency outcomes (e.g., population groups exposed to mustard gas during World War I or the atomic blasts at Hiroshima and Nagasaki). Because of the difficulties just mentioned, the analysis of the data from such studies generally follows the procedures appropriate for open cohorts, focusing on rates rather than risks.

In closed cohort studies, exposed and unexposed persons are ideally derived from the same study base in order to be comparable. This is accomplished when both exposed and unexposed cohorts are representative of the respective groups in the study base, or when all members of the study base are included in the study groups. The study base itself does not have to be representative of any particular broader population. The key issue is *comparability* between or among the study cohorts, and even lack of comparability may be accommodated in the analysis when it is generated only by factors that are confidently known and measured. This is an ideal, however, that is rarely achieved.

There is no validity-serving reason that the compared cohorts should be of any particular relative size; neither do the study groups have to be equal or proportional to the number of exposed and unexposed persons in the study base. However, the statistical power of the study and the precision of the effect estimates (rate or risk ratio and difference) increase not only with increase in the total number of study participants but, for a given total number, when the numbers in the exposed and unexposed cohorts are equal or approximately so. This principle can easily be demonstrated from statistical power formulas, but, in essence, it reflects the fact that the product of two numbers with a given sum is maximized when these numbers are equal (e.g., for a total study size of 20, $10 \cdot 10 = 100$, whereas $15 \cdot 5 = 75$, and $18 \cdot 2 = 36$).

An important factor in the determination of the statistical power of a cohort study is the genuine range of variation in the exposure of interest—the larger the variation in the exposure, the more powerful the study. Genuine variation should not be confused with variation generated by extensive nondifferential exposure misclassification and/or random within-person variability, which tend to bias effect estimates toward the null value and reduce their precision. Moreover, large variation in potentially confounding variables, whether genuine or misclassification-induced, increases confounding and reduces the investigator's ability to account for it in the analysis.

Open Cohorts

Open cohorts consist of persons who may enter or leave the study at any time without compromising the integrity of the study design unless, of course, loss to follow-up is associated with both exposure and outcome. Thus, open cohorts consist of persons whose exposure status, or other characteristics relevant to the disease, may change over time. As a result, exposure does not refer to a particular event but to a state that can change over time. For example, an open cohort that compares smokers with nonsmokers allows for a change in smoking status as it does for a change in age, occupation, or other factors that, by themselves, may affect the risk of the disease under study. In a closed cohort study, the event that signals entry into the cohort occurs only once at a certain point in time. However, changes in covariates of the exposure and nondifferential losses to follow-up necessitate the use of an analytic strategy that is generally reserved for open cohort studies. Just as for closed cohort studies, open subcohorts of exposed and unexposed persons must be derived from the same study base in order to be comparable; however, the study base itself does not have to be representative of any particular population. Similarly, the range of variation of the principal exposure under consideration should be as large as possible, whereas that of poorly identified or measured confounders should be as small as possible. The precision of the effect estimates (rate ratio and difference; see next section) increases when the total number of *outcome events* (rather than the amount of person-time) is higher and the total person-time in the exposed cohort is about equal to that in the nonexposed cohort.

Measures of Effect in Cohort Studies

In a closed cohort study involving an exposed cohort of N_e persons and an unexposed cohort of N_o persons with x_e and x_o persons, respectively, who develop the disease under study over the time period, the cumulative incidence can be calculated in the two groups. The cumulative incidence ratio and difference are derived as follows. The cumulative incidence difference is $\dfrac{x_e}{N_e} - \dfrac{x_o}{N_o}$, and the cumulative incidence ratio is $\dfrac{x_e}{N_e} \bigg/ \dfrac{x_o}{N_o}$. The odds ratio is calculated as $\dfrac{x_e}{N_e - x_e} \bigg/ \dfrac{x_o}{N_o - x_o}$, where, again, N_e and N_o are, respectively, the numbers in the exposed and unexposed cohorts at the start of observation, and x_e and x_o are, respectively, the numbers of cases observed among them.

The odds ratio is somewhat higher than the cumulative incidence ratio, but it approximates the latter fairly well when the greater of the two cumulative incidence proportions in the formulas is below 0.10 (i.e., when the disease is "rare"). The cumulative incidence ratio is, of course, equivalent to the risk ratio, which underestimates but approximates the incidence rate ratio when the same condition is met. One may wonder why the odds ratio should be considered at all when the risk ratio is both intuitively attractive and directly estimable in a consistent, straightforward way. The utility of the odds ratio is that it provides a link between cohort and case-control studies, as well as a link to a mainstream analytical procedure for case-control studies—the logistic regression model. Furthermore, in situations where the interest is not in the occurrence of an event but in the converse of its occurrence, the risk ratio generates incompatible results. For example, when male or female gender is defined as the outcome, if a factor reduces the proportion of males from 0.65 to 0.50, the risk ratio is 0.50/0.65 = 0.77 when male is the outcome, but 0.50/0.35 = 1.43 when female is the outcome; 1.43 is *not* the inverse of 0.77. In contrast, the odds ratio is (0.50/0.50)/(0.65/0.35) = 0.54, in the first instance, and (0.50/0.50)/(0.35/0.65) = 1.86, in the second; 1.86 *is* the inverse of 0.54. More extreme examples would be generated in most instances when the risk ratio refers to survival rather than death, whereas again the odds ratio generates compatible estimates.

In a closed cohort study it is always possible to calculate incidence rates among the exposed and unexposed and, subsequently, their difference or ratio. Indeed, as we have noted, when the follow-up is prolonged and study participants age or change in respect to other risk predictors, or there are losses to follow up or deaths from diseases other than that under investigation, incidence rates and their derivative measures *must* be used according to the following formulas. *Incidence rate difference* is $\frac{\chi_e}{\tau_e} - \frac{\chi_o}{\tau_o}$, and *incidence rate ratio* is $\frac{\chi_e}{\tau_e} \bigg/ \frac{\chi_o}{\tau_o}$, where τ_e and τ_o are the totals of person-time for, respectively, the exposed and nonexposed cohorts, and χ_e and χ_o are the numbers of observed cases that occurred in the person-time attributed, respectively, to exposed and nonexposed persons.

In an open cohort study, persons may enter or exit the study population or change exposure or confounder status at any time. Therefore, the risk that any particular person will become a case depends not only on his or her exposure and status with respect to confounding factors, but also on how long that person was followed. In open cohorts, risks are not directly derived.

In an open cohort study where aging is not an issue (either because of short study span or because incidence does not vary with age) and there are no confounding factors, two cells are created: one for exposed person-time and one for unexposed person-time. In this instance, the indicated simple formulas for rate difference and ratio are used. If the follow-up is long, study persons are of either gender, and their age varies between 40 and 59 years at the initiation of a study that lasted for 15 years, then a three-dimensional matrix of person-time must be created: one for exposure (yes, no); one for gender (female, male); and one for age, usually in 5-year groups (40–44, 45–49 . . . 70–74). A man who was 53 years old and unexposed at the initiation of the study, who became exposed as he was turning 62, and who was followed throughout would contribute 2 years to the cell "man/unexposed/50–54 years," 5 years to the cell "man/unexposed/55–59 years," 2 years to the cell "man/unexposed/60–64 years," 3 years to the cell "man/exposed/60–64 years," and 3 years to the cell "man/exposed/65–69 years." The years following the exposure would generally be counted as exposed, so long as the subject remained in the study and at risk for developing the disease. This individual would contribute nothing to the age groups 40–44 and 45–49. It is obvious that study participants may, and in fact usually do, contribute person-time to more than one exposure category. People who develop the disease under study must be allocated in the same matrix, and a series of incidence rates corresponding to the cells of the matrix are calculated.

Several issues related to the time variables employed in analytic epidemiological studies may be considered here, even though they are relevant to closed cohort and, occasionally, case-control studies as well.

1. The time dimension of the cells just described does not have to be 5 years; it may be shorter if the risk of disease changes rapidly with time or longer if it changes slowly. The general assumption is that the incidence rate is constant for all person-time units encompassed in a particular cell.

2. Time may refer to a chronological period as well as to age because the incidence of many diseases changes over time among persons of the same age. Joint assessment of age and chronological period also takes into account possible cohort or generation effects.

3. For certain occupational and other environmental hazards, cumulative time-weighted exposure is considered to be the critical variable for the causation of disease. In such a situation, a person who is continuously exposed should be allocated to a low exposure category during the initial follow-up period, an intermediate exposure category later on, and a high exposure category as the exposure is accumulated over time. This dual role of time as component of the person-time pool and as semiquantitative indicator of cumulative exposure has not always been adequately appreciated by investigators.[43]

4. The interval between first exposure to a causal factor and the overt occurrence of the corresponding disease is usually termed *latency*, although the same term has been applied to different concepts.[43,466] Latency is only definable when the disease has occurred and, like any other biologic measure, it is subject to considerable interindividual variation. There are several rather complex issues involving latency and its presumed relation to level of exposure,[409] but there are also some straightforward problems that need always be considered in the planning and interpretation of cohort studies. Thus, a cohort study may be noninformative or even misleading when a long latency and residual effects of a past exposure are not adequately accounted for through a sufficiently long period of follow-up and alternative latency assumptions.

5. Cohorts ascertained long after the operation of one or more exposures are *survivor cohorts* and may generate results not applicable to cohorts formed soon after the same exposure(s) became operative.[576] Thus, the lack of association or even a positive association between high blood pressure and survival among the very old may be due to early elimination of individuals susceptible to the harmful consequences of hypertension. This is an example of *effect modification* by age.

Choice of Study Cohorts

Groups of persons may be selected for cohort studies for either of two reasons: (1) they have undergone some unusual exposure or experience of which the effects are to be evaluated; or (2) they offer some special resource that may facilitate ascertainment of their exposure, follow-up, or disease experience.

Special Exposure Groups

Studies of persons with unusually high levels of exposure to a particular substance (or a mixture of chemicals, a special process, or a range of physical factors) are frequently the first step in exploring the possible relationship of the substance to disease. Even if the substance is one to which entire populations are exposed, such as a pesticide, groups with unusually heavy exposures, such as might be received in the manufacture or use of the chemical, would logically be studied first to gain information on the nature and possible ranges of risks that might have to be explored in a broader population study. Thus, nearly all the information available on the risks of ionizing radiation in man comes from studies of groups heavily exposed in the course of war,[249] medical therapy,[77,83,226] occupation,[487,591] or nuclear accidents.[2]

Occupational groups have provided a prime source of cohorts of persons with unusually heavy exposures to chemical, physical, and other disease-producing agents. A classic example is the study of Case et al. on urinary bladder cancer among workers in the dyestuffs industry.[54] As with Case's study, special-exposure cohorts can frequently be assembled retrospectively. For example, Court-Brown and Doll studied the occurrence of leukemia in patients given X-ray therapy for ankylosing spondylitis.[77] The cohort consisted of 13,352 patients treated between 1934 and 1954, and the outcome evaluated was death from leukemia or aplastic anemia between 1935 and 1954. Both the exposures and the deaths had occurred at the time that the study was undertaken in 1955. A prospective component was added to this study by continuing to follow the cohort, as established in 1955, to identify deaths occurring in subsequent years.[83]

The significance of a particular exposure may not be realized or facilities for studying its consequences may not become available until many years after persons were first exposed. Indeed, this is one of the reasons that so many of these studies have been done retrospectively. This may lead to difficulties in identifying the members of a study cohort. Although Court-Brown and Doll were able to enroll persons in the cohort as soon as they became eligible (by receiving radiotherapy), this is not always possible. For example, Wada et al. studied deaths, particularly deaths from respiratory cancer, among former employees of a mustard gas factory that was in operation from 1929 to 1945.[571] The study was begun in 1965, and from a variety of sources it was possible to assemble a list of 2,620 of the 5,000 total number of employees who had worked in the factory during its operation. However, causes of death could not be ascertained prior to 1952, and it was necessary to restrict the observation period to the years 1952 to 1967. Therefore, the study is one of a cohort defined between 7 and 23 years after the exposure and including only a proportion of the exposed persons.

The effect of such losses prior to the formation of the study cohort must be distinguished from the effect of losses after the cohort is defined. Losses before definition of the cohort may limit the generalizations that can be made from the results of the study. For example, negative findings in the study cohort would not exclude the possibility that excess illness occurred prior to the definition of the cohort. However, such losses do not affect the validity of the findings in the cohort itself. In contrast, losses occurring after formation of the cohort *may* affect the validity of the findings, as is discussed later.

Whereas many studies of special exposure groups are conducted retrospectively, studies of survivors of the atomic bombings of Hiroshima and Nagasaki,[249] uranium miners,[572,591] and persons exposed to dioxin following the Seveso chemical accident[27,28] are examples of cohort studies of special-exposure groups that have essentially been prospective throughout. The cohorts were identified shortly after the exposure, or, in the case of the uranium miners, during the exposure, and have been followed continuously.

In some instances, when prospective observations are required and the time during which effects might be expected is very long, the period of required observation can be reduced by admitting to the study persons who are at different stages in the desired observation period. For example, Hutchison wished to observe with semiannual blood counts women who had been given radiation therapy for carcinoma of the uterine cervix.[226] Observation of the outcome of interest—leukemia—was desired over a period of 0–20 or more years after the radiation therapy. The approach was to admit to the study women who at any time in the past had the radiotherapy and who were currently being followed by the clinics involved in the study. In the course of the 5-year study, observations were made on some women from 0 to 4 years after therapy, others from 1 to 5 years after therapy, and so forth, including some who were more than 15 years post-therapy. Thus, observations relevant to an extended period of possible risk were made during a relatively short study period. This approach generates what has been termed an *oblique cohort*.[358] Characteristics of this procedure are that it reduces the length of calendar follow-up time required to capture the latency and the residual effects of the exposure under study, but increases the number of persons that must be enrolled in the cohort.

Most cohort studies that are based on special exposure groups are undertaken in order to exploit the methodological advantages generated by the high levels of exposure. The interrelated advantages of the *extreme points* design[358] are sharper risk contrast, higher precision of rate ratio (or risk ratio or odds ratio) estimates per unit change of the principal exposure variable, and increased overall statistical efficiency. Yet, there are also special exposure groups that are created on the basis of a qualitative characteristic rather than on account of the high level of a particular exposure of quantitative nature. Thus, the risk of transmission of the human immunodeficiency virus (HIV) in general and by type of homosexual practice has been studied prospectively in cohorts of homo-sexual and bisexual men in the United States,[257,601] as has been the transmission of HIV to infants by seropositive women in Zaire.[471] Moreover, the existence of high quality databases and the ability to link them through a unique personal registration number has allowed Swedish investigators to study the long-term conse-quences of several fairly rare conditions or therapeutic interven-tions. For example, Adami et al. studied the effect of alcoholism with or without liver cirrhosis on the subsequent occurrence of primary liver cancer,[5] and Ekbom et al. documented the reduction of risk for extrahepatic bile duct cancer after cholecystectomy.[115] The latter two studies were made possible because special re-sources were available, but they are included in this section be-cause they focus on a special exposure and they require the use of population ("external") rates for their analysis.

Groups Offering Special Resources

Certain groups offer advantages for cohort studies because of special facilities for follow-up or for ways of identifying disease occurrence among their members. Because such groups would only fortuitously also have special exposures of epidemiologic concern, they are most usefully studied when either the exposure of interest is a common one or the group is very large. The available resources may be such as to allow the undertaking of nation-wide retrospective cohort studies by linking health-related data-bases[5,115] or, simply, conveniently located or otherwise accessible general population groups. In contrast to cohort studies on spe-cial exposure groups that are usually driven by a specific hypothe-sis concerning the "defining" exposure, cohorts drawn from groups with special resources often allow the evaluation of several hypotheses. Several examples are given in the following sections.

Groups with Readily Available Health Records

Certain union-sponsored medical care programs and programs such as the Health Insurance Plan of Greater New York, the Kaiser-Permanente Plan, and those of many other Health Mainte-nance Organizations have provided populations large enough for many cohort studies. The prepayment component of these plans not only makes it likely that most members will seek most of their medical care within the program and that their records will therefore be available, but it also provides, through continued membership, a mechanism for periodic follow up.

Workers in industrial plants also provide populations that are readily accessible and easily followed. However, the number of persons in any one plant is unlikely to be large enough for the study of particular diseases, unless specific risks associated with special exposures are present in the plant.

The many studies of life insurance statistics are essentially cohort studies. Persons taking out insurance policies between certain dates constitute the entering cohort, with the subsequent mortality being measured by death claims. An early study utilizing such a population group is that of Dorn and colleagues on the effect of smoking on mortality among holders of US government life insurance.[102,239] The cohort consisted of all such policyholders known to be alive in July, 1954. Thus, entrance into the cohort was determined not by the time the insurance was taken out, but by virtue of its members being alive at a specified time, with the insurance being taken out at some time in the past. As was pointed out in the discussion of special-exposure cohorts, this delayed entry to the study cohort should not affect the validity of the results as they pertain to the relationship between smoking habits of cohort members in 1954 and subsequent mortality. This is so even though it may well be, for example, that smokers, having higher death rates than nonsmokers, were less completely represented in the cohort established in 1954 than they were among the total population that took out this form of life insurance. Thus, the cohort studied by Dorn and his colleagues is a survivor cohort; however, this is hardly unique or unusual. All groups assembled at some point in time after the cohort-defining event (for closed cohorts) or the establishment of a state (for open cohorts) are survivor cohorts. If there is evidence or a reasonable assumption of effect modification with time since exposure, some constraints are imposed on the generalizability of the findings. This is a minor limitation of cohort studies that it is not shared by case-control investigations when the latter cover all incident cases of disease in a defined population.

Certain Professional Categories

Members of the health professions are believed to be more likely than persons in nonmedical-related professions to collaborate in epidemiological investigations, and it is easier to follow up civil servants than members of other large occupational groups. Several investigators have made ingenious use of these opportunities. To study the relationship between cigarette smoking and lung cancer, Doll and Hill studied physicians listed in the *British Medical Register* in 1951.[97–99,101] Because of the legal obligation to maintain registration, the members of this group were relatively easy to identify and trace. Furthermore, they might be expected to receive better than average medical care (and hence diagnosis). Beasley et al. studied Taiwanese male government employees in a cohort study of the relation between chronic infection with hepatitis B virus and mortality from hepatocellular carcinoma.[18] Health care of civil servants in Taiwan is a governmental responsibility and causes of death are accurately recorded.

Several major studies have been, and continue to be, reported from two large cohort studies jointly undertaken by the Channing Laboratory, Harvard Medical School, the Departments of Epidemiology and Nutrition, Harvard School of Public Health, and other collaborating units. The Nurses' Health Study Cohort was initiated in 1976 by enrolling 121,700 female registered nurses 30–55 years old, living in 11 states. The nurses completed a mailed questionnaire that included items about known or suspected risk factors for cancer and cardiovascular diseases. Every 2 years, follow-up questionnaires are sent to cohort members to update exposure information and identify incident cases. In 1980, the questionnaire was expanded to include an assessment of diet.[511,596,597] The Health Professionals Follow-Up Study is based on 51,529 male health professionals who were 40–75 years old in 1986; it has a protocol intentionally similar to that of the Nurses' Health Study.[147,441]

Obstetric Populations

Investigations of the possible roles of prenatal experiences in the production of defect or disease noted at birth are ideally suited to the cohort type of study.[132] In the first place, the period of follow up is short. Second, the delivery and recording of outcome are frequently the responsibility of the same agency (physician or hospital) as that which undertook the measurement of exposure during pregnancy. The two circumstances, indeed, are often recorded in the same medical record.

Volunteer Groups

Hammond and Horn assembled a cohort of 189,854 white men between the ages of 50 and 69 by asking 22,000 American Cancer Society female volunteers to enroll about 10 such men "whom she knew well and would be able to trace."[196] The enrolled men completed a questionnaire, and follow up was through the volunteers as well as more conventional methods. A similar study, undertaken later by the American Cancer Society, enrolled more than one million men and women in 25 states and also covered cardiovascular diseases.[194,195] An attractive feature of volunteer groups such as these is the relative ease of obtaining detailed information; willingness to supply information usually goes along with the person's agreement to enter the study. The possibility of bias resulting from the method of selection of such groups must, however, be considered. For example, it is possible that the American Cancer Society volunteers, having suspicion that smoking was injurious to health, might have tended to select men who not only were agreeable to entering the study, but who also were heavy smokers *and* in lower than average states of health. Although individuals who had gross illness were excluded from the cohort, this might not eliminate the difficulty entirely. Such a bias, if present, should be manifested in the results of early follow-up.

Geographically Identified Cohorts

When a cohort study is to be done of a general population, the cohort may be defined in part on the basis of administrative or geographic boundaries, such as those of a town or county, although it is usually further restricted according to age or other demographic characteristics. Stability of the population, the quality of its medical care, and accessibility to the investigators are important considerations.

In the late 1940s, the US Public Health Service decided to follow a cohort of persons during a period of 20 years to study the occurrence of cardiovascular disease among them. In line with the view prevailing at the time that the study base should be all encompassing and, if possible, representative of the population at large, it was decided to conduct the study in a general population rather than in any special group. The population of Framingham, Massachusetts was selected for the study. Framingham at that time was a fairly stable community of 28,000 persons in eastern Massachusetts. As with other Massachusetts towns, population lists that would facilitate sampling and follow up were kept and updated annually. There was a single general hospital, of high quality, that would simplify surveillance of hospital admissions. To reduce the size of the study group to the desired 5,000, a random two-thirds sample of the population 30–59 years of age was drawn.[85,222,519]

Cohort studies similar in philosophy to that of Framingham have been undertaken in Tecumseh, Michigan,[133] Göthenburg, Sweden,[585] and elsewhere,[155] but they are now being substituted by larger multicentric collaborative studies that utilize population groups of variable origin and characteristics and attempt to collect biological samples as well as questionnaire-elicited information. Such studies currently under way in Europe are the cohort study on diet and cancer in the Netherlands[561,562] and the European Prospective Investigation into Cancer and Nutrition (EPIC). The EPIC study is being carried out in seven countries of the European Union. It will collect data on diet and other lifestyle factors, as well as biological samples from a cohort of more than 300,000 healthy European adults.[438]

Record Linkage

Mention has already been made of the utilization of valuable health databases that exist in Scandinavian and other countries to undertake, through record linkage, retrospective cohort studies.[5,115] College alumni records have also provided the basis for long-term retrospective cohort studies relating experiences and characteristics manifest during the college years to mortality from diseases occurring several decades later.[278,393] The growing number of computerized databases is likely to lead to an exponential increase of cohort studies of various types, covering both rare and common exposures.

Obtaining Data on Exposure

In a study of a cohort that has been defined without prior knowledge of exposure, information must be collected that will allow classification of the cohort members according to the level of exposure to the factor or factors under investigation. When the cohort has been selected because of special exposure, all its members may be considered to have been exposed. Nevertheless, it is usually desirable to classify individuals according to their level or duration of exposure. At the same time that data on exposure are being obtained, information must be sought on differences between exposure categories with respect to demographic variables that might affect the frequency of the disease(s) under investigation. In addition, if the disease under investigation is a common one, it will be necessary to exclude persons who have had it in the past or who already manifest it at the time they are considered for inclusion in the study. This will also require collection of information on eligible persons at the time of enrollment into the study.

Sources of Information

The kinds of information indicated here may be classified into four general categories according to the procedures needed to obtain it: (1) information available from records, (2) information that can be supplied by the individual members of the cohort, (3) information that can be obtained only by medical examination or other special testing of the cohort members, and (4) information that requires testing or evaluation of the working or living environment (present and/or past) of the study subjects. Information from more than one category, or indeed from all four, may be required for a particular study. A comprehensive review of the sources of information used in epidemiological studies has been presented by Armstrong, White, and Saracci.[14]

Information from Records

In some studies, such as of groups exposed to radiotherapy or other medical procedures, or of insured or working populations, the records that are used to determine eligibility for the cohort may include sufficient data to derive crude estimates of level of exposure, as well as demographic and other pertinent information. The studies of ankylosing spondylitis patients,[77] aniline dye workers,[54] and persons exposed to mustard gas[571] relied exclusively on recorded sources of exposure data.

In some situations, records are the *only* reliable source of information. For example, Court-Brown and Doll were able to classify their cohort by dose of radiation received;[77] such information would not have been available from either the patient or any other source but the medical record. Similarly, Feinleib assembled retrospectively from medical records cohorts of women who had undergone various kinds of pelvic surgery, distinguishing groups that had no, one, or both ovaries removed.[122] Although the fact that they had undergone pelvic surgery would be known to most women who have had such procedures, the specific nature of the operation is often not known.

Recorded information has three advantages. First, it can usually be obtained for a high proportion of the cohort. Second, it allows objective classification prior to any knowledge of the outcome that is the focus of the investigation, and thus it provides a built-in protection against information bias in retrospective cohort investigations. Third, the proximity in time between the recording and the information recorded minimizes nondifferential misclassification that tends to reduce statistical power and bias the results, usually toward no association. For these reasons it is usually desirable to assemble whatever information is recorded on cohort members, even if additional sources are also required to obtain data on the exposure that is the primary focus of the study.

Information from Cohort Members

For several exposure characteristics, only cohort members or their next of kin can provide reliable information. Such characteristics, among others, are tobacco smoking and alcohol drinking habits, dietary intakes, residential history, physical exercise, familial pattern of disease occurrence, and personal medical history. In most large cohort studies, in which in-person interviews would be impractical or prohibitively expensive, this information may be obtained through telephone interviews or mailed questionnaires. There are two related concerns: low frequencies of response and poor information quality.

Low response can adversely affect the economics of a study, its statistical power, or both. The cohort design usually protects against selection bias in the estimation of rate ratio (or risk ratio or odds ratio), but measures of disease occurrence themselves (incidence rates) and their differences may occasionally be affected, particularly early in the follow-up period. The factors that affect response frequencies in epidemiological studies are not adequately understood. There appear to be only small differences in response rates according to the length of mail questionnaires (within reasonable limits), the extent to which the accompanying letter is personalized, or other factors pertaining to the questionnaire itself. There are, however, appreciable differences in response rates according to age of the persons to whom the questionnaires are sent and between geographic areas. Perhaps the most important consideration for the investigator who wishes to obtain high response rates is the selection, where feasible, of a study population whose members are likely to have some personal or professional interest in the study.

A serious consequence of poor information quality on exposure is the generation of extensive nondifferential misclassification that tends to bias the respective measure of association toward the null value (1.0 for rate ratio, risk ratio, or odds ratio, and zero for rate or risk differences). Moreover, in unusual situations, such as when the measurement is extremely poor, there are several (rather than only two) levels of exposure, or when the individual exposure is based on an ecologic index reflecting, for example, the proportion of days that a particular concentration is exceeded in the environment, nondifferential misclassification may bias the effect estimates away from the null value.[39,105,199] Equally important and perhaps less recognized is the fact that even modest nondifferential misclassification can severely compromise the investigator's ability to control confounding generated by the misclassified variable.[160,553] Only recently have there been attempts to validate exposure variables, mostly those referring to reported nutritional intakes,[440,595] as well as efforts to correct effect estimates (e.g., rate ratio) and their confidence intervals for nondifferential misclassification error.[459,460]

Information from Medical Examination and Biomarkers

For some exposure characteristics, information can be obtained only by medical examination of the cohort members. Microbiological and serological data have been, and continue to be, extensively used in infectious disease epidemiology, and clinical and biochemical variables (e.g., blood pressure, serum lipoproteins) play a central role in cardiovascular disease epidemiology. With advances in laboratory sophistication and increasing emphasis on the role of viruses in human cancer, traditional sero-epidemiology[401] has grown in importance and has been utilized in several cohort studies that have linked, among others, hepatitis B virus to hepatocellular carcinoma,[18] Epstein-Barr virus to Burkitt's lymphoma,[91] and human T-cell leukemia/lymphoma virus Type I to a rare form of leukemia.[370] Moreover, detection of DNA from human papilloma virus in situ through hybridization techniques has strengthened the evidence linking some types of this virus to cancer of the cervix.[50] The utilization of sophisticated techniques involving nucleic acid macromolecules in epidemiological studies has been heralded as a milestone in the evolution of epidemiology, and the term *molecular epidemiology* was introduced.[343,406] Molecular biomarkers of viral exposures, assessed through traditional serologic procedures, hybridization techniques, polymerase chain reaction, or other methods have led to remarkably successful epidemiological studies in the recent past, and they are likely to be equally useful in the future. Critical factors in the successful utilization of viral biomarkers have been their outstanding specificity and their long-term persistence. Similarly, some organochlorine compounds can persist in the human adipose tissue for long periods and be detected with high specificity through analytic chemistry procedures.[272] By contrast, most molecular biomarkers of chemical exposures, such as DNA adducts,[406] have several shortcomings: (1) they usually reflect recent exposures and, therefore, require repeated samplings over prolonged periods for utilization in cohort investigations; (2) they are rarely highly specific and thus can generate exposure misclassification as well as confounding that would have been avoided with traditional environmental measurements and simple questionnaires; (3) when complex chemical exposures are investigated (e.g., air pollution or environmental tobacco smoke), it is possible that the biomarker would refer to one particular component of the mixture, whereas the biological effect would be due to another;[537] (4) in many situations it is not clear whether a biomarker reflects a relevant exposure, a correlate of the relevant exposure, individual susceptibility, or an early disease stage, thus hindering causal inference; (5) the determination of most biomarkers requires an expensive test or an invasive procedure, or both, thus creating constraints if adequate study size and statistical power are to be achieved; and (6) a biomarker of exposure is no more than a proxy to the real objective of an epidemiological investigation that, as a rule, focuses on an avoidable environmental exposure with disease-producing potential. There is no doubt that the introduction of molecular techniques in epidemiology represents major progress, much as biochemical procedures and metabolic studies have contributed to the expansion of epidemiology in novel areas during the last two decades. The concerns outlined here do not challenge the importance of biomarkers or of molecular procedures for the assessment of various exposures in epidemiologic studies; rather, they point out the methodological complexity of the issues surrounding their introduction into mainstream epidemiology and warn against excessive optimism.

Molecular epidemiology may also lead to the identification of biomarkers of disease susceptibility following a specific exposure; indeed, there are already examples of such undertakings.[267] Whether identification of individualized disease susceptibility patterns will justify epidemiological research or serve the interests of the society broadly remains to be demonstrated.

Information from Measures of the Environment

In some situations, adequate information on exposure levels cannot be obtained from any of the aforementioned sources alone. For example, it may be necessary to measure exposure levels in the environment of various areas in a plant in which individual members of a cohort work. Insofar as present or future exposures are concerned, this may pose no great problem, but if a substantial part of the exposure being assessed has occurred prior to initiation of the study, changes in the conditions of the working environment may make retrospective evaluation quite difficult.

For example, in a study of mortality among US uranium miners, workers were considered eligible for inclusion in the cohort from the time they were first examined by a Public Health Service team.[572,591] These examinations took place between 1950 and 1960, but many of the men had worked in the industry for many years previously and had accumulated a considerable radiation exposure prior to entering the study cohort. Because most of the men had worked in several mines for varying lengths of time and because radiation levels vary quite markedly between mines, an estimate of cumulative exposure could be derived only from a combination of employment records maintained by the mines, detailed employment histories taken from the men, and estimates of radiation levels in individual mines.

In such a situation, there is also a need to summarize the accumulated exposure for each man. In the study just referred to, each mine was characterized as to its average working level—a measure translatable (or at least allowing a ranking) in terms of physical exposure to radon daughter products. The cumulative exposure was measured in working level months (WLM); for example, work for 12 months in a mine with an average exposure of 1 working level contributed 12 WLM. Men were then categorized according to the total WLM accumulated during their mining experience. Measures such as this have obvious drawbacks, both in concept—they imply, for example, that effects are independent of dose rate (i.e., that 12 months of exposure to 1 working level has the same effect as 1 month of exposure to 12 working levels)— and in inaccuracies in the primary measurements that enter into them. Nevertheless, they do provide a basis for formation of broad categories of accumulated exposure and are an essential first step if the data are to be examined for a relationship between level of exposure and extent of risk.

Effect of Nonresponse

When data on exposure must be obtained from the individual members of a study cohort, it is likely that information will not be obtained for some proportion. The Tecumseh study is remarkable in that 88 percent of the selected cohort underwent the initial examination.[133] However, nonresponse proportions of about 30 percent are not unusual. For example, in Framingham, 4,469 (69 percent) of the 6,507 persons in the initial sample actually underwent the first examination.[85] High response proportions have been achieved in cohort studies of nurses[511,596,597] and health professionals.[147,441] In all instances, it is necessary to evaluate the effect of nonresponse on the outcome of the study.

In theory, the true relationship between the exposure and outcome variables will be distorted only if the losses are selective (nonrandom) with respect to both exposure and outcome; for example, when persons with high cholesterol levels and high risk of coronary heart disease for reasons other than their cholesterol levels are more or less likely to be excluded from the study. If the losses are selective only with respect to exposure (e.g., persons with high cholesterol levels fail to cooperate), an incorrect impression of the distribution of cholesterol levels in the population will be obtained; however, the experience of the study cohort will accurately reflect the strength of the relationship between rates of coronary disease and cholesterol levels in the study base. If the losses are selective only with respect to outcome (e.g., persons in poor health fail to respond, as indeed seems to occur in many studies[99]), then disease rates in the study cohort will be lower than in the underlying population; however, the ratio of the rates of persons with high cholesterol levels to those of persons with low levels will be the same as in the study base, although the measures of difference between these rates will be biased. If the loss is unbiased with respect to both exposure and outcome, then, of course, it can be safely ignored.

In practice it is often difficult to know whether the loss is selective with respect to exposure, outcome, or both. To settle this question conclusively, one would have to have the same data for the lost persons as for the study cohort, and in that case the lost persons would not, of course, have been classified as lost. A number of procedures may be followed to allow an indirect assessment. Although each procedure can provide only a partial answer, the results may in sum be convincing. The procedures include:

1. More intensive efforts to obtain exposure data for a small sample of the nonrespondents to determine whether the nonrespondents are different from the respondents in regard to exposure. By means of a second questionnaire sent 10 years after the original inquiry to a sample of some physicians who had previously answered and some who had not, Doll and Hill showed a substantially higher proportion of moderate and heavy smokers among the earlier nonrespondents—a feature that probably contributed to the lower than expected mortality among the respondents.[99]

2. Comparison of nonrespondents with respondents with respect to any ancillary information (e.g., age, gender, ethnic group) that can be obtained from records or resources other than the main source of exposure information.

3. Follow-up of nonrespondents as well as respondents is done so that certain outcomes can be compared in the two groups. For example, if the outcome under investigation is coronary artery disease, it may not be possible to obtain for the nonrespondents the specific clinical information to be obtained for the cohort members, but it may be possible to monitor deaths in both groups.

4. Examination of disease rates in the cohort in different time periods. If the contrast in disease rates between two exposure categories in the study cohort is due in part to selective processes, it will tend to become smaller as the study progresses because the effects of such biases will be strongest in the early years of the study. For example, the mortality of British physicians in the study cohort referred to was estimated to be 63 percent of that of all British physicians during the second year of the study, 85 percent during the third year, and about 93 percent between the fourth and tenth years.[99] However, this procedure should be applied and evaluated with care. With the passage of time, cohort members grow older and the incidence of most diseases, as well as overall mortality, increases rapidly. In this instance, the rate ratio may gradually decline over time, even if the rate difference remains stable or even tends to increase.

Reassignment to Exposure Categories

In studies of closed cohorts, it is not possible, as a rule, to reassign members with respect to the cohort-defining event, but other exposures, that may have confounding influences, may change during the follow-up period. Most important among these confounders is age. Assignment of several cohort members to more than one age category necessitates a similar allocation of their person-time experience and an analytical approach usually reserved for open cohort studies.

In long-term open cohort studies, such as the Framingham Study, the Nurses' Health Study, and the Health Professionals Follow-up Study, periodic interviews or mail questionnaires allow reassignment of cohort members to different exposure categories according to information changes. When the postulated latency for disease occurrence in relation to a particular exposure is long and variable, it may be preferable to utilize the initially determined exposure categories throughout the study.[597]

Changes in a dichotomous exposure that occur but that are not taken into consideration will tend to make the strength of an observed association lower than that which actually existed between exposure and development of the disease. In other words, the true association will be greater than that found. The risk of introducing this kind of error seems more acceptable than that of producing false associations through data-guided latency speculations. Yet, when the duration of follow-up is exceptionally long, this generalization may not be applicable. This is particularly true when the postulated latency is likely to be short, such as in the study of current compared to past smoking in relation to asthma.[547] In this instance, it is preferable to allocate person-time and disease occurrence events between any two consecutive evaluations of cohort members to the most recent among the earlier exposure allocations. Moreover, when there is considerable interest in defining as accurately as possible the amount of exposure associated with a certain level of disease risk, and the exposure accumulates over time during the course of the study (e.g., in the studies of US uranium miners[591] and crocidolite asbestos miners in Australia[213]), then it will be more appropriate to reassess exposure levels periodically during the study.

Separate examination of outcome in those individuals who changed exposure groups during the course of a study is highly desirable. Such examination may assist both in detecting possible biases involved in the reassessment and in allowing an evaluation of real changes in risk associated with change of exposure category (e.g., from smoker to nonsmoker).

Selection of Comparison Groups

Internal Comparisons

In many cohort studies the comparison groups are built in; a single cohort is entered into the study and its members are then classified into exposure categories. For example, the cohorts of Framingham, the Nurses Health Study, and the Health Professionals Follow-up Study were defined without any knowledge of the status of individuals with respect to causal variables. On the basis of information obtained at entry to the study, however, the individuals can be categorized according to smoking habits, dietary habits, and so forth. No outside comparison group is required. In these studies, exposed and unexposed individuals originate by definition from the same study base. Accordingly, other conditions being equal, these studies have stronger claims to validity than cohort studies that depend on external population rates for the derivation of expected numbers of cases in the exposed cohort (see next section).

Comparison with Population Rates

In other studies, particularly when a special-exposure cohort has been assembled, some basis for comparison is required to evaluate whether the outcome observed in the cohort differs from that which would be expected if the members had not been at any special risk. A common comparison is with the experience of the general population at the time the cohort is being followed.

Because most special-exposure cohorts are too small for the derivation of reliable rates specific for age, gender, and cause, the procedure is usually to compare the observed number of cases in the total cohort with the expected number. The expected number is estimated by applying the general population rates, specific for gender, age, calendar time, and cause, to the total person-years in the corresponding age and gender groups in the cohort and summing the expected number of cases over all gender and age groups. It is necessary to take into account the fact that the members of the cohort age as the study progresses, and it may also be necessary to take account of changes over time in the general population rates.

In addition to considering specific items, such as age and gender, the population from which the expected rates are taken should be generally similar to that from which the exposed cohort derived. For example, in the study of US uranium miners, rates for white males in the four states in which most of the mining population was located, rather than in the United States as a whole, were used.[591] In addition, there may be selective factors within the same geographically defined population; for example, a particular ethnic group may predominate in a special-exposure group because the occupation from which the exposure group derived had a predominance of that ethnic group, as was the case with Native Americans in the study of uranium miners.[572,591]

Naturally, comparisons with population rates are possible only for outcomes for which population rates are available. This has limited the method essentially to the study of conditions for which death rates can be used to evaluate risk, and to some studies of cancer incidence, hospitalization for mental illness, and other situations where special data are available.

Comparison Cohorts

Another method of obtaining a basis for comparison is the selection and following of another special cohort, similar in demographic characteristics to the exposed group, but not exposed.

For example, in studies of industrial exposures, persons in other occupations in the same industry may be suitable. To evaluate mortality rates in a cohort of radiologists, Seltser and Sartwell compared them with rates in similarly defined cohorts of internists, ophthalmologists, and otolaryngologists.[487] In some studies of the frequency of neoplasms in children irradiated for thymic enlargement, siblings of the irradiated infants have been used as comparison groups.[413,496]

In theory, an ideal comparison group for the study of patients irradiated for ankylosing spondylitis or thymic enlargement would be patients with the same diseases at similar stages and with similar clinical profiles who were not irradiated, because such comparison would also rule out the possibility that ankylosing spondylitis or thymic enlargement themselves were responsible for any unusual outcome noted. Such groups are rarely available, however, in nonexperimental situations. Indeed, the administration or not of a particular therapy on the basis of specific clinical indications or contra-indications may introduce powerful confounding of the effects of treatment by its own indication or contra-indication. This type of confounding has been termed *confounding by indication*,[177,356] and it is, as a rule, intractable in the analysis. This is the main reason why observational epidemiological studies of cohort or case-control nature are rarely used in "clinical epidemiology" that focus on causal links between disease manifestation or therapeutic interventions on the one hand and disease outcome or prognosis on the other hand. Clinical trials, of course, bypass the problem of confounding by indication through the mechanism of randomization.

Studies of cohorts identified at birth offer favorable opportunities for selection of comparison cohorts because of the ready identification of the related population. Thus, cohorts of birth-injured children might be compared with cohorts of infants selected at random or on a paired basis from the same population of births.

Multiple Comparisons

It may be that, for a specific cohort of exposed persons, neither general population rates nor another special group provide entirely satisfactory conditions for comparison. In such situations, it may be possible to strengthen the evaluation by providing for a variety of comparisons. To illustrate some of the criticisms that can be raised regarding particular comparisons and how these can be countered to some extent by multiple comparisons, the results of the retrospective cohort study referred to previously of children irradiated for thymic enlargement are given in Table 9-1. In this study, a comparison cohort of siblings was used, and, in addition, expected numbers of cases of the diseases of interest, based on general population rates, were calculated for both the exposed and unexposed cohorts.[496] Comparison with general pop-

Table 9-1. Occurrence of Leukemia and Thyroid Cancer among Children Treated by X-ray in Infancy for Thymic Enlargement

Disease	Irradiation (1,722 children)		No irradiation (1,795 siblings)	
	Number observed	Number expected	Number observed	Number expected
Leukemia	7	0.6	0	0.6
Thyroid cancer	6	0.1	0	0.1
All cancer	17	2.6	5	2.7

Source: Adapted from Simpson CL, Hempelmann LH, Fuller LM. Neoplasia in children treated with X-rays in infancy for thymic enlargement. *Radiology* 1955;64 : 840–845.

ulation rates can be criticized on the basis of the variation in incidence of leukemia and thyroid cancer according to geography, ethnic group, economic status, and other variables that were not accounted for in the calculation of the expected number of cases. Yet, comparison with siblings necessitates exclusion of exposed children who have no siblings. Moreover, siblings share many characteristics that are difficult to measure and may be related to the outcome under study; these include genes, diet, and aspects of herd immunity. The fact that the observed cases of cancer other than leukemia and thyroid cancer exceeded the expected number in both the irradiated group and their siblings might be interpreted as evidence of more thorough case finding in the two cohorts than among the general population that furnished the rates for calculation of the expected numbers. However, the extent of this possible bias is by no means large enough to explain the relative excess of leukemia and thyroid cancer in the irradiated group. That the excess for leukemia and thyroid cancer is so much greater than that for the other cancers, whether the basis of comparison is the siblings or the general population, supports the view that the risks of thyroid cancer and leukemia are indeed increased in the irradiated children.

Even in studies where internal categorizations or other special cohorts provide the primary basis for comparison, it is desirable also to compute expected frequencies in the study cohort or cohorts for those outcomes for which population data can be obtained.

Follow-Up

Having defined the study cohorts and obtained data on exposure and other relevant characteristics, there remains the task of determining the outcome among the groups to be compared. Generally, the outcome to be ascertained will be the appearance of either a case of, or death from, a certain disease or group of diseases. The procedures required will of course vary with the outcome to be determined, ranging from routine surveillance of death certificates or disease registries to periodic examination of each member of the cohort.

Many sources are available for following groups of persons. It is obvious that completeness of ascertainment of outcome should be equal in all exposure categories. This objective is most easily attained when the method of ascertainment or follow up depends on a mechanism completely separate from that by which exposure was categorized. Perhaps most satisfactory is reliance on some routine procedure that is applied equally to all persons, regardless of the fact that they are members of a special study group. For example, in the studies of Doll and Hill[99] and Dorn[239] on cigarette smoking, data on exposure were obtained from the individuals constituting the cohort, but knowledge of the outcome—death and death from particular causes—was obtained from routine records. In the former study, copies of all death certificates on which there was indication that the decedent was a physician were sent to the investigators; in the latter, claims for insurance benefits were the primary sources of information. In both studies, these primary sources were supplemented by inquiry of hospitals or physicians caring for the patient prior to death. In many Swedish cohort studies, outcomes (e.g., death or occurrence of cancer) can be traced readily with built-in validity through the existence of a unique personal identification number as well as nationwide databases.[5,115] In the Nurses Health Study and the Health Professionals Follow-Up Study, the use of the highly sensitive National Death Index (referred to in Chapter 8) allows cross-validation of reports from family members, and medical records document information on morbidity provided by cohort members themselves. Routine records of death required for the termination of a pension, those kept by industry, and those kept by treatment centers were the respective mechanisms of follow up for the studies of mustard gas pensioners,[571] dyestuffs workers,[54] and patients with ankylosing spondylitis[77] referred to earlier. Such methods are economical because they do not require location and interview of each individual cohort member.

To be efficient, the routine source of information utilized must be one that will reveal the great majority of the cases of disease or death that actually occur in the cohort. Some of these sources do not provide data on those members of the cohort who, because of emigration, change of occupation, or other reasons, are no longer under the surveillance of the record-keeping agency. Under these circumstances it may not be clear how many cohort members actually are at risk of the outcomes under investigation. This can compromise validity by allowing the operation of undetectable selection bias, as well as limit statistical efficiency through reduction of the number of outcome events.

Although satisfactory as a measure of the occurrence or nonoccurrence of such diseases as cancer of the lung and some other organs, death is often too crude an index of outcome. For example, in the Framingham and Tecumseh studies, indices of heart disease were sought that could be obtained only by periodic clinical examination of individual cohort members. This procedure yields a great deal more information on the individuals examined than would the use of any routine records; however, it has two disadvantages:

1. The proportion of individuals examined decreases with time, and the membership of the cohort on which data are obtained becomes increasingly selected. The possible influence of such selection can be evaluated by comparing cohort members for whom clinical examinations were obtained with those for whom they were not, with respect to their demographic characteristics and crude criteria of outcome not requiring patient contact, by use of such sources of data as records of subsequent hospitalization or death.

2. There is some danger of diagnosis of outcome being influenced by exposure class. This risk might be reduced by such means as not permitting the diagnostician access to past records or by not permitting him or her to delay diagnostic appraisal. Yet, it is difficult for a physician to remain ignorant of the antecedents of a patient or to make a diagnosis in the absence of historical information. "Blind" readings and the use of objective diagnostic tests should be used in such studies whenever possible.

Analysis

The analysis of cohort studies is considered comprehensively by Breslow and Day.[43] Clayton and Hills,[61] Prentice and Thomas,[425] and Greenland[170] discuss some of the outstanding analytical problems. Presentations of the issues surrounding the analysis of cohort studies that are more limited in scope, yet are conceptually sharp, can be found in the texts by Miettinen,[358] Rothman,[466] Walker,[576] Rothman and Boice,[469] and Kahn and Sempos.[240] The purpose of this section is to introduce the reader to some elementary techniques and to the rationale of more complex procedures. The complex procedures depend on statistical regression models, require the use of computer and appropriate software, and usually improve both validity and precision *assuming that the statistical models adequately represent reality.* However, the gain in validity (control of confounding) and precision (reduction of standard error) is usually minor in comparison to those achieved through simpler techniques. The latter are based on stratification by important disease predictors, which are likely to exercise strong confounding influences. Indeed, an investigator should be concerned about possible errors in the modeling process whenever results based on simple stratified analysis, or even crude data, differ sharply from those obtained through regression modeling.

The elementary statistical concepts and formulas used in this text are presented in many of the available books of biostatistics and related fields, for example that of Armitage and Berry.[11] Procedures developed for the purpose of epidemiologic analyses are specifically referenced.

Closed Cohort Studies

The analysis of closed cohort studies is discussed first because they are more simple, deriving essentially from the application of the binomial distribution. One must recall, however, that when studies that were initiated as closed cohort investigations (e.g., the follow-up of persons exposed to potential toxins released in an industrial accident) are continued over periods of years, they will lose some essential characteristics of closed cohorts. This is because even if exposure does not change, risk factors for the disease, such as age, may do so. Furthermore, loss to follow up may make analyses that could be applied to closed cohorts inappropriate. Such studies are more appropriately analyzed by the methods that are described for open cohorts.

Closed Cohorts Without Control for Confounding

An analysis focusing on the directly estimable cumulative incidence is frequently performed in a closed cohort study with a short period of follow up and minimal or no losses during that period. For illustrative purposes, a study is used in which 2,469 homosexual men who were seronegative for human immunodeficiency virus (HIV) at enrollment were followed for 6 months, mainly to ascertain the relative importance of receptive and insertive intercourse for sero-conversion to HIV.[257] Condensed results of this study are presented in Table 9-2.

Cumulative incidence is a proportion (denoted as P), and its standard error is estimated through the binomial distribution formula $\sqrt{\dfrac{P(1 - P)}{N}}$. In the total cohort, the cumulative incidence is 0.0385 and its standard error is:

$$\sqrt{\frac{0.0385(1 - 0.0385)}{2469}} = 0.0039.$$

The 95 percent confidence limits (lower and upper) are estimated by subtracting and adding, respectively, 1.96 times the standard error to the estimated cumulative incidence of 0.0385; these limits are 0.0309 and 0.0461 or, on a percent basis, 3.09 and 4.61.

Cumulative incidence difference between those with none and

Table 9-2. Seroconversion to HIV among 2,469 Homosexual Men
Seronegative for HIV at the Start of a 6-Month Follow Up, According
to Number of Partners with whom Receptive Intercourse or Insertive
Intercourse Was Performed during the Preceding 6-Month Period

Partners for insertive intercourse	Partners for receptive intercourse								
	None			One or more			Total		
	At risk	HIV+	%	At risk	HIV+	%	At risk	HIV+	%
0	471	4	0.85	228	7	3.07	699	11	1.57
1	234	2	0.85	513	20	3.90	747	22	2.95
2+	279	3	1.08	744	59	7.93	1,023	62	6.06
Total	984	9	0.91	1,485	86	5.79	2,469	95	3.85

Source: Adapted from Kingsley A, et al. Risk factors for seroconversion to human immunodeficiency virus among male homosexuals. Results from the Multicenter AIDS Cohort Study. *Lancet* 1987;i : 345–349.

those with one or more partners with whom they engaged in receptive intercourse during the designated 6-month period is, in percent, $5.79 - 0.91 = 4.88$, or, as a proportion, 0.0488. The standard error of this difference, again through the binomial distribution approximation, is the square root of the sum of squares of the component standard errors:

$$\sqrt{\frac{0.0579(1 - 0.0579)}{1485} + \frac{0.0091(1 - 0.0091)}{984}} = 0.0068$$

The 95 percent confidence limits (lower and upper) are estimated by subtracting from and adding to the estimated cumulative incidence difference 0.0488, the standard error of this difference 0.0068, multiplied by 1.96. These limits, 0.0355 and 0.0621, or 3.55 and 6.21 percent, do not straddle the null value of zero; therefore, the difference is statistically significant at the conventional 5 percent level (which corresponds to the normal deviate multiplier 1.96 utilized in this example).

The applicability of the binomial distribution approximation may be compromised when the smallest of the counts involved in the calculations is a single digit number (9 in the previous example) or the outcome under investigation reflects person-to-person transmission *among* the study subjects (as may have happened in this example). Nevertheless, even in this borderline situation the approximation is reasonably good.

As indicated, an analysis tailored to closed cohorts and focused on cumulative incidence is commonly applied when the follow-up period is short and the time element is not explicitly addressed because the follow-up period is assumed to be identical between exposed and unexposed persons. This situation usually arises when the frequency of disease occurrence is relatively high, which, in turn, makes the cumulative incidence ratio and odds ratio poor approximators to the basic measure of effect—the incidence rate ratio. For this reason, the cumulative incidence difference is usually preferred to the cumulative incidence ratio (risk ratio) and odds ratio in studies of, for example, acute outbreaks. When risk ratio or odds ratio are to be used (e.g., in studies of the estimated prevalence at birth of congenital malformations), the appropriate statistical test is based on the hypergeometric distribution and the usual χ^2 test with one degree of freedom. Whether the cumulative incidence ratio or the odds ratio is evaluated, the study persons are cross-classified in the same way in a fourfold table—by exposure status and by outcome status. A simple way of calculating the 95 percent confidence limits of the cumulative incidence ratio or the corresponding odds ratio is to exponentiate them to $\left(1 - \dfrac{1.96}{\chi}\right)$ and to $\left(1 + \dfrac{1.96}{\chi}\right)$ for the lower and higher confidence limits, respectively.[348,349,469] The approximation of the correct limits through this simple procedure is very good when the cumulative incidence ratio and the odds ratio do not deviate greatly from the null value of one. When numbers are relatively small it is preferable to calculate χ (the square root of χ^2 with one degree of freedom) by using the finite sample correction in the formula.[326]

In the example, the cumulative incidence ratio is 6.36, whereas the odds ratio is 6.66. The 95 percent confidence limits for the cumulative incidence ratio are 3.53 and 11.45, whereas for the odds ratio they are 3.64 and 12.17.

Closed Cohort Studies with Stratification for Confounding

A factor is confounding an association between an exposure and a disease when it is independently associated with both the exposure and the disease. The essential approach to eliminate confounding is to stratify the data in such a way that in any particular stratum there is virtually no variability with respect to the potential confounder. In the absence of variability within the confounder strata, there can be no confounding by the stratified factor *within these strata* because there can be no association between any two variables when either of them is kept constant. Indeed, efficient control of confounding by modeling is accomplished through generation of informative fine strata in which paucity of exposed or unexposed subjects is remedied by transfer of information from other strata through model-based intrapolation.

In the example of Table 9-2, the practice of receptive intercourse is positively associated with that of insertive intercourse, with the percentages of men who had not had receptive intercourse being 67, 31, and 27, among those with none, one, or two or more partners for insertive intercourse, respectively. Receptive acts, which appear to strongly affect HIV sero-conversion, are likely to confound the association of insertive acts with HIV sero-conversion, although the reverse or mutual confounding are also possible. To assess the effect of insertive practice, subjects were stratified according to the number of partners with whom they have had receptive intercourse: none and one or more. It is worth noting that in the "one or more" stratum there is residual variability because individuals have all engaged in receptive intercourse, but they may have done so with one, two, three, or more partners. This residual within-stratum variability may allow *residual confounding*; that is, confounding that remains after that attributable to the confounder as classified has been removed, particularly when the crudely stratified factor is a strong confounder (as in the current example). However, this important issue will not be explicitly addressed here, except by emphasizing that residual confounding is minimized when strata are narrow and the potential confounder is accurately measured.[160,553] Instead, we concentrate on the comparison between individuals who had two or more partners in their insertive practice and those who did not engage in such practice, ignoring those in the intermediate category.

When a closed cohort is divided into two or more strata, each containing exposed and unexposed individuals, there may be interest on how the overall cumulative incidence among exposed or among unexposed should be expressed, or on how the overall cumulative incidence difference, cumulative incidence ratio, or cumulative incidence odds ratio should be summarized. Proper expression of the overall cumulative incidence depends on whether there is evidence, or credible assumption, that cumulative incidence among exposed or among unexposed individuals is similar (homogeneity) or different (heterogeneity) across the strata, aside from chance variation. Similarly, correct summarization of measures of association depends on whether cumulative incidence difference, ratio, or odds ratio is similar (homogeneity) or different across the strata of the potential confounder, aside from chance variation. In the latter situation, there exists heterogeneity of the measure of association between the exposure under study and the outcome disease across the strata of the other variable or combination of variables, frequently referred to as *control variable(s)*. The phenomenon is also described as *interaction* between the exposure under study and the control variable(s) with respect to the disease outcome or as *effect modification*[347] by the stratified control variable(s) that may or may not have confounding influence. When there is homogeneity, the objective is to estimate the common cumulative incidence or the measure of or association with maximum precision. When there is heterogeneity, the objective is to standardize the cumulative incidence or the measure of association according to a standard distribution that attributes different importance (explicitly different *weight*) to the various strata of the control variable(s).[354,469] (See also, standardization, Chapter 4.)

Standardization of Effect Measures. The cumulative incidence of HIV sero-conversion among individuals who have had insertive intercourse with two or more partners appears to be different according to whether they had or did not have receptive intercourse during the designated exposure period (7.93 cf. 1.08 percent; Table 9-2). The two cumulative incidence proportions can be "standardized" to the proportional distribution of the exposed individuals themselves by the categories of control variable as follows:

$$\left(1.08 \cdot \frac{279}{1023}\right) + \left(7.93 \cdot \frac{744}{1023}\right) = 6.06 \text{ percent}$$

A standardization in this way leads, of course, to the crude figure itself (6.06 percent). Alternatively, the proportional distribution of all individuals by the categories of the control variable may be used as standard, as follows:

$$\left(1.08 \cdot \frac{984}{2469}\right) + \left(7.93 \cdot \frac{1485}{2469}\right) = 5.20 \text{ percent}$$

In fact, any distribution proportionally expressed with proportions adding to 1 can be used as standard, although the first of the indicated approaches is usually preferable. Confidence intervals can be set by subtracting and adding 1.96 times the corresponding standard error, calculated as explained below.

Because a standardized cumulative incidence is simply the *weighted average* of a series of proportions, its standard error can be estimated as the square root of the sum of squares of the standard errors of the contributing components weighted with the corresponding weights. Therefore, the standard error of 6.06 percent, when viewed as a crude cumulative incidence proportion, is:

$$\sqrt{\frac{0.0606 \cdot 0.9394}{1023}} = 0.0075$$

whereas, when viewed as the standard error of the standardized cumulative incidence using the proportional distribution of the exposed individuals themselves as the standard is the square root of:

$$\left(\frac{279}{1023} \cdot \sqrt{\frac{0.0108 \cdot 0.9892}{279}}\right)^2 + \left(\frac{744}{1023} \cdot \sqrt{\frac{0.0793 \cdot 0.9207}{744}}\right)^2$$

which is 0.0074—virtually identical to the previous result. However, in epidemiological studies, there is usually more interest in the difference or the ratio of standardized cumulative incidences, rather than on standardized cumulative incidences per se.

Using as the preferable standard the proportional distribution of the exposed individuals themselves (two or more partners in insertive intercourse) by the categories of the control variable (none, or one or more partners in receptive intercourse), the difference of the standardized cumulative incidence of sero-conversion is:

$$\left(1.08 \cdot \frac{279}{1023}\right) + \left(7.93 \cdot \frac{744}{1023}\right) = 6.06 \text{ percent}$$

minus

$$\left(0.85 \cdot \frac{279}{1023}\right) + \left(3.07 \cdot \frac{744}{1023}\right) = 2.46 \text{ percent}$$

or $6.06 - 2.46 = 3.60$ percent.

The standardized difference, 3.60 percent, is smaller than the crude difference, $6.06 - 1.57 = 4.49$ percent, which indicates that part of the crude difference in HIV sero-conversion between the compared categories of insertive practice is due to confounding by receptive practice. In contrast, the association with receptive intercourse remains largely unaffected when insertive practice is standardized.

The standard error of the cumulative incidence of HIV sero-conversion among those with two or more partners in their insertive practice has been estimated as 0.0074. The cumulative incidence of those with no insertive practice, adjusted for receptive practice according to the proportional distribution of this practice among individuals in the selected standard, is 2.46 percent, with standard error equal to the square root of the sum:

$$\left(\frac{279}{1023} \sqrt{\frac{0.0085 \cdot 0.9915}{471}}\right)^2 + \left(\frac{744}{1023} \sqrt{\frac{0.0307 \cdot 0.9693}{228}}\right)^2$$

which equals 0.0084.

The standard error of the difference between the standardized cumulative incidence in the two compared groups is therefore:

$$\sqrt{0.0074^2 + 0.0084^2} = 0.0112, \text{ or } 1.12 \text{ percent}$$

The difference of the standardized cumulative incidence in the two groups is 3.60 percent with 95 percent confidence interval $3.60 \pm 1.96 \,(1.12)$ or 1.40 to 5.80. Because this interval does not straddle the null value of zero, it might be concluded that insertive intercourse independently of receptive intercourse increases the risk of HIV sero-conversion. However, the demonstrable confounding influence of receptive intercourse in spite of the crudeness of classification with respect to this variable strongly suggests that the adjusted difference may still reflect to a substantial extent residual confounding.

Pooling. Calculation of the standardized cumulative incidence difference, as the difference between two cumulative incidence measures adjusted to the same standard, accommodates confounding by the control variable(s). Standardization does not presuppose homogeneity or lack of interaction of cumulative incidence difference (or ratio, or odds ratio) with the control variable(s). Instead, standardization weights the stratum-specific cumulative incidence difference (or ratio or odds ratio) according to the relative size of the corresponding stratum in the chosen standard. By contrast, *pooling* accommodates confounding but at the same time assumes that there is no heterogeneity of cumulative incidence (or ratio or odds ratio) across the strata of the control variable(s). In pooling the common (average) effect measure is estimated by weighing the stratum-specific estimates according to their precision (i.e., on the basis of the number and the balance of observations in every stratum). Moreover, in pooling the null hypothesis is that *in every stratum* the cumulative incidence difference is zero or, *equivalently*, the cumulative incidence ratio or odds ratio is one. In this situation, an appropriate statistical test is the Mantel-Haenszel χ^2 with one degree of freedom over several two by two tables, as many as the required strata.[326] This procedure represents a generalization of the simple χ^2 test in a single fourfold table and assesses the statistical significance of the deviation of the *pooled* overall odds ratio from the *null hypothesis*-based value of one, which applies to every stratum-specific fourfold table. Therefore, the Mantel-Haenszel procedure provides a valid test against the null hypothesis that the cumulative incidence difference is zero or the cumulative incidence ratio or odds ratio is one, although it can generate a pooled overall estimate only with respect to the odds ratio. The latter property makes the Mantel-Haenszel test particularly useful in case-control studies

(Chapter 10), but the Mantel-Haenszel χ (the square root of χ^2) can also be used to set approximate confidence limits around the pooled estimates of cumulative incidence difference and cumulative incidence ratio that must be derived in some other way.[348,349,469]

A fair approximation to the pooled estimate of cumulative incidence difference weights the stratum-specific estimates according to their precision (inverse of their variance) using the following as weights:

$$\frac{N_e \cdot N_o \cdot (N_e + N_o)}{(x_e + x_o) \cdot (N_e - x_e + N_o - x_o)}$$

In the example (Table 9-2), the cumulative incidence difference of sero-conversion between those who had two or more partners in their insertive practice and those who did not engage in such practice was $1.08 - 0.85 = 0.23$ percent among those who did not engage in receptive practice, and $7.93 - 3.07 = 4.86$ percent among those who had one or more partners in their receptive practice. The corresponding weights are

$$\frac{279 \cdot 471 \cdot 750}{7 \cdot 743} = 18950$$

for the 0.23 percent estimate and

$$\frac{744 \cdot 228 \cdot 972}{66 \cdot 906} = 2757$$

for the 4.86 percent estimate.

To simplify calculations, weights should be expressed proportionally and their sum should equal one. Therefore, the weight of 0.23 percent becomes

$$\frac{18950}{18950 + 2757} = 0.87$$

and the weight of 4.86 percent becomes

$$\frac{2757}{18950 + 2757} = 0.13$$

The pooled cumulative incidence difference is simply:

$$(0.87 \cdot 0.23) + (0.13 \cdot 4.86) = 0.83 \text{ percent}$$

The Mantel-Haenszel χ^2 is 6.22 and the Mantel-Haenszel χ is 2.49, corresponding to $P \sim 0.013$. Test-based 95 percent confidence limits[348,349,469] for differences are symmetrical around the point estimate 0.83 percent and are calculated by multiplying this estimate with $\left(1 - \dfrac{1.96}{2.49}\right)$ for the lower limit and with $\left(1 + \dfrac{1.96}{2.49}\right)$ for the upper limit. This process contrasts with the exponentiation that is required for ratios in order to generate log symmetrical limits. Therefore, the 95 percent confidence limits of the pooled estimate of the cumulative incidence difference are symmetrically set at 0.18 and 1.48 percent.

The simple procedure for the calculation of the pooled estimate of cumulative incidence difference is attributed to Miettinen[469] and can be inaccurate when numbers are very small in any particular stratum. The Mantel-Haenszel χ^2, on the contrary, does not require large numbers in any particular stratum, but the test-based limits are not accurate when the observed data are sharply incompatible with the null hypothesis.

It has already been pointed out that cumulative incidence ratio and odds ratio are not conceptually appealing measures of effect in studies of acute outbreaks and most other situations that can be legitimately analyzed as closed cohorts. However, if these ratio measures are to be used and stratification is necessary for control of confounding, the Mantel-Haenszel χ^2 with one degree of freedom over several two by two tables represents the test of choice. As indicated, this test assesses the statistical significance of the deviation of the observed overall odds ratio from the null hypothesis-based value of one, which is assumed to apply to every stratum.[326] The Mantel-Haenszel procedure generates a pooled estimate of odds ratio, around which test-based confidence limits can be set directly, using the Mantel-Haenszel χ. Test-based confidence limits using the Mantel-Haenszel χ also can be set around the pooled estimate of cumulative incidence ratio. This latter estimate, however, is not generated by the Mantel-Haenszel procedure, but can be approximated by weighing the natural logarithms of the stratum-specific estimates using the following as precision-maximizing weights:

$$\frac{N_e \cdot N_o \cdot (x_e + x_o)}{(N_e + N_o) \cdot (N_e - x_e + N_o - x_o)}$$

This weighing was suggested by Miettinen,[469] whereas log-transformation is regularly used for ratio measures to normalize their inherently skewed distributions.

When there is evidence that the cumulative incidence ratio or the odds ratio varies across strata substantially more than could be explained by chance, then pooling may not be appropriate and standardization should be the preferable summarizing procedure. Standardization of cumulative incidence ratio or odds ratio is no different and no more demanding than standardization in any other context; however, setting confidence limits around a standardized cumulative incidence ratio or odds ratio is a more complicated procedure.

Open Cohort Studies

Open Cohort Studies Without Control for Confounding

In open cohorts and in most closed cohorts with variable period of follow up for cohort members or losses during that period, the appropriate measure of disease frequency is the incidence rate and the appropriate measures of association are the incidence rate difference and the incidence rate ratio. In this section, we frequently use, for purposes of illustration, data from a small cohort study that examined the predictors of further survival of elderly Greeks in three small villages.[546] The study was chosen because raw data were available and because the incidence of death is relatively high among elderly persons, allowing for substantial statistical power even in a small series for which very simple calculations are required. The analyses shown are restricted to men, who have substantially higher mortality than women. Only two of the possible mortality risk factors are examined: (1) being or having been a smoker compared to never having been a smoker at the time of cohort recruitment, and (2) age at the time of cohort recruitment. Tobacco smoking is considered the main exposure variable, whereas age is considered a possible confounder. Time of enrollment was different in the three villages (between October 1988 and June 1990) and so was the end of the follow-up period (between April 1993 and January 1994). The outcome was death from any cause, and in this small study losses to follow-up were due only to censoring because of study termination. The data to be used are presented in Table 9-3.

The incidence rate is defined as the number of new cases divided by the person-time in the study population. The standard error of the incidence rate is:

$$\sqrt{\frac{\text{incidence rate}}{\text{person-time}}} = \sqrt{\frac{\text{new cases}}{(\text{person-time})^2}} = \frac{\sqrt{\text{new cases}}}{\text{person-time}}$$

The formula reflects the fact that the numerator in the incidence rate (number of cases) is a Poisson variable with standard error estimated by its square root, whereas the denominator (person-time) is arbitrarily defined and has no sampling variation.

Table 9-3. Deaths from Any Cause during a Variable Follow-Up Period (mean 60 months) Among 92 Men 70 Years or Older in Three Greek Villages, by Smoking History and Age at Enrollment

Age	Number	Smokers	Nonsmokers
70–74	Dead	6	1
	Persons	28	10
	Person-months	1,535	516
	Mortality (months^{-1})	0.0039	0.0019
75–79	Dead	9	1
	Persons	27	8
	Person-months	1,321	448
	Mortality (months^{-1})	0.0068	0.0022
80+	Dead	8	5
	Persons	10	9
	Person-months	367	362
	Mortality (months^{-1})	0.0218	0.0138
Total	Dead	23	7
	Persons	65	27
	Person-months	3,223	1,326
	Mortality (months^{-1})	0.0071	0.0053
	Mortality per 1,000 pm	7.1	5.3

Source: Adapted from Trichopoulou A et al. Diet and survival of elderly Greeks: a link to the past. *Am J Clin Nutr* 1995;61 : 1346s–1350s.

The overall incidence of death (mortality) among smokers is 0.0071 months^{-1} with standard error:

$$\sqrt{\frac{0.0071}{3,223}} = 0.0015 \text{ months}^{-1}$$

or

$$\sqrt{\frac{7.1}{3.223}} = 1.5 \text{ per 1,000 person-months}$$

Similarly, the overall mortality among never smokers is 0.0053 months^{-1}, with standard error 0.0020.

The incidence rate difference is 0.0071 − 0.0053 = 0.0018 months^{-1}. The standard error of the difference is the square root of the sum of squares of the two standard errors, that is:

$$\sqrt{(0.0015)^2 + (0.0020)^2} = 0.0025 \text{ months}^{-1}$$

The 95 percent confidence interval of mortality difference is 0.0018 ± 1.96 · 0.0025 = −0.0031 to 0.0067. Therefore, the difference is not statistically significant and the χ value (normal deviate) is 0.0018/0.0025 = 0.72, corresponding to a two-tailed P of 0.47. However, the crude rate difference may be affected by negative confounding by age because never smokers are on the average older than smokers. Confounding is termed as *negative* when it tends to obscure, rather than exaggerate, a relation.

The incidence rate ratio is:

$$\frac{X_e}{\tau_e} \bigg/ \frac{X_o}{\tau_o}$$

Ratio measures as a rule should be log transformed for statistical handling and then back transformed into arithmetic scale for descriptive purposes and biomedical interpretation. It can be shown easily by invoking the properties of the Poisson distribution that the standard error of the natural logarithm of incidence rate ratio is

$$\sqrt{\frac{1}{X_e} + \frac{1}{X_o}}$$

Therefore, the incidence rate ratio (mortality ratio) between smokers and nonsmokers is $0.0071/0.0053 = 1.34$. The natural logarithm of 1.34 is 0.29, and the standard error of the latter quantity is:

$$\sqrt{\frac{1}{23} + \frac{1}{7}} = 0.43$$

The 95 percent confidence interval of the natural logarithms of the incidence rate ratio is $0.29 \pm (1.96 \cdot 0.43)$ or -0.55 to 1.13. By taking antilogs, the 95 percent confidence interval of the incidence rate ratio 1.34 is 0.58 to 3.09, straddling the null value of one and, therefore, indicating the lack of statistical significance. The same conclusion can be reached with $0.29/0.43 = 0.67$, which is a χ value (normal deviate) corresponding to a two-tailed P of 0.50. These χ and P values are similar to those obtained through assessment of the incidence rate difference (the minor discrepancy is due to approximations and rounding errors). It is useful to remember that for ratio measures the square of the point estimate equals the product of the lower and upper limit—a convenient check for possible arithmetic errors.

Open Cohort Studies with Stratification for Confounding

The data in Table 9-3 indicate that age may confound the association between smoking and mortality because age is independently associated with both the risk of death (positively) and the probability of being a smoker (inversely, although not in a regular way).

Moreover, there is a suggestion that age may be an effect modifier in the association between smoking and mortality because the incidence rate difference, as contrasted to the ratio, appears to increase with age. Therefore, standardization of age-specific incidence (mortality) rates need to be considered, although the collective epidemiologic and biologic evidence does not provide strong support for a powerful modification by age of the association between smoking and total mortality. Standardization of incidence rates and incidence rate differences is quite analogous to standardization of cumulative incidence proportions and cumulative incidence differences, with substitution of the standard error of an incidence rate $\left(\dfrac{\sqrt{\text{new cases}}}{\text{person-time}}\right)$ for the standard error of a cumulative incidence proportion $\left(\sqrt{\dfrac{P(1-P)}{N}}\right)$.

Pooling. In most instances, the likelihood of interaction between the control variable(s) and the principal exposure under study with respect to the outcome of interest should not dominate the analysis unless the study is large and powerful, existing evidence for interaction is quite strong, and there is a sound biomedical hypothesis to account for genuine effect modification. This is because the appearance of interaction depends on the nature of the measure of effect (difference or ratio) and because the statistical documentation of genuine interaction requires a statistically powerful study. By ignoring interaction, the problem becomes one of pooling the stratum-specific estimates (incidence rate differences or ratios) and setting appropriate confidence limits around the pooled estimate. In the section dealing with closed cohort studies with stratification, we have pointed out that the Mantel-Haenszel χ^2 provides a valid test against the null hypothesis that odds ratio is equal to one, cumulative incidence ratio is also one, and cumulative incidence difference is zero in every stratum. Similarly, a modification of the Mantel-Haenszel χ^2 for open cohort data provides a valid test against the null hypothesis that the incidence rate ratio is one and the incidence rate difference is zero in every stratum.[389,466,469,494] The Mantel-Haenszel χ can then be used to set test-based approximate confidence limits.

The Mantel-Haenszel χ modified for data in open cohorts is calculated by summing over all strata the observed exposed cases Σx_e, summing over all strata the exposed cases that would have been expected if the null hypothesis of no association were true in every stratum $\Sigma(x_e + x_o) \cdot \dfrac{\tau_e}{\tau}$, and dividing their difference by its standard error, which equals the square root of the sum over all strata of the quantity $\dfrac{(x_e + x_o) \cdot \tau_e \cdot \tau_o}{\tau^2}$ (symbols as on page 170, τ equals the sum of τ_e and τ_o). For the data in Table 9-3:

$$\Sigma x_e = 23$$

$$\Sigma \frac{(x_e + x_o) \cdot \tau_e}{\tau} = \frac{7 \cdot 1535}{2051} + \frac{10 \cdot 1321}{1769} + \frac{13 \cdot 367}{729} = 19.25$$

$$\text{Standard error} = \sqrt{\Sigma \frac{(x_e + x_o) \cdot \tau_e \cdot \tau_o}{\tau^2}} = 2.54$$

Therefore, Mantel-Haenszel $\chi = \dfrac{23 - 19.25}{2.54} = 1.48$, corresponding to two-tailed P ~ 0.14.

An approximate pooled estimate of incidence rate difference can be calculated by weighing the stratum-specific estimates according to their precision and using as weights $\dfrac{\tau_e \cdot \tau_o}{(x_e + x_o)}$.

For the age group 70–74, incidence difference is 0.0020 months^{-1}, the weight is 113,151, and the relative weight is 0.62. For age group 75–79, incidence difference is 0.0046 months^{-1}, the weight is 59,181, and the relative weight is 0.32. For age group 80+, incidence difference is 0.0080 months^{-1}, the weight is 10,220, and the relative weight is 0.06. Therefore, the pooled incidence rate difference is 0.0032 months^{-1}. Test-based 95 percent confidence limits are derived by multiplying the pooled estimate with $\left(1 - \dfrac{1.96}{1.48}\right)$ and with $\left(1 + \dfrac{1.96}{1.48}\right)$, which results in −0.0010 and +0.0074. Because the age-adjusted incidence rate difference (0.0032) is substantially higher than the crude incidence rate difference (0.0018), it is concluded that age in this setting was a negative confounder of the association between smoking and mortality. It is worth noting that inference about confounding does not depend on statistical significance but only on the comparison between adjusted and unadjusted measures of association.

Pooling the incidence rate ratio across several strata represents a procedure far more common than pooling incidence rate differences because the former measure varies less than the latter by age, gender, and other major covariates, particularly in studies of cancer epidemiology.[42,576] The modified Mantel-Haenszel χ^2 for open cohorts provides again a valid test against the null hypothesis of a uniform rate ratio of one across all strata. Moreover, an appropriate pooled estimate of incidence rate ratio has been proposed by Rothman[466,469] as equal to the sum across all strata of $\frac{X_e \cdot \tau_0}{\tau}$ divided by the sum across all strata of $\frac{X_0 \cdot \tau_e}{\tau}$. In the example of Table 9-3, the pooled rate ratio equals 1.94.

The standard error of the pooled incidence rate ratio has been derived by Greenland and Robins,[179] but test-based confidence limits are reasonably accurate unless the rate ratio is much higher or much smaller than the null value of one. For the data in Table 9-3, the Mantel-Haenszel χ is 1.48 and the 95 percent confidence limits are calculated by exponentiating the pooled rate ratio estimate 1.94 to $\left(1 - \frac{1.96}{1.48}\right)$ and to $\left(1 + \frac{1.96}{1.48}\right)$; the lower limit is 0.81 and the upper limit is 4.67.

Standardization. In many special-exposure cohorts, the observed number of cases or deaths are compared to the number of cases or deaths that would have been expected if rates concerning the mostly nonexposed general population were applied to the exposed person-time. This is a process of standardization using as standard the distribution of person-time in the exposed population by gender, age, calendar period, or any other variable that happens to be available and retrievable for both the exposed and the general population. The validity of the process depends on three assumptions: (1) that the exposed person-time is accurately recorded (see next section), (2) that the diagnosis of cases and the attribution of deaths is made with adequate and similar criteria in the exposed and the general population, and (3) that the exposed and the general population represent the same study base and therefore are comparable (a frequently dubious assumption).

The ratio of observed (symbolized by O) to expected (symbolized by E) cases is an estimate of the incidence rate ratio if the general population contains a negligible proportion of exposed individuals (as is usually the case). The ratio is frequently referred to as standardized morbidity (or mortality) ratio, or simply as SMR. The standard error of the natural logarithm of SMR can be approximated by $\frac{1}{\sqrt{O}}$ (i.e., by the inverse of the square root of the observed number of cases). In the data of Table 9-1, among the 1,722 irradiated children, 17 cases of cancer were observed, whereas 2.6 were expected for an SMR of 6.54. The natural logarithm of SMR (ln SMR) is 1.88, with standard error 0.24 and 95 percent confidence limits of ln SMR 1.41 and 2.35. After exponentiation, the approximate 95 percent confidence limits of SMR are 4.10 and 10.49, indicating a highly significant excess incidence. The exact 95 percent confidence limits[469] are 3.94 and 10.26, suggesting that the approximation is satisfactory. Among 1,795 nonirradiated siblings of the irradiated children, five cases of cancer were observed, whereas 2.7 were expected for an SMR of 1.85 and approximate 95 percent confidence limits of 0.77 and 4.45. These limits do not adequately approximate the corresponding exact limits 0.68 and 4.11, and they indicate that an exact approach should be used when the number of observed cases is smaller than approximately 10.

Calculation of Person-Years of Observation

Person-years are regularly used as denominators in analyses of open cohort studies in chronic diseases. As indicated in Chapter 5 of this text, this concept simultaneously takes into consideration the number of persons under observation and the duration of observation of each person. For example, if 10 persons remain in the study for 10 years, there are said to be 100 person-years of observation. The same figure would be derived if 100 persons were under observation for 1 year or 200 persons for 6 months. The use of person-time accommodates the fact that most cohorts do not retain the same strength during the period in which outcome has been recorded. There are two main reasons for this.

1. Entrance dates may vary. For example, veterans answering Dorn's second mail questionnaire on smoking entered the cohort some 3 years after those answering the first.[102] Patients with ankylosing spondylitis entered the British cohort at various times between 1935 and 1954.[77]

2. During the course of the study, some individuals will drop out from the "under observation" category because of death, loss from the cohort, or other reasons.

In addition to changes in numbers under observation, changes in the age distribution of the cohort and perhaps exposure status of some members will occur as individuals are followed in time. If there are no alterations in exposure status and changes in numbers and age occur equally in the various exposure groups, they might, for purposes of comparison between exposure groups, be ignored. However, an assumption that all groups are equally affected is rarely sound. Separate calculations of rates that take into account differences due to both changing strength and age are indicated.

Data from the early years of the study of Doll and Hill[98] shown in Table 9-4 illustrate the person-years method. No new physicians were admitted to the study cohort after the beginning date (November 1, 1951); therefore, the changes in age distribution are

Table 9-4. Number of Men Under Observation at Successive Anniversaries of Entering the Study, by Age, in a Cohort Study of British Physicians

Age (years) at specified date	Number of men under observation by date							Person-years*
	Nov. 1, 1951	Nov. 1, 1952	Nov. 1, 1953	Nov. 1, 1954	Nov. 1, 1955	Apr. 1, 1956		
Under 35	10,140	9,145	8,232	7,389	6,281	5,779		35,489
35–44	8,886	9,149	9,287	9,414	9,710	9,796		41,211
45–54	7,117	7,257	7,381	7,351	7,215	7,191		32,156
55–64	4,094	4,212	4,375	4,601	5,057	5,243		19,909
65–74	2,694	2,754	2,823	2,873	2,902	2,928		12,462
75–84	1,382	1,433	1,457	1,485	1,483	1,513		6,431
85+	181	200	223	256	278	296		1,028
All ages	34,494	34,150	33,778	33,369	32,926	32,746		148,686

Source: Adapted from Doll R, Hill AB. Lung cancer and other causes of death in relation to smoking. A second report on the mortality of British doctors. *Br Med J* 1956;2 : 1071–1081.
*See text for method of calculation.

due solely to the aging of the cohort and the occurrence of deaths. The derivation of this table did not involve repeated censuses of the cohort but was based on extrapolation from the known ages of its members in 1951 and on the data that were being routinely assembled on decedents.

The person-years of observation, shown in the last column, were derived as follows: In the age group under 35 years, there were 10,140 men alive on November 1, 1951, and 9,145 alive on November 1, 1952. Therefore, if death occurred evenly through the year, there was an average of 9,643 men alive during the first year of the study, and these contributed 9,643 person-years of observation. Similarly, during the second, third, and fourth years, there was an average of 8,688, 7,811, and 6,835 men, respectively, under observation. During the last period (5 months), the average number under observation was $6,030 \cdot 5/12 = 2,512$ person-years. The person-years of observation during the entire period was, therefore, $9,643 + 8,688 + 7,811 + 6,835 + 2,512$ or a total of 35,489 person-years.

Such calculations can be made for each exposure category, and they are shown for this study in Table 9-5. The summary rate (total) for all ages for each exposure group was derived by standardizing rates for each exposure group to the age distribution of the population of the United Kingdom in 1951.

Losses to Follow-Up

In most types of cohort study, particularly those in which follow-up information is obtained by periodic medical examination or other contact, a number of members of the cohort will be lost to trace. Such individuals can no longer be considered under observation, and some adjustment of the denominator is required. The difficulty raised by persons lost to follow-up is that the probability of loss may be related to the exposure category, the outcome being measured, or both. Thus, it is possible that cohort members who develop the disease under study may tend to migrate to some other geographic area for treatment, or they may tend to move less than those not affected. Furthermore, smokers, for example, may be more or less "restless" than non-smokers. Because it is extremely difficult to detect all such possibilities that might have relevance in a particular study, it is of paramount importance to minimize losses to follow-up. However, this objective is rarely achieved, at least in countries with high population mobility, such as the United States. Even if some persons are not completely lost (i.e., it is known that they are still

Table 9-5. Death Rates from Lung Cancer According to Smoking Habits of British Male Physicians Age 35 and Over, 1951 to 1956

Age group (years)	Nonsmokers			Light smokers*			Moderate smokers*			Heavy smokers*		
	Person-years	Number of deaths	Death rate per 1,000 per year	Person-years	Number of deaths	Death rate per 1,000 per year	Person-years	Number of deaths	Death rate per 1,000 per year	Person-years	Number of deaths	Death rate per 1,000 per year
35–54	11,266	0	0.00	23,102	2	0.09	23,751	4	0.17	15,248	4	0.26
55–64	1,907	0	0.00	6,333	2	0.32	6,514	6	0.92	5,155	16	3.10
65–75	1,078	0	0.00	5,201	7	1.35	3,893	13	3.34	2,290	11	4.80
75+	856	1	1.17	3,950	11	2.78	1,931	4	2.07	722	3	4.16
Total†	15,107	—	0.07	38,586	—	0.47	36,089	—	0.86	23,415	—	1.66

Source: Adapted from Doll R, Hill AB. Lung cancer and other causes of death in relation to smoking. A second report on the mortality of British doctors. *Br Med J* 1956:2 : 1071–1081.

*Smoking categories: Light: 1–14 g daily; Moderate: 15–24 g daily; Heavy: 25 g or more daily

†The rates for all ages are standardized by applying the age-specific rates to the total United Kingdom population in 1951.

alive), they may still be lost insofar as determination of an outcome other than death is concerned.

The consequences of having a proportion of persons lost to follow-up are similar to those of failure to obtain exposure information on some members of the entering cohort. In theory, the losses will affect the relative rates for exposure categories only if they are associated with both exposure category and outcome. Losses to follow-up that are only associated with exposure (e.g., heavier for smokers than for nonsmokers) should not affect the rates of the outcome if proper allowance is made for the loss in the analysis. Losses in follow-up that are selective with respect to outcome alone will affect the absolute levels of the outcome measures but not their relative levels between different exposure categories. However, if the follow-up losses are at all substantial, they may produce considerable distortion of the actual rates and risks and will be undesirable, even if their ratios between various exposure categories remain unaltered.

Methods of dealing with the problem of losses to follow up in the analysis depend on the method of obtaining the outcome information.

1. When follow up depends on a regularly scheduled examination and ascertainment of the outcome depends on detecting a change in status between one examination and the next, the most accurate procedure is to assume that persons lost to trace between two examinations were lost immediately after the first examination. The denominator will then be the number of persons actually examined on each occasion (or the number of person-years experienced between two examinations by persons having the second). The reasoning behind this procedure is that persons lost between the two examinations cannot figure in the numerator of the rate and should therefore not be included in the denominator.

2. When follow up depends on a certain event occurring between two dates and ascertainment of the events takes place at the time of their occurrence (e.g., when deaths are being ascertained through some reporting system), a number of alternatives are possible.

a. If the exact date at which the person leaves the cohort is known, an adjustment can be made for the length of time he or she was under observation.

b. If it is known only that a person disappeared at some time between the two dates, it can be assumed that he or she was under observation for half the period between the two dates.

c. Two denominators can be calculated—one based on the assumption that all persons were lost immediately after the last date they were known to be present, and one based on the assumption that they were all lost immediately prior to the first date on which they were known to be absent. The correct rate must lie somewhere between the rates based on the two assumptions. This procedure is an elementary form of *sensitivity analysis*.

By use of one or the other of these methods, it is usually possible to evaluate the effect of follow-up losses in the various exposure groups. However, the problem resulting from the possibility that loss to follow up is associated with both exposure category and outcome remains. It may again be possible to make two assumptions: (1) none of the persons lost to follow up developed the specific outcome, and (2) all the persons lost to follow up developed the specific outcome. This yields an estimate of the range of rates possible in each exposure category. Unfortunately, this procedure is useful only in studies in which the proportion lost to follow up is small and the frequency of specified outcome is high (e.g., in studies of case fatality in severe diseases). In most epidemiological studies, the frequency of the outcome measured is commonly smaller than the proportion of persons lost to follow up, and the range between the estimates of outcome frequency will be too large to be of practical value.

Bias, Confounding, Synergism, Monotonic Relations, and Misclassification

Establishment of causal relations is a principal objective in epidemiology. It requires assessment of the role of chance in the generation of empirical associations and documentation that bias and confounding are unlikely to explain these associations. Although there are fewer possible sources of selection and information bias in cohort than in case-control studies, these should always be carefully explored, particularly when there are substantial losses to follow up, when information concerning exposure and outcome is retrospectively ascertained, when outcome definition is socially conditioned (e.g., when the diagnosis depends on autopsy or sophisticated tests that are more frequently performed in certain health care settings), and when external rates are used for the calculation of expected number of cases or deaths in a specially exposed group of individuals.

Confounding is equally important in cohort and case-control studies and it is generated by factors that are *independently* associated with both the exposure and the outcome under investigation. This occurs when the putative confounding factor is associated with the disease among nonexposed individuals, is associated with the exposure among nondiseased persons, and does not represent an intermediate step in the chain of events and conditions that link exposure to outcome. Confounding depends on the prevalence of the confounding factor(s), and factors with low prevalence in a particular research setting rarely create noticeable distortions. An association generated by confounding is *always* less strong than the association of the confounding factor with the disease under study *and* less strong than the association of this factor with the exposure under investigation.[576] When confounding is evaluated and controlled for in the analysis, three points need to be remembered: (1) confounding by a certain factor can only be evaluated by descriptively comparing the effect measure (rate ratio or difference) before and after adjusting for this factor and never by means of statistical testing,[358,466] (2) confounding by any particular factor can be substantially reduced when other confounding factors that are strongly correlated with it have already been accounted for, and (3) confounding is not adequately controlled when there is substantial random misclassification in the confounding factor(s).[160,553]

Synergism implies that a certain factor has a different effect in the presence of another factor rather than in its absence. In other words, the joint effect of two factors is different (e.g., larger) than the effect that would have been predicted on the basis of the effects of the two interacting factors individually. However, the "prediction" may be based on either the addition of the effects of the two factors (additive model) or on their multiplication (multiplicative model). Many procedures used in epidemiology, including the Mantel-Haenszel method, logistic regression, and the proportional hazards model assume multiplicative effects. Therefore, a positive interaction in such a model implies that the joint effect of the two factors is more than multiplicative. Conversely, in a multiplicative model, similar to proportional hazards, absence of interaction indicates that the joint action of two factors generates a multiplicative effect.[466]

Synergism is conceptually similar to *effect modification*, the latter term being used frequently in the epidemiologic literature.[132] Other conceptually similar terms are interaction, heterogeneity of effect measure, and lack of homogeneity of effect measure. When there is heterogeneity of the measure of effect of a particular factor (e.g., incidence rate ratio or cumulative incidence difference) across a number of strata of another factor, it makes little sense to calculate a "pooled" common estimator because this estimator could not properly apply to any one stratum. Indeed, in the presence of interaction it may not be useful to examine whether the stratified factor confounds the overall effect of the main study factor because this effect is demonstrably different in different strata. If an overall effect measure needs to be calculated for public health reasons, a standardization procedure should be used by applying arbitrary weights to the different stratum-specific effect measures. It should be pointed out that demonstration of interaction requires large numbers, probably four times as many as those required for the demonstration of a single-factor association. In the absence of the required statistical power, many of the interactions that are unexpectedly identified in epidemiological studies are probably due to chance and should be interpreted with caution.

Although multiplicative models are flexible and convenient, comparison of observed associations in additive models provide a sense of synergism that is intuitively more appealing, as well as more relevant for public health policies.[470,474] For example, in a study of male asbestos workers, the cumulative incidence of lung cancer among exposed individuals who were smokers was found to be much greater than the sum of the risks associated with asbestos and cigarette smoking alone.[486] Thus, the risk ratio of lung cancer in smokers compared to nonsmokers was about 10. The risk ratio associated with 20 years of exposure to asbestos dust was found to be of the same order of magnitude. However, asbestos workers who smoked were estimated to have 92 times the risk of dying of lung cancer as men who neither smoked nor worked with asbestos. In these data, multiplicative models would imply no interaction, whereas comparison to additive models would imply substantial interaction.

If A signifies the presence of a factor and $\overline{A}$ its absence, and B signifies the presence of another factor and $\overline{B}$ its absence, then RR (AB) is the rate ratio generated by the joint action of these factors, whereas RR $(A\overline{B})$ and RR $(\overline{A}B)$ are the rate ratios generated by only one of these factors, in comparison to the rate in the absence of both factors. The synergy index beyond additivity S has been defined by Rothman[466] as:

$$S = \frac{RR(AB) - 1}{RR(A\overline{B}) + RR(\overline{A}B) - 2}$$

S equal to 1 implies absence of interaction *in an additive model*, higher values imply positive interaction, and lower values imply negative interaction (antagonism). Statistical issues concerning synergism in epidemiological studies have been addressed by

Rothman[462,464] and Greenland,[162,170] whereas the biological phenomena underlying synergism have been considered by Koopman,[265] Rothman,[463] and Greenland.[164]

In many instances, exposure is not dichotomous (exposed, nonexposed), but it extends over several categories that are formed
naturally (e.g., number of sexual partners: 0, 1, 2, 3 . . .) or after
some convenient grouping (e.g., nonsmokers, smokers of up to
one pack per day, smokers of more than one pack per day). It is
always possible to consider every category of exposed individuals
as a distinct entity and compare it with the nonexposed category
using one of the methods previously indicated, usually a variant
of the Mantel-Haenszel procedure. However, this approach does
not take into account the natural order of the exposure categories,
and it can generate a series of regularly increasing (or decreasing)
effect measures, the confidence intervals of which straddle the
null value at every exposure level. A powerful alternative that is
available in multivariate modeling and in stratified analysis is the
evaluation of a linear trend in the response proportion or rate with
increasing exposure level. In stratified analysis, the appropriate
procedure is the Mantel extension test[322] and represents a generalization of the Armitage test for trends in proportions and frequencies in a single $2 \cdot K$ table, where K is the number of exposure
levels.[10] The Mantel extension test is a χ^2 test with one degree
of freedom, and it is powerful because it harvests the available
quantitative or semiquantitative information about increasing or
decreasing trends. However, the test does not evaluate linear
exposure–response because demonstrably irregular patterns and
even nonmonotonic relations can generate significant results in
the Mantel extension procedure.[306] Maclure and Greenland have
suggested alternative methodologic approaches for assessing exposure–response patterns,[306] but a simple piece of advice is to
infer a linear (or log-linear) pattern only when the Mantel extension test (or an equivalent test in a multivariate model) is significant *and* the data are descriptively compatible with such a pattern. As a minimum, Miettinen has suggested that exposed
individuals should be categorically compared with nonexposed
individuals, and a trend test should be applied only among the
exposed.[358] Greenland pointed out that fractional polynomial regression and spline regression can provide flexible tools for the
description of nonmonotonic trend analysis and exposure–
response patterns.[172,582]

Differential misclassification of exposure is frequently manifested as information bias, but a careful study design can minimize it. By contrast, nondifferential misclassification of individuals by exposure status is generally unavoidable in observational

studies. The usual consequence of nondifferential misclassification in the principal exposure variable is attenuation of the measure of effect estimate; that is, bias toward the null. Exceptions do occur, however, particularly when there are several exposure categories, parameters of misclassification are inordinately high, errors are inversely associated with the corresponding exposure variable(s), or exposure is defined through ecologic means and expressed as a proportion.[39,105,565] Nevertheless, in most situations, nondifferential misclassification of the principal exposure variable leads to an underestimation of the effect measure in both cohort and case-control studies.[13,461] Correction for misclassification tends to increase the effect estimate but does not affect the significance level.[593] A crude method for correction of the cumulative incidence ratio or the incidence rate ratio is available when the correlation coefficient r between the real and the actually utilized exposure is known from a validation study or some other source.

$$\text{true rate ratio} = \text{exponent} \left[\frac{\ln(\text{observed rate ratio})}{r} \right]$$

Thus, if the observed rate ratio is 2 and the correlation coefficient is +0.6 (as it is, for example, in many studies of nutritional and environmental epidemiology), the true rate ratio would be estimated as 3.2. The confidence limits for the corrected estimate can be approximately set through the test-based procedure[348] using the χ value (normal deviate) that corresponds to the original statistical assessment because statistical significance is not affected when the effect estimate is corrected for misclassification. Methods for derivation of more accurate confidence limits also are available.[461]

Correction of the observed rate ratio may be necessary if one wishes to calculate to what extent the difference in the incidence of a particular disease between two populations can be explained on the basis of the known differences between these populations on a series of accurately measured risk factors that were identified with nondifferential misclassification in analytic epidemiological studies.[220]

Nondifferential misclassification in a confounding variable severely limits the ability to control for this confounding in the analysis, whether this is attempted through stratification or through modeling.[160,553] When misclassification is limited in only one of the strata (e.g., in the open-ended categories of the very old or the very poor), residual confounding may be concentrated in this stratum and give the erroneous impression of effect modification.[417]

Life Tables

An alternative way of analyzing data from cohort studies, whether closed or open, is through the technique of clinical life tables, or simply life tables, as distinct from the demographic life tables. Conceptually, life tables are more closely related to open cohorts in the sense that the relevant effect measure is the incidence rate ratio. However, they also are applicable to closed cohorts, particularly when losses to follow up or, equivalently, deaths of study participants from diseases unrelated to the one under investigation must be accounted. The tables are frequently used in clinical follow-up studies for estimation of survival from cancer or other diseases and for documentation of how prognosis is affected by a particular treatment or other factors. Clinical follow-up studies are essentially cohort studies with subjects restricted to patients with a certain diagnosis. In such studies, exposure may be a particular treatment or a certain clinical characteristic and outcome may be death, recurrence of cancer, or another relevant health event. These studies are the focus of *clinical epidemiology*[583] and they differ from more traditional epidemiological investigations of disease causation in two main ways. First, the incidence of the study outcome over a period of several years is usually higher in clinical follow-up studies, making the life tables procedure more convenient to use and easier to interpret in a clinical context (e.g., generation of 5-year survival proportions by stage of diagnosis for various cancers). Second, in most instances, the principal exposure under investigation is a treatment with the potential to reduce the incidence of the study outcome, making it ethically acceptable to consider randomized intervention protocols. Thus, life tables are the standard analytical procedure in clinical trials with prolonged follow up.

The layout for a life table analysis is shown in Table 9-6. The data are from a study of survival through the first 2 years of life of 218 children born to HIV-1 positive mothers and another 218 children born to HIV-1 negative mothers, individually matched for maternal age and parity.[281] In cohort studies, matching exposed with unexposed individuals allows control of confounding by the matching variables even when the matching process is not accounted for in the analysis. However, a matched analysis (through stratification or modeling) usually generates slightly more precise effect estimates (i.e., a more narrow confidence interval around the effect measure).

In life table analysis, there are four main questions of increasing complexity: (1) how to calculate probability of survival at the end of a series of successive intervals;[80,111,116,245,293] (2) how to set confi-

Table 9-6. Survival Over 2 Years of Children Born to Human Immunodeficiency Virus Type 1 (HIV-1) Positive and Negative Mothers, Kigali, Rwanda, 1988 to 1991

	Children born to HIV-1 positive mothers						
Months since birth (i)	Children alive at the start of interval (O)	Deaths during interval (d)	Losses during interval (W)	Children at risk of death during interval (O' = O − W/2)	Probability of death during interval (q = d/O')	Probability of survival through this interval (p = 1 − q)	Cumulative survival probability to the end of interval (π)
0–2.99	218	11	0	218	0.0505	0.9495	0.9495
3–5.99	207	4	4	205	0.0195	0.9805	0.9310
6–8.99	199	4	5	196.5	0.0204	0.9796	0.9120
9–11.99	190	8	3	188.5	0.0424	0.9576	0.8733
12–14.99	179	4	1	178.5	0.0224	0.9776	0.8538
15–17.99	174	5	0	174	0.0287	0.9713	0.8293
18–20.99	169	1	5	166.5	0.0060	0.9940	0.8243
21–23.99	163	3	3	161.5	0.0186	0.9814	0.8090
24	157						

	Children born to HIV-1 negative mothers						
Months since birth (i)	Children alive at the start of interval (O)	Deaths during interval (d)	Losses during interval (W)	Children at risk of death during interval (O' = O − W/2)	Probability of death during interval (q = d/O')	Probability of survival through this interval (p = 1 − q)	Cumulative survival probability to the end of interval (π)
0–2.99	218	4	0	218	0.0183	0.9817	0.9817
3–5.99	214	2	1	213.5	0.0094	0.9906	0.9725
6–8.99	211	1	1	210.5	0.0048	0.9952	0.9678
9–11.99	209	2	2	208	0.0096	0.9904	0.9585
12–14.99	205	0	4	203	0	1	0.9585
15–17.99	201	0	1	200.5	0	1	0.9585
18–20.99	200	0	5	197.5	0	1	0.9585
21–23.99	195	1	1	194.5	0.0051	0.9949	0.9536
24	193						

Source: Adapted from Lepage P, et al. Mother-to-child transmission of human immunodeficiency virus type 1 (HIV-1) and its determinants: a cohort study in Kigali, Rwanda. *Am J Epidemiol* 1993;137 : 589–599.

dence limits around the point estimates of survival probabilities;[187,410,465] (3) how to compare overall survival patterns of two groups, that is, the survival curves of exposed and unexposed persons;[78,323,410] and (4) how to adjust for confounding variables.[78,323,410] The issues surrounding survival analysis are lucidly reviewed by Peto et al.[410] and Kahn and Sempos.[240]

In Table 9-6, during the first of the successive time intervals of 3-month duration, among 218 children born to HIV-1 positive mothers 11 have died with a probability of death equal to 0.0505. Among the 207 children that have survived to the start of the next time interval, 4 children were withdrawn from the study or were lost to follow up during this interval. Therefore, children at risk of death were 207 at the beginning of the second interval but only 203 at the end of it, implying that only 205 children born to HIV-1 positive mothers were actually at risk of death during the second 3-month interval. Among these effectively at-risk children, four died with a probability of death 0.0195. Survival probabilities during a particular time interval among children who have survived to the beginning of that interval (conditional survival probabilities) are complementary to the corresponding probabilities of death. The last column gives cumulative survival probabilities to the end of any particular interval. Because survival to the end of the third interval, for example, requires survival to the end of the first and the second and the third interval, the cumulative probability equals the product of the three conditional probabilities of survival to the end of the third interval $(0.9120 = 0.9495 \cdot 0.9805 \cdot 0.9796)$. Therefore, the probability of survival at the end of the twenty-fourth month of life is 0.8090 for children born to HIV-1 positive mothers and 0.9536 for children born to HIV-1 negative mothers.

When there are very few persons whose survival is investigated, it is not possible to group deaths, losses, or survivors by interval as in Table 9-6. An elementary life table can still be constructed, however, using a very simple method devised by Kaplan and Meier.[245] This method is frequently used in small-scale clinical investigations.

The standard error of cumulative survival probability (π) at the end of a particular interval can be approximated by multiplying π with $\sqrt{\dfrac{(1 - \pi)}{O}}$, where O is the number of individuals *alive at exactly that time*, which is, of course, the number of individuals alive at the start of the next interval.[410] Thus, the standard error of 0.8090 (Table 9-6) is $0.8090 \sqrt{\dfrac{(1 - 0.8090)}{157}}$ or 0.0282, and the 95 percent confidence limits are $0.8090 \pm 1.96 \cdot 0.0282$ or 0.7537 and 0.8643. The standard error of 0.9536 (Table 9-6; HIV-1 negative mothers) is $0.9536 \sqrt{\dfrac{(1 - 0.9536)}{193}}$ or 0.0148, and the 95 percent confidence limits are 0.9246 and 0.9826. An alternative method proposed by Rothman has better properties but is more complicated; its use could be reserved for studies with small sample size.[465]

Knowledge of cumulative survival probabilities and their standard errors at a certain point of time in the follow-up period allows the undertaking of statistical testing. In the example of Table 9-6, at the end of the twenty-fourth month of life the difference in cumulative survival probability between children born to HIV-1 positive and negative mothers is $0.9536 - 0.8090 = 0.1446$ with standard error

$$\sqrt{0.0282^2 + 0.0148^2} = 0.0318$$

The standard normal deviate, or χ, is 4.55 corresponding to $P < 10^{-5}$. However, evaluation at a certain point of time does not reveal how the survival curves compare throughout the follow-up period. This is of obvious importance because two survival curves with a certain cumulative survival probability difference at the end of the follow-up period may have deviated soon after the start of follow up (too many early deaths in one of the groups), or they may have run very close to each other until very late in the follow-up period (too many *late* deaths in one of the groups).

There are two tests suitable for the overall comparison of two survival curves: (1) the logrank test,[410] and (2) a slight modification of the Mantel-Haenszel procedure for several two by two tables[326] introduced by Mantel.[323] Both tests require that the two survival curves do not cross and, indeed, do not have widely dissimilar shapes. The Mantel-Haenszel procedure is described in Chapter 10, and, for all practical purposes, it is equivalent to the logrank test. The procedure generates a summary χ^2 with one degree of freedom and a pooled odds ratio over several two by two tables. For the comparison of two survival curves, each successive interval is considered as a distinct two by two table with cell counts d and $(O' - d)$ for exposed and unexposed groups, respectively (Tables 9-6 and 9-7).

For the cohorts of children born to HIV-1 positive and negative mothers,[281] the Mantel-Haenszel χ for comparison of their overall survival to the end of the twenty-fourth month since birth[323] is again 4.55 (the exact equality to the standard normal deviate based on comparison of cumulative survival proportions at the end of the twenty-fourth month is a coincidence) with $P < 10^{-5}$. The Mantel-Haenszel odds ratio, an estimate of the incidence rate ratio, is 4.40 with test-based 95 percent confidence limits 2.32 and 8.32. In this instance, however, the test-based confidence interval may be too narrow in comparison to that estimated through an exact method because the odds ratio is substantially elevated and the level of significance rather striking.

The Mantel modification for comparing survival curves through the Mantel-Haenszel procedure can also be used to control confounding.[323] If survival curves of children born to HIV-1 positive and negative mothers were estimated separately for mothers with none or some formal education, then instead of the eight fourfold tables (Table 9-7) there would be 16 such tables, but the procedure would be otherwise identical and just as simple. Note again that in this matched for maternal age cohort study, there can be no confounding by this variable even if maternal age were a risk factor for infant mortality and matching were not accounted for in the analysis.[466]

Comparison of overall survival patterns of the two groups, point and interval estimation of the rate ratio between exposed and unexposed groups, and adjustment for confounding for non-matched factors can also be efficiently accomplished through multivariate modeling, specifically through the proportional hazards or Cox model.[78]

Multivariate Analysis and Cox Regression

Control of confounding and, to a lesser extent, evaluation of interaction among the study variables is a central objective in epidemiological research. Stratification and the statistical techniques that were developed to address testing and estimation in stratified analysis are usually straightforward. However, stratification by several control variables, or even by a few variables with several categories each, can generate strata with sparse and grossly unbalanced data (several exposed but few or no unexposed persons and vice versa) that provide little or no information. Moreover,

Table 9-7. Data Layout for Application of the Mantel-Haenszel Procedure for the Comparison of Overall Survival Curves of Children Born to HIV-1 Positive (Exposed) and Negative (Unexposed) Mothers to the End of the 24th Month Since Birth

Months since birth (i)	Exposed dead (d)	Exposed, at risk, but alive $(O' - d)$	Unexposed dead (d)	Unexposed, at risk, but alive $(O' - d)$
0–2.99	11	207	4	214
3–5.99	4	201	2	211.5
6–8.99	4	192.5	1	209.5
9–11.99	8	180.5	2	206
12–14.99	4	174.5	0	203
15–17.99	5	169	0	200.5
18–20.99	1	165.5	0	197.5
21–23.99	3	158.5	1	193.5

Source: Adapted from Lepage P, et al. Mother-to-child transmission of human immunodeficiency virus type 1 (HIV-1) and its determinants: a cohort study in Kigali, Rwanda. *Am J Epidemiol* 1993;137 : 589–599.

even when a study is so large as to allow the creation of many informative strata, few investigators are able to decipher patterns spread across more than 20 strata; therefore, stratification loses its main appeal—to keep the investigator in touch with his or her own data.

Modeling the data appropriately through one of the multiple regression procedures can enhance statistical power, improve control of confounding, and vastly increase flexibility by allowing transfer of information through model-based intrapolations. However, misspecification of the model (inappropriate or inefficient model design) can have the opposite effect, notably inadequate control of confounding and even introduction of bias. Moreover, model misspecification, possible procedural errors, and arithmetic mistakes may remain undetected because few investigators have adequate feeling of model-processed data.

The basic regression equation is:

$$Y = \alpha + \beta_1 X_1 + \beta_2 X_2 \ldots + \varepsilon$$

where Y is the dependent variable, which, in epidemiology, is usually a suitably transformed metric of disease occurrence (e.g., the natural logarithm of the incidence rate); α is the regression intercept or regression constant or corner parameter and is of little interest because it depends on study design and background disease characteristics; X_1, X_2, and so forth are the predictor (independent) variables that may have genuinely causal impact or reflect confounded associations; ε is the unavoidable random error term; and β_1, β_2, and so forth are the partial regression coefficients (i.e., the all important effect measures). Each of the partial regression coefficients indicates how much the disease metric will change when the respective predictor variable (possible cause or risk factor) increases by one unit and all other variables in the model remain constant. Partial regression coefficients are appropriate measures of effect because their magnitude does not depend on the frequency or range of variation of the respective predictor variable. Moreover, these coefficients are in theory unconfounded by the effects, if any, of the other predictor variables that are included in the model, assuming that the latter variables are accurately measured and the statistical model is appropriately designed. By contrast, partial correlation coefficients and standardized regression coefficients should not be utilized as effect measures because they depend on the range of variation and the overall frequency, respectively, of the corresponding predictor variables and are therefore dependent on design factors.[181,466]

Both open and closed cohort studies can be analyzed in terms of the incidence rate ratio, which is, in fact, the central measure of effect in epidemiology. Cox regression is tailored to cohort studies, including clinical trials with prolonged follow up, because the partial regression coefficients in the model are the natural logarithms of the respective rate ratios.[78] When the respective predictor variable takes only two values (e.g., 0 for nonexposed and 1 for exposed), the antilog of the partial regression coefficient is the desired rate ratio. If the predictor variable is quantitative (e.g., diastolic blood pressure in mm Hg), the antilog of the partial regression coefficient is the rate ratio per unit of increase in diastolic blood pressure. If the investigators prefer to estimate the rate ratio per 10 mm Hg of increase in blood pressure, the partial regression coefficient must first be multiplied by 10 and then be exponentiated. Similarly, confidence limits must be set around the logarithm of the ratio and subsequently exponentiated.

Cox regression is also called proportional hazards model because it makes no assumptions as to how the baseline disease incidence (hazard) changes over time among totally unexposed persons. It assumes, however, that every categorical exposure (no, yes) and every increase in a quantitative predictor variable by a certain magnitude (e.g., by 10 mm Hg in diastolic pressure) has the same proportional effect (rate ratio) irrespective of the level of the baseline incidence (hazard). The Cox model is inherently multiplicative because it involves logarithms, and it is inherently exponential for quantitative variables such as age or diastolic pressure. This may be undesirable in certain situations, but the model can be designed in a way that bypasses the problem.[466]

Independent variables of nominal nature (e.g., blood groups, occupation, gender) require as many model terms as there are categories minus one (which is used, by default, as the reference category). Ordinal variables (e.g., nondrinkers, light drinkers, moderate drinkers, heavy drinkers, or 0,1,2,3) and continuous variables (e.g., height, diastolic blood pressure) of principal interest may be entered as one log-linear term each or be transformed into several categories and dealt with as nominal variables. The latter approach avoids forcing the data into particular model assumptions, including the exponential increase of rate ratio. Occasionally, both approaches may be used in alternative models, continuous terms allowing more powerful testing of trends, and categorical representation permitting an assumption-free examination of exposure-response patterns and better model fit.

For confounding variables (e.g., social class) and recognized selection factors (e.g., residence), it is better to use as many categorical terms as practical for each variable because this improves the model fit and there is little interest in interpretability. However, if data are very sparse or a monotonic relation with disease is well established, there may be an advantage in using an ordinal or continuous term, and thus preserving degrees of freedom. Stepwise regression procedures are not appropriate in epidemiology because they may leave room for residual confounding. It is important to remember that confounding cannot be assessed with statistical testing.

Interaction terms among confounding and selection variables may be used extensively and freely because they improve the model fit and do not generate interpretation problems. Extreme caution is needed, however, when interaction terms are introduced that involve the main exposure variable of interest. Regression coefficients of single terms are no more interpretable—all of the terms that involve the main exposure variable must be simultaneously assessed.

When rates in population groups are to be modeled, rather than data based on individuals as in most cohort studies, the appropriate procedure is Poisson regression because occurrence of events in person-time is a Poisson variable.[43,61] As discussed at the beginning of this chapter, the experience of an open cohort can be allocated in a matrix of person-time. For a study with exposure (yes, no), gender (female, male), and age (40–44, 45–49, etc., up to 70–74) as the only variables, a three-dimensional matrix would have $2 \cdot 2 \cdot 7 = 28$ groups of person-time.

With additional study variables, this matrix can be further expanded. The effect of all the study variables on the disease incidence rate can be studied simultaneously in a Poisson regression model. In situations where estimation of the baseline disease incidence over time is of interest (as in an occupational cohort where follow-up time might be a measure of latency), Poisson regression, in contrast to Cox regression, can be applied to assess different intervals of follow-up as one of the classification variables for person-time. The proportional hazards model focuses on proportional changes of the baseline rate under the influence of the study variables, but ignores the pattern of change, over follow-up time, of the baseline rate.[78]

Interpretation

Interpretation of the results of a cohort study will generally center on two problems: (1) evaluation of the extent to which methodologic problems contribute to differences (or lack of differences) in outcome rates between exposure categories, and (2) whether observed differences in outcome between exposure categories are likely to reflect causal relationships between the exposure and the outcome under investigation. Considerations relevant to the first problem have been touched on throughout this chapter, and those relating to the second were discussed in Chapter 2. Only two particular aspects are elaborated on here: exposure-response relationship and inferences from different measures of risk.

Exposure-Response Relationship

The existence of an exposure-response relationship (i.e., an increase in disease rate with increase in amount of exposure) supports the view that an association is a causal one. The consistent increase in mortality from lung cancer with increase in cigarette consumption has played a major role in acceptance of this relationship as causal.[99,101] However, the lack of an exposure-response relationship does not rule out the possible causal nature of an association. The presence of diseases dependent on a single major gene, for example, show no exposure-response relationship, unless it is one modified by other causal components.

Inferences from Different Measures of Risk

In interpreting the findings of cohort studies, one may find that rate ratios and rate differences give different impressions as to the importance of a particular exposure. If several factors that are etiologically important for the same disease are being compared, the same order of importance of the factors will be suggested whether rate ratio or rate difference is examined. However, when the importance of the same exposure is assessed for several different manifestational entities, this may not be the case. For example, data from Doll and Hill's study (shown in Table 9-8) indicate that the mortality rate ratio from heavy cigarette smoking is far greater for lung cancer and chronic bronchitis than for deaths from other causes, but the rate difference (attributable mortality) is greater for cardiovascular disease than for lung cancer. Each of these observations contributes to the evaluation of the findings.

1. The size of the rate ratio is a better index than is the rate difference of the likelihood that a causal relationship exists between the exposure and the disease involved. Thus, a difference of 10 per 100,000 per year (rate difference or attributable rate) noted between two exposure categories would be less likely to be an error of measurement if it occurred between rates of 1 and 11 than between rates of 110 and 120. It would take less bias to raise a rate from 110 to 120 than to raise it from 1 to 11, just as it is easier to make an error of 1 inch in measuring a mile than in

Table 9-8. Relative and Attributable Mortality from Selected Causes Associated with Heavy Cigarette Smoking by British Male Physicians, 1951 to 1961

Cause of death	Death rate* among nonsmokers	Death rate* among heavy smokers†	Death rate ratio	Attributable death rate*
Lung cancer	0.07	2.27	32.4	2.20
Other cancers	1.91	2.59	1.4	0.68
Chronic bronchitis	0.05	1.06	21.2	1.01
Cardiovascular diseases	7.32	9.93	1.4	2.61
All causes	12.06	19.67	1.6	7.61

Source: Adapted from Doll R, Hill AB. Mortality in relation to smoking: ten years' observations of British doctors. *Br Med J* 1964;1399–1410, 1460–1467.
*Death rates per 1,000 per year
†Heavy smokers are defined as smokers of 25 or more cigarettes per day.

measuring a foot. Furthermore, the likelihood that an association between two variables results from association of both with a third variable would appear to decrease as the rate ratio increases because the higher the rate ratio the stronger, and, therefore, presumably more obvious, must be the association between each of the variables and the third variable. Thus, in the present example, on the basis of the evidence in Table 9-8 alone, one would be inclined to accept the associations with cigarette smoking as evidence of a causal relationship more readily for lung cancer and for chronic bronchitis than for cardiovascular disease.

2. Yet, if it is accepted that the observed association is a causal one, then the rate difference (attributable rate) gives a better idea than does the rate ratio of the impact that a successful preventive program might have. Because the associations of cigarette smoking with lung cancer and with cardiovascular disease are both causal in nature, then elimination of cigarette smoking would prevent even more deaths from cardiovascular disease than from lung cancer.

10 Case-Control Studies

A case-control study is an inquiry in which groups of individuals are selected based on whether they do (the cases) or do not (the controls) have the disease of which the etiology is to be studied. The two groups are then used to evaluate the relation to the study disease of existing or past characteristics (states, events, or other exposures) among the individuals.

Definition of the measure *odds* as distinct from *risk* is essential to the description of the basis of case-control studies. In an odds, the number of individuals with a characteristic (e.g., an exposure or a disease) is expressed relative to the number without the characteristic. Thus, if 2 of 10 people receive a particular exposure, the *exposure odds* are 2 : 8, or 0.25, whereas the exposure *risk* is 2/10, or 0.2. Similarly, if 3 of 10 people develop hypertension, the *disease odds* are 3 : 7, or 0.43, whereas the disease *risk* is 3/10, or 0.3. The odds (whether of exposure, disease, or another variable) can be computed either from the numbers (number affected divided by number not affected) or from proportions (proportion affected divided by proportion not affected).

The traditional conceptualization of case-control studies has been that cases are compared to controls with respect to exposure frequency via the exposure odds *ratio*,[74,326] which is the exposure odds among cases divided by the corresponding odds among controls. In general, there is more concern about the likelihood of disease given exposure than about the likelihood of exposure given disease. However, the exposure odds ratio derived from case-control studies *equals* the disease odds ratio derived from cohort studies, and both measures approximate the disease risk ratio when the disease is uncommon, as is usually the case. Examples of exceptions when it would be unwise to assume that the disease is uncommon would be death as the outcome in old persons or the number of cases in an acute infectious disease outbreak. This conceptualization is still acceptable and served well in hundreds of case-control studies that generated much of what became known about the etiology of chronic diseases in the three decades after 1950.[65,124,216,229,288]

In the 1970s, the concept was advanced that case-control studies should be viewed as efficient sampling schemes of the disease experience of the underlying open or closed cohorts.[349,358,466] This approach allows an integrated view of cohort and case-control epidemiological designs.

Theoretical Foundation of Case-Control Studies

Consider a well-defined dynamic population in a stable "steady state" situation, such as women 30 years old or more who are residents of a particular town, continuously or during a certain fraction of the calendar period 1 January 1990 to 31 December 1994. During this period, x_e parous and x_0 nulliparous women were diagnosed for the first time with breast cancer. If we knew how long every parous and nulliparous woman who had not previously had breast cancer was a resident of this town during this calendar period, we would have a typical "open" cohort study and we would be able to calculate breast cancer incidence rates among exposed (parous) and unexposed (nulliparous) women, as well as the resulting difference and ratio measures of association. Such information, however, is rarely available.

The person-time denominator in an incidence rate equals the sum of the time contributed by every individual person at risk, or, equivalently, the product of the number of individuals at risk by the average time they were actually at risk of developing the disease, or, equivalently, *the product of the total study period (in this example, 5 years or 5 · 365 days) by the average number of persons at risk at any particular day during the study period* (for practical purposes, a day can be thought of as a moment in time).

The equivalency of these statements does not depend on the frequency of the disease under consideration (common or rare disease), but it relies on the steady population concept that is approximately fulfilled in many situations.[576] Using the latter formulation, the total person-time equals the product of 5 · 365 days by the average prevalent number of women at risk.

Let τ_e be the person-time contributed by those exposed (parous) and τ_0 the person-time contributed by those unexposed (nulliparous). The incidence rate ratio $\dfrac{x_e}{\tau_e} \Big/ \dfrac{x_0}{\tau_0}$ can also be written as

$\dfrac{x_e}{x_0} \Big/ \dfrac{\tau_e}{\tau_0}$. In a case-control study based on a dynamic population, x_e and x_0 (exposed and unexposed cases) are directly ascertained, and the ratio $\dfrac{\tau_e}{\tau_0}$ can be estimated in an unbiased way not dependent on any rare disease assumption by the ratio of exposed versus unexposed prevalent individuals at risk in the study base (the total study period cancels out). Accordingly, any particular group of prevalent individuals at risk for the disease in the source population during the study period (i.e., the "study base") that correctly reflects the ratio of exposed to unexposed person-time in this population over this period can be used for this purpose. These unaffected individuals (y_e for exposed and y_0 for unexposed) are the controls in a case-control study. To the extent that y_e/y_0 (the exposure odds among controls) is an unbiased estimate of $\dfrac{\tau_e}{\tau_0}$, controls may be viewed as reflecting the person-time by exposure status, and case-control studies can be considered as unbiased and efficient sampling processes to study the incidence rate ratio in the underlying dynamic cohort. By sampling "prevalent" exposed and unexposed individuals as controls, one is taking into account not only their relative numbers but also the duration of the time spent by them in the exposed or nonexposed state (i.e., the person-time in the study base).[182,183,349,549,576]

In the preceding example, the case-control approach is clearly more feasible than an analysis covering the total dynamic cohort that represents the primary study base for the cases. Because all cases are included and the controls are a representative sample of the study base, cases and controls are comparable.

In many instances, the cases of the disease under study can be identified in one or more collaborating hospitals or other health establishments. If there are other nonparticipating hospitals that also serve the same population (e.g., of a particular town or county), it may not be possible to identify the primary study base that gave rise to the cases that found their way into the participating hospitals. Indeed, strictly speaking, there is no definable primary base. In such situations, a study base can only be conceptualized as comprising the persons who, had they developed the disease under study, would have been admitted to the collaborating hospitals. This *secondary* or *case-defined* study base must be properly sampled to provide a suitable control series.[349,358,576]

A general rule is first to exclude from the case series patients who were not residents of the area served by the collaborating hospitals, but were admitted because of unusual circumstances or the reputation enjoyed by one or more of these hospitals for their effective treatment of the study disease. Next, residents of the area giving rise to the cases who were actually admitted to the participating hospitals *for a disease or diseases unrelated to the exposure under investigation* are considered an appropriate sample of the secondary study base if the assumption is reasonable that, had they developed the disease under study, they would have been admitted to the same hospitals. A comparison disease unrelated to the exposure under investigation affects exposed (y_e) and unexposed (y_o) persons in the secondary study base in numbers proportional to the corresponding person-time.

When several diseases are used for the accrual of a control series, it is possible to evaluate the assumption that all of them generate, as they should, similar exposure odds. Harder to evaluate is the assumption that controls do indeed come from the elusive secondary study base. The best empirical evidence in support of this assumption is that the case-control study demonstrates previously established risk factor(s) for the disease under investigation. This is discussed further later in this chapter.

A legitimate concern in case-control studies, particularly those relying on a secondary study base, is that the comparison disease or diseases or any other control-generating procedure, although in principle unrelated to the exposure under study, may generate biased exposure odds as a result of the selection process (that favors, for example, women or persons of lower socioeconomic class). Controlling for the suspected selection factor (e.g., gender, socioeconomic class) through stratification or modeling will rectify this problem *provided that the selection factor can be identified and accurately measured.*[42,417]

Nested case-control studies are usually undertaken within closed cohorts. In a frequently used sampling scheme, all cases are utilized in the design; however, for every case only a small number of controls, perhaps one to five, are chosen from among those who have survived, remain under observation, and are free of the disease of interest *at the time the corresponding case was diagnosed.* In this instance, controls are matched to cases on the follow-up time, not necessarily in a constant ratio. This procedure is sometimes referred to as *incidence density* or *risk set sampling.*[549,576] Because time is incorporated in the design, person-time is inherently accounted for in the analysis and the odds ratio is an unbiased estimate of the incidence rate ratio without any rare disease assumption. It is worth noting that controls for early occurring cases may become cases at a later time.[549,570]

In other types of case-control studies nested in closed cohorts, all cases that have occurred by a certain point in time within a closed cohort are included and controls are sampled from the individuals who have remained noncases by the same point in time *without any reference to follow-up time at which the cases occurred* (*cumulative incidence sampling*). Because the time dimension is not incorporated, the incidence rate ratio cannot be estimated in an unbiased way. The calculated odds ratio, however, represents a good approximation to the risk ratio when the risk (cumulative incidence) is low. Alternatively, in a *case-base* or *case-exposure* design, controls are chosen not among noncases but from the whole population at risk. The risk ratio then can be directly estimated in an unbiased way, although, again, the time dimension is not accounted for and incidence rate ratio can only be approximated. As previously indicated, the risk ratio is conceptually appealing but statistically less tractable than the odds ratio.[126,549,570]

In certain special exposure cohort studies that use external rates to calculate expected numbers of cases or deaths, it may be difficult to collect detailed exposure histories from the total cohort. Instead, a subcohort is chosen randomly from the cohort of exposed persons and detailed information on exposure is collected from them as well as from all the cases that have occurred in the total cohort. Time is not usually incorporated in the analysis, and this design, which is termed *case-cohort*, resembles the case-base approach.[268,423,549,567,570] In contrast to the case-base approach, however, the case-cohort design allows integration of external data (rates used to calculate expected number of cases in the cohort) and internal information (more detailed aspects of exposure). For example, Bergkvist et al.[23] studied a cohort of 23,244 women who were prescribed menopausal estrogens in the Uppsala region of Sweden and compared the number of breast cancer cases (N = 253) that occurred in a 5-year follow up with the number expected (N = 222.5) on the basis of the Uppsala County breast cancer incidence rates among nonexposed women. They then used detailed information from a subcohort of 653 women, randomly selected from the total *exposed* cohort, to study the effect of duration of exposure to menopausal estrogens and differential effects of estrogens used alone or in combination with progestins. This information was available only for the "exposed" breast cancer cases and the "exposed" subcohort.

Selection of Cases

In assembling a group of cases for study, consideration must be given to the diagnostic criteria for definition of the disease, to the source of the cases, and to the question of inclusion of incident or prevalent cases.

Diagnostic Criteria

Criteria are usually specific to each investigation and few generalizations are possible. Criteria that provide clear and reproducible applications of definition are obviously desirable, and decisions that tend to provide manifestationally more homogeneous groups of cases are usually preferable. If time and funds are available, establishment of a number of groups of cases based on variously defined manifestational criteria is desirable, providing the possibility of separate examination of cases defined by each group of criteria. Depending on similarities or differences of the group-specific association patterns with the suspected cause, such groups will assist in judging whether or not certain clinical syndromes should or should not be regarded as part of the disease under investigation.

Walker has pointed out that for certain diseases with frequently mild symptoms, such as cholelithiasis or endometriosis, definitive diagnosis is more likely when special tests are done, which, in turn, are more likely to be performed for individuals with higher socioeconomic status and better health insurance coverage.[576] In such situations, the disease under study is, for example, "cholelithiasis in wealthy persons" rather than "cholelithiasis." In other words, improved diagnostic criteria and better diagnostic validity violate the correspondence between the study group and the study base because not all persons with cholelithiasis in the source population are wealthy and thus eligible for the study.

Source of Cases

Series of affected individuals in a case-control study commonly are one of the following:

1. All persons with the disease occurring in a clearly defined population, such as that of a city or county, during a certain time period (primary study base)
2. All persons with the disease seen at a particular medical care facility or group of facilities in a specific period of time (secondary or case-defined study base)

The second type of series is commonly used because the procedure is relatively easy and inexpensive to undertake. The first procedure, although more laborious because it involves special efforts to locate and obtain the necessary data from all affected individuals in a defined population, is generally more satisfactory because (1) it avoids the bias that may arise from the selective factors that guide affected individuals to a particular medical care facility or physician, and (2) it allows computation of incidence rates of the disease in the total population and in exposure-defined subgroups.

It should be apparent that the challenge in the first approach is to achieve complete ascertainment of cases and adequate collaboration from a high proportion (for reasonable credibility more than 80%) of cases and controls. In principle, there should be no difficulty in drawing a random sample from the primary study base.[358,466] In contrast, the challenge in the second procedure is to conceptualize the secondary study base that gave rise to the study cases and draw a random sample from what is, in essence, an imaginary construct.

In certain situations the advantages of both types of procedures may be obtained. For example, when a defined population is served by a single medical facility or by a group of facilities sharing common record-keeping procedures (e.g., the population of a pre-paid medical care plan), all cases may be readily identifiable and yet still related to the source (base) population of which the size, age, gender, and other demographic characteristics are known. The study base need not, of course, be defined in geographic terms. Closed populations, such as those of schools, military establishments, and certain places of work, may offer the same advantages if they are large enough. In the investigation of congenital defects or of disorders of parturition, the related population will then be a certain number of deliveries, and the births occurring in a certain hospital or combination of hospitals may provide all the cases occurring in what may be regarded as a clearly defined population.

Incident or Prevalent Cases?

Whether the cases have come from selected facilities or from a defined population, it is preferable that they be limited to those that were newly diagnosed within a specific period. Although the inclusion of all cases existent during the period may, in a chronic disease, greatly increase the number of cases available for study, the inclusion of patients undergoing recurrences or of long-term survivors will complicate the interpretation of the findings. For patients in advanced states of the disease, it may be difficult to differentiate past events causally related to the disease from those consequent to it. In addition, in studies of prevalent cases, even if the exposures clearly antedated the onset of the present disease, it may not be possible to determine to what extent a particular characteristic noted in excess in the cases has relevance to the duration and course rather than to the etiology of the disease.[451]

Considerations for Selection of Controls

Control selection is guided by four objectives: (1) elimination of selection bias, (2) minimization of information bias, (3) minimization of residual confounding by unidentified or poorly measured variables (confounding by accurately measured factors can be controlled in the analysis), and (4) maximization of statistical power under the limits imposed by validity requirements and logistical constraints. In the previous edition of this book, MacMahon and Pugh recommended four types of considerations in the context of these objectives,[314] which are similar to the four principles proposed more recently by Wacholder and his colleagues for control selection in case-control studies.[568] These principles or considerations are outlined here.

Selection bias is not present when cases and controls are strictly comparable with respect to study base. This is achieved when controls are a representative sample of the study base that generated the study cases.[357,568] The study base itself need not be representative of any particular population.

Information bias that leads to differential misclassification can, as a rule, be avoided when the exposure of interest is measured with the same accuracy among cases and among controls; however, only optimal accuracy among both cases and controls can eliminate bias generated by nondifferential misclassification. The latter type of bias is generally considered less pernicious because, as a rule, it tends to attenuate an existing association.[108,593] As discussed in Chapter 9, exceptions do occur, but they tend to arise in rather unusual situations.[39,105,565]

Residual confounding by poorly defined or measured variables (e.g., environmental pollution, genetic background, quality of medical care) can be minimized by matching controls to cases, individually or in larger groups, with respect to one or more clearly identifiable variables that are thought to reflect the poorly defined or measured ones (e.g., neighborhood for environmental pollution, kinship for genetic background, hospital or primary care physician for quality of medical care). Because matching must almost always be accounted for in the analysis through stratification or modeling, the "within strata" variability of the poorly defined or measured variables is seriously restricted, and so is their potential for residual confounding. In other words, residual confounding is always *conditional* on the variables that are accounted for in the analysis.

Whereas minimization of the conditional variability of confounding variables minimizes their uncontrollable (residual) confounding, the statistical power of a study is higher when the conditional "within strata" variability of the principal study exposure is substantial. Matching and controlling for confounding variables through stratification or modeling usually reduces the variability of the principal exposure under study, but this is an acceptable loss in the pursuit of validity as the primary objective. If, however, matching and the subsequent stratified or model-based analysis were undertaken for factors that were not disease predictors, but only correlates of the exposure under study, then the whole process would slightly reduce statistical power without improvement in validity, a common but relatively benign and frequently unavoidable form of overmatching.[87,353]

Of the four considerations outlined, the first, which was termed by Wacholder and his colleagues[568] the *study-base principle*, is the most subtle. A few examples, provided here, help to illustrate this. Comparability of information is discussed in the exposure section of this chapter, and issues of confounding and power are discussed in the section on matching and in other parts of this book.

In the early 1970s, a case-control study was undertaken in Athens, Greece to assess the role of induced abortions in the etiology of ectopic pregnancy.[395] For each of 26 women with an ectopic pregnancy and at least one previous pregnancy, three controls were chosen from the maternity hospital, with matching for husband's education, as well as age during a pregnancy whose order corresponded to the ectopic pregnancy in the case. The three matching factors (i.e., husband's education, maternal age, and pregnancy order) were thought to be likely confounders. A highly significant odds ratio of 10 was estimated. Several years later, Weiss and his colleagues correctly pointed out that controls in that study were not representative of the study base.[584] This was not because matching was utilized. The problem was that controls were generally *completing* a pregnancy corresponding to the order of the ectopic pregnancy in the matched case. Other factors being equal, women completing a pregnancy were less likely to have an induced abortion at an earlier pregnancy. Such implicit restriction was not present among cases because ectopic pregnancy is usually diagnosed very early in the gestation period.

A new study of similar design was undertaken in a similar population in Athens in the late 1980s.[242] The new study used as controls women with a *newly diagnosed* pregnancy of the same order as the ectopic pregnancy in the corresponding case. In this instance, the odds ratio was 1.87. It is apparent that the controls were a genuine sample of the study base only in the latter study; in the former study, gestation was already beyond the stage at which an ectopic pregnancy is diagnosed. This by itself would not have made the control group of the former study unsuitable. Had the odds for a history of induced abortion(s) been similar among women in the early and the late stage of a pregnancy of a particular order, both control groups would have been appropriate; however, this was not the case.

The example presented in the section for *selection of cases* illustrates how diagnostic criteria change the study base and, accordingly, impose constraints on control selection so that the control group represents the altered study base. Similarly, an evaluation of the causes of male infertility must take into account that the study base comprises only heterosexual, mostly married, men who are attempting to father children. A control group comprising spouses of infertile women would be suitable for the evaluation of male factors, unless these factors were also associated with female infertility. Clearly, sexually transmitted diseases *are* associated between spouses and cannot be validly studied through such a control group.[477,568]

In general, selection bias will be introduced whenever controls are chosen through a process that, for whatever reason, is associated with the exposure under consideration in the study base. Thus, if thick and dense electrical distribution lines are more prevalent in low socioeconomic status neighborhoods, and less affluent young persons are less eager to participate as controls in epidemiological studies, selection bias will be introduced in a population-based study of adult cancer in relation to proximity to electrical distribution lines (an important source of exposure to magnetic fields). This is because cancer cases are usually independently ascertained through population-based registries or hospital discharge data. Controlling for all the selection factor(s) (i.e., socioeconomic status, age, gender) will eliminate the associated selection bias *for all other variables*, including exposure to thick and dense electrical wires (magnetic fields). Therefore, an appropriate stratified analysis or an adequately specified statistical model will generate unbiased estimates of the odds ratios for these other variables. The problem is that although age and gender may be accurately measured, socioeconomic status is not, and there may remain substantial selection-generated residual confounding by socioeconomic status.[42,417]

Occasionally, investigators may decide to restrict their case series to residents of a selected number of towns, to exclude patients older than 79 years, or to limit their study to the gender with the higher incidence of disease or the most common ethnic group(s). Exclusion and inclusion criteria for cases affect the designation of the respective secondary study base, and, accordingly, they should also apply to the controls. The process may occasionally follow the opposite direction: difficulty of identifying or enrolling controls of particular sociodemographic characteristics may lead to a changed study base and exclusion of both cases and controls that belong to groups with: (1) very low disease rates; (2) limited variability with respect to the principal exposure; (3) no opportunity for the disease (e.g., women with hysterectomy in a study of endometrial cancer); (4) questionable reliability of exposure information (e.g., the elderly); or (5) individuals exposed to a factor of overwhelming importance in a study of an exposure with weak etiologic potential (e.g., smokers in a study of lung cancer in relation to passive smoking). Exclusions of certain groups usually enhances feasibility and administrative efficiency and does not compromise internal validity.[458,568] The possibility of effect modification in the excluded groups can no longer be examined. However, the statistical power for assessment of effect modification is generally limited, and biological considerations offer better guidance in most instances. *Opportunity for exposure* should never be an exclusion criterion for particular cases and controls[416] because conditions that increase or reduce the likelihood of an exposure play an essential role in the causal process.

It has already been stated that, in principle, controls should form a representative sample of the study base for the case series. It has also been indicated that intentional or unintentional operation of selection factors during control recruitment (e.g., selection of more female than male controls for a disease that affects equally the two genders) will not affect the odds ratio estimates for other study variables if the selection factors are correctly identified, accurately measured, and appropriately controlled. The flexibility of the case-control method is further increased by the realization that even a control series *outside the study base* does not necessarily invalidate the study results.[357,358] Thus, in a hypothetical investigation of the association between blood group A (or histocompatibility antigens, or several other gender-independent genetic markers) and testicular cancer in young men, a control group of young women from the same population, clearly outside the study base but of the same ethnicity, might be acceptable because the exposure odds for blood group among young women should not be different from the corresponding exposure odds among young men in the same population. Robins and Pike[446] have shown that deterministic selection of controls (e.g., cases' best friends, cases' closest neighbors, a newborn delivered immediately before or after the birth of an affected newborn) can generate valid odds ratio estimates for most exposures if the case-defined mini-strata do not overlap, all subjects in every mini-stratum are utilized, and an analysis preserving the mini-strata structure is performed (stratified analysis or conditional logistic regression). Yet, if the exposure under study was itself involved in forging the friendship that made cases choose the friends they chose (e.g., drinkers tending to select drinkers and smokers tending to select smokers), or if the study factor is of a contagious nature, selection bias of unpredictable direction may ensue.[127]

Information on Exposure

Sources

The most common sources of information on the past experiences and characteristics whose etiologic relevance is examined in case-control studies are interviews with the patient or, in the case of diseases of children, with the parents. Other sources include interviews with relatives, hospital records, birth certificates, employment records, environmental data, and so forth.[14,199] Biomarkers are also being used with increased frequency. Case-control studies of serologic biomarkers of chronic infection with hepatitis B and C viruses have contributed to elucidation of the etiology of hepatocellular carcinoma,[241,544] and case-control studies of human papilloma virus detected through molecular hybridization techniques have pointed out the role of certain types of this virus in the causation of cervical cancer.[432,433,481] Strengths and limitations of biomarkers of exposure have been discussed in Chapter 9 and are considered in some detail by Pearce et al.[404]

Two characteristics of the information on exposure are important—comparability in cases and controls and validity. Information validity is a general concept but it usually applies to qualitative (categorical) exposures or dichotomized (or polychotomized) quantitative variables; for continuous untransformed variables the term information accuracy is commonly used.

Comparability of Information

If data on the exposure under study are inaccurate or incomplete, a spurious association may be introduced between the exposure and the disease when the inaccuracy or incompleteness affects cases and controls to a different degree (*information bias*). If only a fraction of the relevant events is reported (e.g., if only half the women who took a particular drug in early pregnancy can remember doing so), but this proportion is the same in both the cases and the controls, there will, if there is a true association, still be an association between the reported drug intake and the study disease. If there is no true difference, no apparent difference will emerge except in unusual situations (which are discussed later). However, if, for example, among subjects who took a medication, half the cases and only a quarter of the controls have the recollection of taking it, an erroneous conclusion will be reached. If there was no true association, one will appear, and if there was a positive association between the drug and the disease, it will be exaggerated. Conceivably, also, a higher frequency of taking the drug among the controls could be hidden. Lack of comparability between the accuracy or completeness of information in cases and controls is one of the common and serious criticisms that can be leveled against a case-control study.

There is little empirical evidence that information bias has compromised the results of properly designed and executed case-control studies, and it is a fair assumption that selection bias is a more serious problem than information bias in such studies.[106,136,302,427,570,586] Nevertheless, information bias must be carefully considered in the interpretation of results of even well-conducted studies, particularly when (1) questions are asked about exposures of a delicate nature, such as sexual practices, induced abortions, or income, because patients with serious diseases may be more forthcoming on such subjects than control subjects;[82,292] (2) the exposure information is based on sera or tissue samples collected over a long time period, because the duration of storage may differ between cases and controls or test results may have different time-dependent properties in cases and controls;[188,241] and (3) the questionnaire is so extensive and time consuming that less motivated persons, presumably more of them in certain categories of control subjects, provide less complete information. This appears to be the situation in several case-control studies of cancer in relation to diet, as assessed through semiquantitative food frequency questionnaires.[225] However, overreporting or more complete reporting by cases is likely to cover foods in general, rather than specific food items with a particularly high or low content of specific nutrients. When overreporting is general and the study focuses on particular nutrients or food groups, as is almost always the case, adjustment for reported energy intake[593,594] that is obviously associated with completeness of food reporting or overreporting substantially reduces the consequences of information bias from this source.[545] Clearly, the role of energy intake per se cannot be assessed with confidence in case-control studies, but the interpretation of this variable is difficult even in cohort investigations.[593,594]

Avoidance of Bias

Although it may be possible to determine that differences in accuracy or completeness of information exist between cases and controls, it is rarely possible to evaluate the extent of such differences and to take account of them adequately in the comparison. Therefore, every effort must be made to achieve comparability during the process of assembling the data. There are two basic considerations:

1. Achieving similarity in the procedures used to obtain information from cases and controls: To the extent possible, staff engaged in abstracting information from records should be unaware whether they are dealing with a case or a control. If the information to be obtained is of a medical or personal nature, it is unusual that an interview can be conducted without the interviewer becoming aware of the general state of health of the person being interviewed, but it may sometimes be possible to arrange that the interviewer does not know whether he or she is interviewing a case or a control. When this is arranged, it is useful for the interviewer to record at the end of the interview whether he or she became aware during the course of the interview whether the subject was a case or a control. To the extent possible, the place and circumstances of the interview should be similar. A given interviewer should interview equal proportions of cases and controls. As much effort should be made to gain cooperation and accurate response from controls as from cases.

2. Use of information recorded prior to the time of diagnosis of the present illness, wherever possible: For example, in a comparison of birth weights of children and controls with mental disabilities, birth certificates or hospital records would be superior to the mothers' memories as sources of information on birth weight, not only because of the ordinary deficiencies of human memory, but also because the hospital records were made prior to the identification of the child as having a disability. Although there is no more prolific source of data relative to a person's past experience than his or her own memory, this source suffers not only from people's propensity to forget or distort past events, but, most important in the present context, from the fact that such losses and distortions may be affected by subsequent events. For example, the fact that she, or her child, currently has a serious illness may alter a woman's recollection of the events that preceded the illness. In using data from interviews in which the case has a serious illness and the control does not, only factors of a highly objective nature can be compared with confidence.

Evidence of Comparability

Certain analytic procedures can be undertaken to evaluate to what extent a particular result could be explained by lack of comparability between cases and controls. Although one can never establish that two series are truly comparable, the greater the number and relevancy of the tests that can be applied without revealing lack of comparability, the greater the confidence in the belief that it is present in sufficient degree.

First, certain analyses can be conducted to determine whether the procedures planned to ensure comparability in the data collection have indeed been carried out. It is revealing evidence of compromised comparability between two series when a substantial difference is present in the proportions of individuals for whom data were not obtained. In the case of interview data, the times of the beginning and end of interviews can be recorded and the durations compared for evidence of greater interest on the part of the interviewers in one group than in the other. Interviewers, at the end of the interview, can be asked to classify each respondent with respect to level of reliability of his or her responses.

Second, cases and controls can be compared with respect to frequency of reporting of experiences or characteristics that seem unlikely to be relevant to the etiology of the disease under investigation. Such factors are sometimes referred to as validation or dummy variables. For example, in a case-control study of pancreatic cancer,[244] lack of association of the study disease with tonsillectomy, appendectomy, gastric ulcer, duodenal ulcer, gastritis, hemorrhoids, and hypertension was interpreted as evidence that the information provided by cases and controls was comparable *and* that the series were representative of the same study base. This, in turn, increased the confidence of the investigators that the apparent associations with diabetes mellitus, pancreatitis, and cholelithiasis were genuine.

It is, of course, difficult to be sure that any particular characteristic does not have etiologic relevance. At the same time, cases and controls would not be expected to differ with respect to a large number of such dummy variables, particularly if the difference always appeared in the direction explicable in terms of more complete reporting by the cases.

In addition to dummy variables, it may in some circumstances also be possible to examine what might be called a dummy disease; that is, a disease (or group of patients) that would not be expected to share the etiologic background of the true cases although they went through the same study procedures as the cases. For example, in a study of 1,465 patients with lung cancer, Doll and Hill[96] noted that the lung cancer patients differed from their controls in (1) giving a higher percentage of histories of smoking and in particular of heavy smoking, and (2) reporting a higher frequency of pneumonia and chronic bronchitis in the past. During the course of the same study, 335 patients with chest disease were interviewed in the belief that they had lung cancer. These patients were subsequently found not to have lung cancer and were excluded from the lung cancer series. Nevertheless, their histories were compared with those of the lung cancer patients and with those of the controls (patients with diseases other than lung cancer). It was found that, with respect to smoking habits, the incorrectly diagnosed group resembled the controls and not the lung cancer cases, but with respect to history of pneumonia and chronic bronchitis, they resembled the lung cancer cases rather than the controls. These comparisons suggest that: (1) the difference between the lung cancer cases and the controls in smoking habits was not the result of the patient or the interviewer knowing that the patient had lung cancer, and (2) there was a tendency for patients with diseases of the chest of all forms to report more pneumonia and chronic bronchitis than did patients with other diseases. "Unresolved" pneumonia was, at that time, a frequent misdiagnosis in early lung cancer, and its more frequent reporting among lung cancer cases, as among patients with other chest diseases, is readily explicable in nonetiologic terms.

A similar approach has also been followed in a planned systematic way. In the 1970s, an association between chronic infection with hepatitis B virus (HBV), ascertained through the detection of hepatitis B surface antigen (HBsAg) in the serum, and hepatocellular carcinoma (HCC) was demonstrated. However, there was no agreement as to whether the association was causal or a reflection of immunosuppression of the seriously sick HCC patients. HCC patients are also frequently hospitalized for preexisting chronic liver disease; therefore, they may acquire etiologically irrelevant but serologically indistinguishable HBV infections during late-life hospitalizations. To discriminate between these alternative interpretations, a case-control study was undertaken in Greece of 80 HCC cases, 160 hospital controls with diagnoses other than cancer or liver disease, and another series of 40 controls comprising patients with metastatic liver cancer (MLC).[544] The latter controls were valuable because patients with MLC share with HCC patients clinical symptomatology, clinical severity, potential for immunosuppression, and repeated adult-life hospitalizations, although their primary malignancy was probably unrelated to HBV. Frequency of detection of antibodies to hepatitis B antigens, indicating past but not chronic active infection with HBV, was equally elevated among patients with HCC and MLC in comparison to other hospital controls. This finding confirmed that HCC and MLC patients were indeed excessively exposed to HBV, probably during their previous hospitalizations, but indicated also that the detectable serologic pattern of *antibody* response to HBV is not crucial to HCC causation. In contrast, seroprevalence of HBsAg was much higher among HCC patients than among MLC patients or the other hospital controls. The value of a control series comprising patients with disease "imitating" or "phenocopying" the disease under investigation but having independent etiology(ies) has also been pointed out by other authors;[358,569] however, the procedure is not often used and its value has perhaps not been adequately appreciated.

If the disease under investigation is a common one, persons may be interviewed as controls but subsequently become cases because controls represent a sample of the study base from which the cases arise. For example, in a study of coronary heart disease in the population of the Health Insurance Plan of Greater New York (HIP), information on exposure variables (smoking, history, physical exercise, etc.) was obtained from the patients in a clinical setting after diagnosis of their illness, whereas for the controls—a randomly selected sample of the population—the information was sought by mail questionnaire. It was, therefore, important to assess the comparability of the data obtained on cases and controls, both because there was a nonresponse rate of 17 percent in the control series and because of the possibility that persons report differently in a clinical interview than in a mail questionnaire. The study report[491] contains many examples of the ways in which this comparability may be and was assessed, but, in the present context, the comparison of the two sets of information obtained for 156 persons who both answered the mail questionnaire and underwent interview is of particular interest. Similarly, Giovannucci et al.[148] compared prospectively and retrospectively assessed diets of women before and after they developed breast cancer in the Nurses Health Study cohort and demonstrated overreporting, or more complete reporting, of dietary intakes by the women after the diagnosis of breast cancer.[596,597] It is clearly important, although not always practical, for an investigator to contrive such dual sets of data; for example, reinterview at a later date a sample of one or both groups (cases or controls) under the circumstances that prevailed in the other group at the time of the original interview.

Lack of comparability can rarely be adequately addressed in the analysis. If cases and controls were interviewed in different proportions by interviewers with distinct operational styles that could have introduced *systematic* differences, controlling for interviewer identity in the analysis can minimize the associated bias. However, creation of different strata on the basis of presumed information quality (e.g., directly versus proxy-interviewed cases and controls) is generally ineffective.[178,568,578]

Validity of Information

Validity refers to the extent to which a situation as observed reflects the true situation or the situation as evaluated by other criteria that are thought to reflect the true situation more closely. In the present context, the term is used to refer to the extent to which subjects in a case-control study are correctly classified as to the presence or absence, or level, of an exposure of interest.

Sensitivity and Specificity

The concepts of sensitivity and specificity are illustrated by reference to the data in Table 10-1 taken from the study of Dunn and Buell[108] on the relation of circumcision of the sexual partner to risk of cancer of the cervix uteri. To evaluate the validity of histories of circumcision, a group of men was asked whether or not they had

Table 10-1. Comparison of Study Participants' Statements as to Circumcision Status with Physician's Findings at Examination

	Participants' statements			
	Completely circumcised		Partially or not circumcised	
Physician's findings	Number	Percent	Number	Percent
Completely circumcised	21	47.7	8	6.6
Partially or not circumcised	23	52.3	114	93.4
Total	44	100.0	122	100.0

Source: Adapted from Dunn JE Jr, Buell P. Association of cervical cancer with circumcision of sexual partner. *J Natl Cancer Inst* 1959;22 : 749–764.

been circumcised, and they were examined by a physician, whose opinion was assumed to represent reality. Of the men who said they had been circumcised, 52 percent were found to have at least some foreskin; of those who said that they had not been circumcised, 7 percent were found to have no foreskin. *Sensitivity* is the extent to which subjects who truly manifest a characteristic, or have truly experienced a certain exposure, are so classified. In the present example, the sensitivity of self-assessed complete circumcision is 21/29, or 72 percent. *Specificity* is the extent to which subjects who do not manifest a characteristic, or have not really experienced a certain exposure, are correctly classified. In this instance, it is 114/137, or 83 percent. Sensitivity and specificity are the essential components of information validity for qualitative variables because they incorporate the reproducibility (repeatability) of the reported, or otherwise assessed, information on exposure. The *predictive value* of a positive statement or finding is the proportion of persons who are truly exposed among those who declare themselves, or are otherwise identified, as such. The predictive value of a test depends not only on the sensitivity and specificity of the test, but also on the prevalence or incidence of the disease in a specific population. Unlike sensitivity and specificity, predictive value cannot be assumed to apply to populations other than that in which it is estimated. The predictive value provides little additional insight in the context of a case-control study that focuses on the odds ratio (rate ratio or risk ratio). By contrast, the predictive value of a positive finding or a statement is of major importance in screening programs or when rate differences (attributable rates) are the focus of an investigation.[69,139,455,456,564]

When the exposure variable is of quantitative or semiquantitative nature, such as nutritional intakes, validation requires the estimation of a suitably adjusted correlation coefficient between the interview-derived values of a particular nutrient and those based on a more reliable "standard" method that is presumed to reflect reality adequately (e.g., diet records over an extended time period).[440,593,595]

Reduced information validity implies more extensive exposure misclassification. If the parameters of misclassification differ between cases and controls then the issue is lack of comparability, a serious and frequently intractable problem. When the parameters of misclassification (sensitivity and specificity for qualitative variables; correlation measures for quantitative variables) are similar among cases and controls, the resulting misclassification is referred to as nondifferential. Nondifferential misclassification in the principal exposure variable *does* create information bias, but this bias has, as a rule, a predictable direction toward the distribution pattern predicted by the null hypothesis (no association between the principal exposure variable and the disease under study). The predictable direction of this bias, its tendency to obscure or hide genuine associations rather than exaggerate existing ones or create spurious relations, and the availability of methods for assessing the magnitude of this bias and properly correcting the empirical effect estimates[13,460,461] have all contributed to the consideration of nondifferential misclassification bias as a more benign form among the various types of possible biases in epidemiological research.

The text on nondifferential misclassification in Chapter 9 applies to case-control studies as well because case-control designs are alternative sampling approaches of underlying cohorts. The next section demonstrates the most common consequence of nondifferential misclassification using as an example a case-control study.

Nondifferential Misclassification of the Main Exposure

This section discusses the effects of nondifferential misclassification in a primary exposure variable of binary nature; that is, cases and controls can be either exposed or nonexposed, and both sensitivity and specificity are the same. Not considered here are situations in which the main exposure variable is multilevel or quantitative rather than binary, and situations in which the nondifferential misclassification applies to covariates (confounding variables) rather than the main exposure variable. In this circumstance, unless misclassification is so bad that the truly unexposed are labeled as exposed more frequently than the truly exposed, an association between the disease and the misclassified principal exposure will not be generated if a true association did not exist. Thus, if an association is observed, and one can be confident that misclassification errors apply equally to cases and controls, one can conclude that a true association exists that is *at least* as great as that observed. Indeed, random misclassification may reduce the association to a level so low that the particular study is unable to demonstrate it. Thus, nondifferential misclassification errors may lead to a false negative conclusion—a conclusion that no association exists when in fact one does.

We shall use as an example the previously introduced study of Dunn and Buell[108] on the relation of circumcision of the sexual partner to risk of cancer of the cervix. These authors calculated the effect of this misclassification on studies designed to evaluate various circumcision-focused hypotheses. For example, the rate ratio of cervical cancer in non-Jewish, compared to Jewish, white women in the United States is about five. If this ethnic difference is explained in terms of circumcision of Jewish males, the rate ratio associated with lack of circumcision must be at least five. Suppose that only complete circumcision—as is characteristic of Jewish males—confers protection, and that both partial and complete lack of circumcision are associated with a five times higher risk of cervical cancer. Then the apparent rate ratio of cervical cancer in their sexual partners associated with men's *statements* of not being circumcised can be calculated as follows:

$$\text{Apparent rate ratio} = \frac{(5w) + (1x)}{(5y) + (1z)}$$

where w is the proportion of men who say they are not completely circumcised and indeed are not

x is the proportion who say they are not completely circumcised but have complete circumcision

y is the proportion who say they are completely circumcised but are not

z is the proportion who say they are completely circumcised and indeed have complete circumcision.

Thus,

$$\text{Apparent rate ratio} = \frac{(5 \cdot 93.4) + (1 \cdot 6.6)}{(5 \cdot 52.3) + (1 \cdot 47.7)} = 1.5$$

Whereas an association could still be found between lack of complete circumcision and cancer of the cervix, it is much more difficult to document an association with a rate ratio of 1.5 than one with a rate ratio of 5.

Early work on the consequences of nondifferential misclassification in case-control studies can be found in papers by Rogot[452] and Newell.[382] More recent studies allow investigators to measure misclassification error on the basis of parallel *validation studies* and to correct relative measures of effect in cohort and case-control investigations for the consequences of this error on point and interval estimates.[13,460,461] The use of validation studies, their design, and their desirable size, are considered in several recent papers and texts.[168,440,593,595] Even when formal validation studies have not been undertaken, repeating interviews after a lapse of time, making multiple measurements of biochemical or environmental exposures, checking interview information against records, comparing different records against each other, and other such procedures can provide a useful insight on the nature and extent of misclassification errors. The simple but crude method to correct the estimated rate ratio for nondifferential misclassification error, described in the corresponding section of Chapter 9, is equally applicable in case-control studies.

In certain, rather unusual, situations, nondifferential misclassification in the main exposure variable can bias the corresponding odds ratio *away from the null value* (i.e., tends to exaggerate a real but weak association or a weak association that was generated by chance). There are four such types of situations, and they may be encountered in either cohort or case-control studies.

1. Misclassification is so extreme that an apparently "exposed" person is, in fact, more likely to be unexposed, and vice versa. This situation is very unlikely, except when a signal is systematically misinterpreted or a coding error is made.

2. There are several, rather than just two, levels of exposure. Depending on the level-specific sensitivity and specificity values, the exposure–response pattern may take different shapes, and the overall regression coefficient may overestimate the true regression coefficient.[105] This coefficient is an effect estimator and in logistic regression equals the natural logarithm of the odds ratio. Although distortion of the exposure–response curve is common, gross overestimation of effect is probably rare.

3. Exposure is expressed as a proportion or fraction, ranging from zero to one.[12] In this situation, true extreme values (near zero or near one) can only be misclassified toward the middle of the distribution. The resulting "contraction" in the independent variable (exposure) scale increases the slope of the exposure–response trend (regression coefficient, odds ratio). The phenomenon is more common in ecological studies,[39] but it may also be encountered in analytical investigations.

4. Measured exposure is a quantitative or semiquantitative variable, and the nondifferential (among cases and noncases) error is strongly *inversely* associated with the true exposure value.[565] This may occur when, for instance, people who drink too much tend to underreport consumption, whereas people who drink very little or not at all tend to overreport their intake. Again, in this situation, "contraction" in the exposure scale will increase (exaggerate) the slope of the exposure–response curve.

Nondifferential misclassification of covariates (control variables, confounding factors) reduces the ability to control confounding, and, depending on the direction of confounding, it can lead to either over- or underestimation of the effect, if any, of the main exposure variable.[160,459,553]

Confounding and Statistical Power

In the section on control selection, the four relevant considerations were presented and the most important among these—focusing on the need for cases and controls to share the same study base—was discussed in some detail. In the section on exposure information, procedures to avoid, evaluate, and correct for information bias were presented. In this section, the remaining two considerations are examined briefly.

There are important common elements in most aspects of design and analysis of cohort and case-control studies, but issues of genuine confounding (i.e., excluding those due to faulty study design or implementation and manifested as selection or information bias) are identical in both study types. Accordingly, the principles discussed in the context of cohort studies are equally relevant for case-control investigations.

In practice, likely confounders are identified among the risk factors for the disease under study, that is, on the basis of a priori information. However, their actual role in any particular research situation is assessed by comparing the effect estimate (odds ratio) before and after adjustment for the putative confounder. If one or more confounding factors have been identified, the confounding influence of additional factors should be assessed conditionally on (controlling for) the previously identified factors.[358,359,466,576]

The magnitude of confounding that is generated by a certain factor depends on: (1) the strength of the association of the factor with the disease under study among individuals (cases and controls) who have not experienced the principal exposure under investigation; (2) the strength of the association of the factor with the principal exposure under investigation among persons who have not experienced the disease under study (i.e., among controls); and (3) the prevalence of the factor. The confounding impact of the prevalence of a confounding factor is not easily discernible, but it has been elegantly demonstrated by Walker through three-dimensional diagrams.[576] As a rule, a factor with a very low (less than 0.05) or very high (more than 0.95) prevalence rarely generates substantial confounding.

Occasionally an attempt is made to interpret the results of a study in which a presumed confounding factor has not been accounted for. Estimation of the likely confounding influence of the unaccounted factor can be made on the basis of assumed values in the three previously indicated parameters, and a sensitivity analysis can provide some evidence about the robustness of the estimate.[16,495] This is an inexact approach that is compounded by the fact that the uncertainty added by the external variable(s) is not reflected in the effect estimator (e.g., the odds ratio). Nevertheless, control of confounding on the basis of external information can be useful in meta-analyses in which several studies have controlled for a likely confounder but a few have not. In those instances, none of the alternatives (i.e., exclusion of the latter studies, combining effect measures with different levels of adjustment, or attaching quality scores to the individual effect measures) is particularly attractive.[166,171] Exercises on the degree of confounding likely to be generated under various assumptions have demonstrated that, unless the omitted variables are both common and extraordinary powerful risk factors for the disease under study (e.g., age or tobacco smoking in the instance of cancer of the lung), the apparent odds ratio (confounded odds ratio) will rarely overestimate (or underestimate) the true odds ratio by more than a factor of two.

The statistical power of a case-control study with a binary exposure (yes, no) and without identifiable confounding can be easily calculated.[11,469,479] In general, the power is higher when the study is larger, although not proportionally so. For a given total study size, the power is higher when the numbers of cases and controls are about equal, and it is substantially lower when the numbers are very different. For a certain number of cases, a larger number of controls is associated with higher statistical power, but the degree of power increase declines as the ratio of controls to cases increases from 1 : 1 to 2 : 1 to 3 : 1, and so forth, so that, in general, beyond a ratio of about 6 : 1 there is little justification for increasing the number of controls. When the exposure is a multilevel ordered variable or a quantitative one (e.g., number of cigarettes smoked per day, an antibody titre), the power of the study can be substantially higher if there is indeed a monotonic exposure–response relation to the occurrence of the disease. Finally, an increased range of variation of the principal exposure variable in the study base is reflected in higher statistical power in the corresponding case-control study.

The requirements for statistical power must be judged in conjunction with practical and economic considerations. Certain sources of controls are more easily and cheaply accessible than others. Greater amounts of information would be obtained if data were obtained for as many controls as possible in the selected source, but economic considerations usually force compromise between what is desirable and what is feasible.

Confounding variables are, by definition, correlated with exposure, and an appropriate analysis should control for them through stratification or statistical modeling. Within any particular stratum of a confounder, the range of the principal exposure is reduced, more so when the confounder is an important one. Therefore, the presence of confounding variables and the contemplated stratified analysis impose power restrictions. To compensate for confounding-imposed power reduction, the number of cases and/or controls should be increased. A rule of thumb that is difficult to defend except by invoking "experience" is that for every recognizable major confounder the study size should be increased by about 10 percent to preserve statistical power at the level that would have been achieved in the absence of the confounder.

Nondifferential misclassification of any confounding variable results in reduced ability to control adequately for the confounding influence. Therefore, the odds ratio for the principal exposure under study remains partially confounded, even though stratification or modeling has been undertaken to control for the (misclassified) confounding variable.[160,553] The direction of residual confounding is the same as that of the confounding that was originally present, that is before stratification or modeling were introduced, and its size depends on the extent of the nondifferential misclassification. Indeed, residual confounding must always be suspected whenever control for an apparently misclassified variable changes the deviation of the crude odds ratio from the null value of 1 by more than, perhaps, 2/3 (e.g., from 2.0 to 1.3, or from 0.4 to 0.8).[542] A method to correct odds ratio estimates and their confidence limits for nondifferential confounder misclassification has been presented by Rosner, Spiegelman, and Willett.[459]

Sources and Methods for Control Selection

In discussing sources and methods of selection of control groups, reference will be made to the four objectives previously indicated. We must stress, however, that the weighing of the many separate aspects of these broad questions to arrive at specific decisions in a particular study is difficult. The decisions are often the ones most critical to the establishment of confidence in the results of case-control studies.

Before selecting individual controls, it is necessary to establish the source of the cases, that is, the person-time study base from which cases are generated and from which controls must be selected. An important consideration is whether or not the cases represent all the newly affected individuals over a specified time period in a defined population (primary study base). If they do, then the control group should also be drawn from that population over the same time period. They should either be representative of the primary base or the ways in which they are unrepresentative should be known—either because they have been deliberately introduced or because they follow from the method of selection from the population. If the cases are selected because they attended a particular hospital or clinic, then it is preferable to find a source of controls that shares as far as possible those selective processes by which the cases came to attention; for example, persons who, if they had the disease under investigation, would also be likely to attend the same hospital or clinic. The most common types of study bases and, accordingly, sampling frames for control selection are considered.

Controls from a Population Explicitly Defined

A population that can be defined with criteria external to the particular case-control study may be an administratively defined population or an otherwise identified primary study base (e.g., all live births in a community or in a single maternity hospital). This is an appropriate source only when the cases represent all, or the great majority, of cases occurring in this population. When this situation exists, this source is in theory one that can be sampled with assurance that it represents the study base that gave rise to the patients. Moreover, the definition of the study base can accommodate any exclusions that the investigator wants to apply in case ascertainment, such as exclusion of men and very young women in a study of breast cancer. In addition, the distribution of the primary exposure and other covariates among controls reflects the situation in the primary study base and allows calculations of absolute incidence rates among exposed and unexposed persons, as well as incidence differences. However, the use of population controls also poses certain difficulties. If the information of interest must be obtained from the persons themselves, nonresponse rates are nearly always appreciably higher in randomly or otherwise selected members of the general population than in persons under medical care. In addition, the usual concerns regarding differences in quality of information provided by cases and controls will be reinforced if the circumstances of the interview are different; for example, if cases are interviewed in the hospital and controls must be interviewed at home. Furthermore, selection and interview of a sample of the population are generally more expensive and time consuming than use of other potential sources of control groups.[276,569]

When the likelihood of seeking or receiving medical care depends on socioeconomic factors, the externally defined population may not represent the primary study base for cases brought to medical attention. In this instance, a case-defined (secondary) study base must be conceptualized and implicitly sampled, possibly through accrual of hospital controls.[66,576]

Having established the source from which the controls will be drawn, it is necessary to decide whether the data from the cases will be compared with data on all the individuals who might be available from the primary base or whether a sample will be selected. If a sample is decided on, a choice must be made between the sampling options available. It has been said that the selection of the source of a control group is more important than the method of sampling individuals from that source.[62] Although this may be true, it is also true that, however satisfactory its source, the usefulness of a control group can be seriously impaired by unsatisfactory sampling or selective yield.

Total Population—No Sampling

When the base population can be identified and is chosen as the source of a control group, it may be possible to use data on the total population. Clearly, this is practical only when data on the frequency of the factors under examination (primary exposures and confounders) are recorded routinely for the total study base. For example, in studies of diseases of early life (or of diseases of later life for which influences operative in early life are suspected), it may be possible to obtain, for all the cases in a defined base population, information on such variables as birth weight, parity, and age of parents. The information may be compared with data for the same variables routinely published in vital statistics for all births in the same area.[313] Computerized files increase the opportunities for studies of this type. However, the kinds of detailed historical information required in case-control studies is rarely available on a routine basis.

Random and Systematic Sampling

A random sample is one that was drawn in such a way that each member of the total group to be sampled had an equal chance of being represented; for example, each individual may be numbered and the persons for the study selected through a table of random numbers. A systematic sample is one in which the group to be sampled is placed in some sort of order and then individuals are selected systematically throughout the series, such as every second, hundredth, or thousandth individual. Provided the order in which the group is placed prior to systematic sampling is not structured with respect to some variable directly or indirectly important to the study, the characteristics of a systematic sample are similar to those of a random sample, and similar tests of statistical significance may be applied. The distinction between these two methods, therefore, is not of great importance in most situations, and the choice of one of the other methods depends primarily on the practicability of each in a given situation. This is contrary to the situation in clinical trials where, because of the greater opportunities for subversion of a systematic sampling procedure, random sampling is preferred over systematic methods.

Random or systematic samples are often used in the selection of controls when a listing of all the potential controls is available. Various types of listings with national coverage have been developed in Scandinavian countries and have been used for the undertaking of large nested case-control studies.[4] In the United States, such listings, regularly revised, exist for the residents of the state of Massachusetts,[68] for Medicare recipients nationwide,[200] and, increasingly, for subscribers to major managed care organizations.

To obtain a representative sample, the procedures for random or systematic sampling must be followed explicitly and carefully. No confidence can be placed in a sample that is selected haphazardly. Bias resulting from haphazard selection is frequent and has long been recognized.[320,587] For example, haphazard selection from lists of names may be influenced by the length of the name (relating to ethnicity), its position on the page, or the legibility of the handwriting (possibly related to hospital service and hence to diagnosis). Haphazard selection from files of cards or records may select those that are thicker or more worn and, therefore, of greater medical interest.

When a listing of persons in the primary study base is not available, an attempt can be made to generate a random sample of population controls through the procedure of random digit dialing (RDD). The premise of RDD is that in a population with virtually complete telephone coverage, every individual has, or can be made to have through a preliminary contact assessing household structure, an equal probability of selection.[159,197,198,276,569] It should be obvious that this premise is difficult to fulfill; answering machines, call forwarding, socioeconomic and lifestyle factors, and the attitude toward what may be perceived as an intrusion can all generate selection bias of unknown magnitude and direction. In defense of RDD, one may argue that it represents one of the few realistic options in the quest for a random sample of population controls. Whether the option is satisfactory for epidemiological investigations remains unresolved. It is worth recognizing that the lineage of RDD as an epidemiological tool can be traced to telephone-based market research and electoral surveys. In none of the latter situations does misrepresentation of the study base have the long-lasting impact that the results of an epidemiological study of compromised validity can have.

Paired Sampling

When an externally defined population serves as the primary study base but no listing of persons in the base is available, an alternative to RDD is to utilize paired sampling. Pairing does not imply that just one control will be chosen for each case, nor does it necessitate that the same number of controls will be available for every case, as long as the varying ratio can be accommodated in the analysis. Pairing is regularly used in *matched designs*, but the two concepts are not equivalent. Whereas matching explicitly identifies matching variables and values, the objective of pairing is to provide a scheme for control selection that minimizes subjectivity and arbitrariness during this process and, accordingly, guards against selection bias. Pairing is also commonly applied when a secondary or case-defined study base is conceptualized as the sampling frame for control selection; therefore, it is used when hospital patients, associates of the cases, or relatives of the cases are used as controls. It is worth noting that although no specific matching factors are involved in simple pairing, there may be implicit indirect matching on some factor(s), usually of a vague socioeconomic nature, that could impose consideration of matched analysis.

As indicated, pairing may be required as a process for control selection when a listing of individuals does not exist in the primary or the secondary study base and a procedure such as RDD is considered unreliable or ineffective (e.g., when telephone coverage is incomplete). For example, if the controls are to be drawn from persons living in the same neighborhoods as the patients, how far do these neighborhoods extend? Similarly, if the sample is to be drawn from other patients attending the same hospital as the cases, it may not be realistic or desirable to wait until the total number of such patients is known before beginning to assemble the control sample. In these situations, paired sampling involves the selection from the sampling frame of one or more controls for each case. Individuals are selected by virtue of some defined temporal or geographic relationship to the case, such as the next patient (or next two patients, etc.) admitted after the case, the person living in the nearest residence to that of the case, or the student next to the case in an alphabetical class listing.

The rules for selection must be clearly defined and adhered to. For example, in the selection of a neighborhood paired sample, it will be necessary to specify whether the interviewer goes to the right or the left of the patient's house, what the procedure is in the case of two-family and apartment houses, and so forth. The fact that nobody is at home at the time the interviewer calls is not an adequate reason for rejection of the selected control because the probability of all members of a family being away from home at any moment is highly correlated with family size and other demographic characteristics. Once an individual has been selected, the use of alternative selectees always raises the question of whether the omission of the difficult-to-locate group biases the sample.

Controls from a Secondary Study Base

Whenever the cases in a case-control study are derived from a person-time base population that cannot be administratively circumscribed or otherwise explicitly defined, controls must be representative of the secondary or case-defined study base. This condition arises, for example, when the cases are identified from hospitals whose catchment area(s) cannot be specified, from disease registries that are not population based, and from medical practices or clinics serving patients with variable place of residence, health insurance, or referral pattern. In situations such as these, controls may be chosen from among other hospital (or registry, medical practice, or clinic) patients; friends, neighbors, or associates of the cases; or the patients' relatives. In all these instances, pairing or another algorithm is commonly used for actual control selection.

Patients of Hospitals or Other Health Care Institutions

Other patients attending the same hospital or institution as the cases may be used as a source of controls. One assumption underlying this choice is that patients with other diseases are subject to the same selective factors that influenced the cases to utilize this particular institution. For example, if the cases in the study are taken from a hospital located in an area inhabited by a particular ethnic group, the control group drawn from other patients attending the same hospital is likely to have the same ethnic distribution as the study group. Of course, ethnic group can be identified through interview and, even if cases and controls differed in their distribution by this variable, there would have been no confounding by it if ethnic group were taken into account in a suitably stratified analysis or statistical modeling of the data. However, other variables that may be related to the principal exposure(s) under study may not be so easy to identify and measure (e.g., socioeconomic characteristics, environmental conditions, distance from the hospital). Control selection from among other patients of the same hospital increases the likelihood that cases and controls share the same study base.[311] Nevertheless, complete confidence that selection bias did not affect the results of a particular study is rarely warranted; it is always possible that the catchment area of a certain hospital is different for some diseases because of the reputation, or lack thereof, of the institution or its staff.

Even when all cases in a defined population can be studied and facilities for population sampling are available, the question of whether apparently healthy members of the population are preferable to hospital patients as a source of controls is by no means clear. The major disadvantage of hospital controls is, of course, that they are ill and may therefore be unrepresentative of the study base with respect to disease-causing exposures and other variables associated with these exposures.[357,358,568] However, controlling for the selection factors in the analysis will remove selection bias for all other variables, assuming that the selection factors can be identified and accurately measured.[41,42,358,446,568] Moreover, response proportions and validity of exposure information are likely to be superior as well as comparable if both cases and controls are interviewed in the hospital than if they are interviewed under different circumstances. For any particular study, these advantages and disadvantages must be weighed in light of the nature of the cases, their source, and the type of information to be collected.

The question will arise whether a control group should be drawn from all patients attending the hospital or only from patients with certain diseases that are believed not to be associated with the factors being studied. For example, should the dietary habits of a series of patients with colorectal cancer be compared with those of a sample of all patients in the same hospital or with those of a particular diagnostic group, such as accident cases? The appeal of the second course is that if there are diseases other than colorectal cancer that are influenced by diet, the all-patients-in-the-hospital group will be unrepresentative of the study base with respect to diet, and an association between colorectal cancer and diet could partly or wholly reflect the effect of diet on diseases other than colorectal cancer. By contrast, if a diagnostic category can be identified that is known not to be influenced by diet, then the control group having that diagnosis can be assumed to represent the base population in this respect, and an association between colorectal cancer and diet can be presumed to be a true reflection of the influence of diet on cancer of the large bowel. The practical difficulty of this approach is that of identifying a diagnostic category that is firmly known to be representative of the base population with respect to study factors. Consequently, if a difference is found in a situation where the controls were drawn from a single diagnostic category, it may become difficult to decide with confidence whether it is the cases or the controls that differ from the base population.

On the whole, it is preferable to include in the control group patients with several diseases that are believed to be unrelated to the exposure under study. Inclusion of several rather than only one or two such diagnoses in the control group minimizes the impact of any possible future report implicating the principal study exposure in the etiology of one of the control diseases. In addition, patients diagnosed with one or more diseases known to be related to the principal study exposure could be included as an additional control group; they would be as useful to the epidemiological study as are "positive control samples" in laboratory analyses. Given the wealth of information already available about the risk profile of many chronic diseases,[543] it makes sense to stress inclusion criteria more than exclusion criteria for the choice of diagnostic categories in the control series.[358]

The temptation to use persons who have no known disease but are examined at the hospital (e.g., healthy individuals attending a screening or cancer detection clinic) should be resisted. Such persons are usually markedly different with regard to socioeconomic status, ethnic background, and other such factors from patients who come to the same hospital because of illness. Healthy "patients" should be distinguished from the healthy hospital visitors who have been used as controls in some studies.[244,251] Visitors to hospital patients have several advantages: they are apparently healthy, able to be interviewed in the hospital setting, likely to represent the same study base as the patients, and more cooperative than general population controls. However, their availability and cooperation may depend on cultural norms, and there have been few studies documenting their utility.

Inclusion or exclusion of several diagnoses from the control series should always refer to admission diagnoses for the current hospitalization and not to past diagnoses, whether these required hospitalization or not. Thus, in a study focusing on diet in relation to colorectal cancer, patients currently admitted for diabetes mellitus (who are likely to have a diet that does not accurately represent the dietary intakes in the study base) should not be included in the main control group. However, patients with a *history* of diabetes mellitus should not be excluded from the control series, unless a decision is made to exclude them from the case series as well.[299,358] The latter option may have to be considered when there is suspicion that patients with a control disease diagnosis (e.g., osteoarthritis) are more likely to be hospitalized when they also have a history of diabetes mellitus than when they do not (leading to overrepresentation, among controls, of the dietary habits that are associated with diabetes). This is an example of the bias pointed out by Berkson, which is a form of selection bias.[24]

When cases with a particular type of cancer are identified through a cancer registry, controls are sometimes chosen from among those registered with other types of cancer. A similar approach may be used for case-control studies based on other types of disease or death registries. In such instances, proportional incidence or mortality analyses have been utilized. It has been pointed out[360] that the case-control method represents an improvement over the traditional proportional mortality analysis,[269] although neither approach can distinguish between the alternative interpretations imposed by the proportional allocation of all deaths to mutually exclusive and collectively exhaustive diagnostic categories of causes of death. In more general terms, use of dead controls challenges the principle that controls should be representative of the study base that has generated the corresponding cases because the dead are not at risk for developing the disease under study. Only when there is positive evidence that the distribution of the relevant exposures is the same in a series of decedents as in the properly identified study base can the series be used as a control group.[154,276,341,342,569]

When cases are dead or seriously incapacitated, interviews with proxy respondents may be obtained. Because live controls are generally more appropriate than dead controls, the question arises of whether the controls should be interviewed or proxy respondents should be obtained for them as well. Proxy interviews should be used for both dead cases and their living controls in the following situations: (1) when proxy respondents systematically overestimate or underestimate the exposures of living controls, (2) when the responses of living controls and their proxies are poorly correlated, and (3) when there is no information available about the nature and strength of the association between responses provided by the living controls and their proxies. When some cases and their controls are directly interviewed, while proxy respondents are used for the rest of the cases and their controls, stratification by respondent type is likely to demonstrate an apparent effect modification (the odds ratio is likely to be closer to the null value in the proxy respondents stratum because nondifferential misclassification of exposure is more extensive among them), but the overall odds ratio will not be noticeably affected.[282,341,342,568,569,578] The relevant issues are sufficiently complex to justify the advice that proxy respondents should be avoided whenever possible.

More than one control series is rarely justified, unless the different series serve different research objectives. For example, in a study of viral and nutritional factors in the etiology of hepatocellular carcinoma,[188] it became apparent that no single hospital control group could satisfy both objectives. As indicated in the exposure section of this chapter, patients with metastatic liver cancer form an appropriate control group for assessing the importance of viral exposures; however, several types of cancer have nutritional component causes, and a control group of patients with metastatic liver cancer is clearly not suitable for evaluating the importance of diet in the etiology of hepatocellular carcinoma.

Many epidemiological studies of the etiology of cancer and other chronic diseases have been of case-control design and have utilized hospital controls. Even during the relatively recent period 1980–1984, half of all case-control studies of cancer have relied on hospital controls.[291] It is fair to say that much of what is currently known about the epidemiology and etiology of cancer and other chronic diseases has first been reported from hospital-based case-control studies. Yet, these studies have occupied a prominent role in many of the past and current controversies, and they have also generated results that have not been subsequently confirmed. The collective evidence, therefore, highlights both the substantial potential of these studies and their enormous complexity.

Deterministic Selection of Controls

A deterministic selection of controls involves choosing every case's best friend(s), every case's closest neighbor(s), or every case's siblings, for example, as controls. The theory for valid deterministic selection of controls has been explored by Robins and Pike.[446] It requires that the secondary study base is divided into nonoverlapping mini-strata (each including a case and his or her best friend(s), a case and his or her closest neighbor(s), etc.); that all subjects in every mini-stratum be utilized; that the exposure under study (e.g., tobacco smoking or alcohol drinking) is not itself a contributor to the formation of the friendship or neighborhood mini-strata; and that the analysis preserves the mini-strata structure. Some of these requirements are difficult to satisfy; for instance, friends and neighbors may belong to overlapping strata.[15] Moreover, case-control mini-strata are frequently formed under the influence of factors that may themselves be the exposures under study (e.g., occupation, tobacco smoking, alcohol drinking). In this situation, selection bias of unpredictable direction is likely to be introduced, and this cannot be easily evaluated.[127] Finally, precision-reducing overmatching may be introduced during the formation of the mini-strata, but this is rarely a major concern and does not compromise validity if an appropriate analysis is undertaken (matched analysis or conditional logistic regression). Although there are several subtle issues in the theory of deterministic control selection, it appears that gross errors can be avoided if the exposure under study is not instrumental to the formation of the case-defined strata and the analysis takes into account the implicit matching process.

Neighborhood Controls. Neighborhood controls can be identified through residents' lists or local inquiry and may be used in studies with either a primary or a secondary study base. They have some advantages, including an implicit control for confounding socioeconomic factors that may be hard to identify and/or measure and apparent freedom from health-related selection factors. However, they also have several drawbacks: cooperation may be limited and refusal proportions high; hospital catchment areas may not be congruent with neighborhood definitions; cost may be high; and the ability to identify neighborhood controls contemporaneously with cases may be compromised by delays in case identification, population mobility, and absence of suitable directories.

Friends and Associates. Friends and associates may be identified by the cases or be selected on the basis of having shared with the cases attendance at the same school, similar place of employment, and so forth. Controls of these types are likely to have similar socioeconomic profile with cases and similar access to health care. Moreover, they are likely to be healthy and willing to cooperate. Nevertheless, friend controls and, to a lesser extent, controls among cases' associates are likely to introduce selection bias and some degree of overmatching.[127,446] Selection of friends by cases on the basis of presumed willingness to cooperate may also introduce sociability-related and gregariousness-related bias that could be reflected in some of the study exposures. Finally, it is doubtful that friends or work associates meet the deterministic control selection assumptions previously indicated.[276,446]

Relatives of the Cases. Two types of relatives are commonly used as sources of controls—spouses and siblings. Both groups are generally similar in ethnic and social background to the cases. This is usually an advantage because it eliminates certain spurious associations. However, if the study factor itself is one in which close relatives are likely to be similar, for example, diet, smoking history, or genetic background, they will not constitute a suitable control group.[127]

Use of sibling controls allows unusual control over genetic and socioeconomic factors that may be confounding.[411] Sibship relationships form strata that fully satisfy the criteria for deterministic control selection.[446] Conditional logistic regression modeling makes it possible to analyze data dispersed in many strata, each comprising one case and a variable number of sibling controls while allowing for control of additional variables such as age and gender. Clearly, cases with no siblings cannot contribute in this analysis, and factors such as sibship size or stable parental characteristics cannot be evaluated because of extreme overmatching. In general, the feasibility of using sibling controls will depend on the average family size, population mobility, the sources of the information to be assembled, and other factors that will determine whether at least one sibling control will be available for an adequate proportion of the cases.

Matching

In the context of a case-control study, matching describes a pairing recruitment process to select controls identical to the cases with respect to one or more potentially confounding variables. Matching is usually undertaken by tying one or more controls to every individual of the case series in what is described as *individual matching.* A process that is conceptually and methodologically similar but considerably less practical is *frequency matching.* In frequency matching, the study base to be sampled is divided into subgroups according to the chosen variables, and different proportions—corresponding to the distribution in the case series—are selected from each subgroup. For example, if the cases contain four times as many males as females, four times as many individuals would be selected from the male subgroups of the base population as from the female subgroups. The use of frequency matching (or stratified matching) in case-control studies has some considerable disadvantages. In the first place, because of lack of the necessary information, it is often very difficult to subdivide the population to be sampled. Second, the necessity to know the final composition of the patient series means that the controls cannot be assembled until after the case series is complete. This may mean that all the controls would be interviewed after the cases were interviewed, which could be undesirable. For these reasons, frequency matching is unusual in case-control studies.

Matching can also be employed in cohort studies by matching individually or collectively (frequency matching) unexposed to exposed individuals. In cohort studies, individual matching with constant ratio of unexposed-to-exposed individuals (or similarly balanced frequency matching) eliminates confounding by the matching variables *even when a crude analysis is undertaken* that takes no account of the matching process. An analysis that takes matching into account (through stratification or through suitable modeling of the data) is needed (1) when there is variability in the matching ratio, in order to achieve validity; and (2) always, in order to maximize study efficiency (i.e., to minimize the standard error of the effect estimates).[179] Readers familiar with analysis of variance (ANOVA) procedures will recognize the analogy with the two-way ANOVA methods.[11,175,505] Moreover, in matched cohort studies, it is always possible to evaluate the main effect(s) of the matching factor(s) on disease outcome, as well as possible effect modification(s) involving the matching factor(s).

Matching in Case-Control Studies

Matching has different objectives in case-control studies than in cohort studies, and these have been lucidly described by Rothman.[466] Control of confounding in case-control studies *requires stratification by levels of the confounding variable(s) (or appropriate modeling of the data) whether or not matching has been undertaken.* This is because matching introduces in case-control studies, *but not in cohort studies*, a bias toward the null that can only be removed through stratification. In other words, matching has different implications in cohort and case-control studies. In the former, it can achieve control of the original confounding even in the absence of stratification; in the latter, it can accomplish control of the original confounding, but, at the same time, it introduces a novel confounding, always toward the null, that can only be removed through stratification. The different consequences of matching on cohort and case-control studies are due to the fact that in cohort studies matching imposes a constraint on exposure through the confounder-exposure association, but not on outcome that has yet to occur. By contrast, in case-control studies, matching is constrained by both exposure and disease status and tends to force the association under study toward the null. Stratification eliminates the within-strata association between the confounder and exposure and "frees" the exposure-disease association from the design-imposed bias toward the null. It should be stressed that the matching-generated bias in the crude analysis is always toward the odds ratio value of one, irrespective of the nature of the association under study (positive or inverse) or the association between exposure and the confounder(s).

Given the complexity of matching in case-control studies, the additional effort and time needed to identify matching controls, and the requirement for stratified analysis (or appropriate modeling of the data) whether or not matching for particular confounder(s) has been undertaken, one may wonder why should matching even be considered? The answer is that in a stratified analysis there should be a balanced number of cases and controls in all or most of the strata in order for the study to retain the highest statistical power that can be expected on the basis of the available number of cases and controls. For instance, if age and gender are recognized confounders of an association, there would be little power in a large study in which most cases were very old men whereas most controls were very young women. This is an unrealistic example, but realistic ones abound. Thus, gravidity (number of pregnancies) is a risk factor for ectopic pregnancy and is positively associated with number of induced abortions. In an unmatched study of induced abortions in relation to ectopic pregnancy, a very large number of control women would be needed to have a few with gravidity sufficiently high to serve as appropriate controls for the numerous high gravidity cases, unless individual matching for gravidity were employed.[242] The situation is more extreme when there is reason to believe that confounding could be generated by so-called *random factors*.[260] A random factor is a variable that can take a very large number of nominal values that cannot be logically grouped and cannot be accommodated in a stratified analysis unless the variable were explicitly or implicitly matched for during the paired sampling of controls. Such variables are neighborhood, sibship, date, hospital ward, and so forth. Thus, the objective of matching in case-control studies is improvement of efficiency (statistical power, precision of estimates) and not assurance of validity—only adequate stratification (or appropriate modeling of the data) can safeguard validity.

The Matching Process

When it is decided to select an individually matched series, it is usually preferable to use the method of paired sampling as described previously, with the additional requirement that the individuals selected from the base population must match the corresponding case with respect to specified criteria. The selected control would then be, for example, not necessarily the next person admitted to the hospital but the next person admitted who satisfied the defined criteria.

If it is decided to match on a quantitative variable, it is also necessary to specify how close the match must be. For example, must age match within 1 year or 5 years? The decision is based partly on matters of practicality. If a large sampling frame is available, quite narrow limits may be specified, and close similarity with respect to the matched variable may be achieved. However, criteria that are difficult to satisfy lead to added expense and loss of study material because cases that cannot be matched must be excluded. Yet, if the matching variable is a strong confounder, loose matching may allow room for residual confounding.[160,553]

Indications and Contraindications

On the basis of the outlined theory, there are several situations, not necessarily mutually exclusive, for which matching should be considered in case-control studies.

1. The more unusual the distribution of cases with respect to a particular confounding variable, the less overlap there will be in unmatched groups and the less efficient the approach of controlling confounding factors will be in the analysis.

2. Matching may be useful in small studies of rare diseases with several confounding variables of nominal value, each of them with several categories.

3. Only matching can accommodate confounding by unmeasurable variables or random factors;[260] these variables can be implicitly matched for during paired control selection (e.g., neighborhood or sibling controls).

4. Exact matching for a continuous variable allows optimal control of the associated confounding, whereas logistic regression of unmatched data may fail to stipulate the most appropriate model.[42,570]

5. Matching tends to increase efficiency per subject studied, but the gain is substantial only when the matched factor is a strong confounder.[176,466,529,570]

There are also considerations weighing against matching in case-control studies:

1. The main effects of matched variables cannot be evaluated, so that matching should be restricted to either established risk factors for the disease or random factors such as neighborhood, sibship, or date.

2. Control of additional confounders, beyond those already matched for, cannot be accomplished through stratification; it requires either modeling of the data through conditional logistic regression or breaking the matching and applying de novo stratification or unconditional logistic regression, with some loss of statistical efficiency.

3. Modification of the effect of the main study variable(s) by any of the matched variables can only be evaluated in multiplicative models (a minor drawback because the analytic procedures of choice, the Mantel-Haenszel method and logistic regression, are inherently multiplicative).[530]

4. When matching on several variables is attempted simultaneously, matching controls may not be available for some of the cases, which, accordingly, will have to be excluded.[533]

5. Matching usually introduces cost and complexity and may considerably prolong the duration of a study. Indeed, the improved statistical power per study subject (increased size efficiency) may be negligible in comparison to the additional cost required for the implementation of a matched design (reduced cost efficiency). In such a situation, it is preferable to avoid matching and, instead, to attempt to reach the necessary statistical power by increasing the total study size in an unmatched design.[466,570]

6. The consequences of nondifferential exposure misclassification are more serious in matched than in unmatched studies.[161]

Overmatching

When considering whether or not to use a matched control sample and which variables, if any, should be used in the matching process, it is important to note that, although often helpful, matching can also be harmful in some circumstances,[353,358,466] *even when matching is accounted for in the analysis through stratification or conditional logistic regression* (see the relevant discussions in the analysis section). There are two particular situations in which matching should not be undertaken in order to avoid overmatching. First, variables intermediate in the causal pathway between the study factor and the disease should not be matched. For example, if smoking alters blood cholesterol, which in turn is causally associated with cardiovascular disease, smoking would be considered a cause of cardiovascular disease. Yet, in a case-control study, if cases and controls were matched on cholesterol levels, no association of the disease with smoking would emerge. Indeed, substantial reduction of the odds ratio linking a certain exposure to a particular disease after matching for a suspected "intermediate" factor represents powerful circumstantial evidence that the factor represents an intermediate step in the causal or pathogenetic process. Second, factors should not be matched that are related to the suspected cause but not to the disease. For example, if contraceptive use were related to religion but religion were not related to the disease under study, it would be inappropriate to match on religion. The consequences of matching in this situation would be some loss of statistical efficiency of the study, although the odds ratio estimate would not be changed in a predictable way. It is, of course, not always clear whether a factor that is known to be strongly associated with the exposure of interest is also related to the disease. In such a circumstance, the decision to match may be made on the basis that the risk of loss of statistical efficiency (if the factor turns out not to be related to the disease) is more acceptable than the risk of introducing spurious associations (if the factor is indeed related to the disease).

Table 10-2 summarizes the impact of matching and subsequent stratification (or conditional modeling of the data) in case-control studies, according to the associations or lack thereof, of the external factor with either or both the exposure under study and the disease. Overmatching is present in situations four and five.

Two other issues need to be considered in the context of matching. First, if the matching factor (e.g., neighborhood, friendship) was implicitly associated with the exposure under study (e.g., residential outdoor pollution, drinking habits), selection bias may ensue because of misrepresentation of the study base,[127] in addition to overmatching of the type indicated in situation number four of Table 10-2. Second, matching on an alternative indicator of the exposure under study (e.g., matching for particulate air pollution when atmospheric sulfur dioxide is examined as an air pollution indicator in relation to chronic obstructive pulmonary disease) or matching for an alternative indicator of the disease (e.g., matching for forced vital capacity that is part of the definition of chronic obstructive pulmonary disease) can also lead to bias.[41,570] This is because matching for particulates removes from sulfur dioxide concentration its original meaning as an air pollution indicator (particulates and sulfur dioxide should now be evaluated jointly to indicate air pollution), and matching for forced vital capacity removes from the label "chronic obstructive pulmonary disease" its original and generally understood conceptual content. Situations such as these, however, are uncommon.

Analysis

The introduction to the analysis section of the chapter on cohort studies (Chapter 9) and many of the issues considered in that section are also relevant to case-control studies because investigations of the latter design are only sampling alternatives to investigations of the former type. Detailed expositions of available procedures can be found in the books by Breslow and Day,[42] Kleinbaum, Kupper, and Morgenstern,[259] Schlesselman,[480] and Clayton and Hills,[61] whereas several other texts focus on the con-

Table 10-2. Impact of Matching and Subsequent Stratifying for an External Factor (F) in a Case-Control of Disease (D) in Relation to a Certain Exposure (E), According to the Nature of Association of the External Factor with Either or Both the Exposure and the Disease

Situation	Design	Analysis	Validity	Efficiency	Remarks
1 D ⟵ E / F	Not matched	Not stratified	Bias	Irrelevant	Incorrect analysis
	Not matched	Stratified	Valid	Reduced	Appropriate; possibly inefficient
	Matched	Not stratified	Bias to null	Irrelevant	Incorrect analysis
	Matched	Stratified	Valid	Better	Appropriate
2 D ⟵ E / F	Not matched	Not stratified	Valid	Better	Appropriate
	Not matched	Stratified	Valid	Slightly reduced	Appropriate; possibly inefficient
	Matched	Not stratified	Valid	Better	Wasted resources
	Matched	Stratified	Valid	Slightly reduced	Wasted resources
3 D ⟵ E / F	Not matched	Not stratified	Valid	Better	Appropriate
	Not matched	Stratified	Valid	Slightly reduced	Appropriate; possibly inefficient
	Matched	Not stratified	Valid	Better	Wasted resources
	Matched	Stratified	Valid	Slightly reduced	Wasted resources
4 D ⟵ E / F	Not matched	Not stratified	Valid	Better	Appropriate
	Not matched	Stratified	Valid	Slightly reduced	Appropriate; possibly inefficient
	Matched	Not stratified	Bias to null	Irrelevant	Incorrect analysis
	Matched	Stratified	Valid	Reduced	**Overmatching:** reduced precision
5 E→F→D	Not matched	Not stratified	Valid	Better	Appropriate
	Not matched	Stratified	Bias to null	Irrelevant	Incorrect analysis
	Matched	Not stratified	Bias to null	Irrelevant	Incorrect design
	Matched	Stratified	Bias to null	Irrelevant	**Overmatching:** bias

Symbols: → Established association (causal or risk indicating)
⋯→ Causality under investigation (not established)
↔ Established association (irrespective of nature, directionality, or sign)

ceptual foundations of analytic procedures rather than on the actual handling of complex numerical data.[240,358,466,469,576] The purpose of this section is to introduce the reader to available simple techniques and to the rationale for more complex procedures.

Case-Control Studies with Two Exposure Levels and No Stratification

As noted earlier, in a case-control study with just two exposure levels (exposed, unexposed), the exposure odds among cases (x_e/x_0) divided by the exposure odds among controls (y_e/y_0) gives the odds ratio (OR). The OR is the essential measure of effect in case-control studies—it is an unbiased, consistent estimate of the incidence rate ratio between exposed and unexposed persons when the case-control study is based on incident cases and suitable controls from a dynamic population, irrespective of the frequency of the disease. The OR also is a very good approximation of the cumulative incidence ratio between exposed and unexposed persons when the case-control study is based on a closed cohort and the cumulative incidence of the disease in any of the compared groups is lower, or not much higher, than 10 percent. Just as important, the OR is a valid measure of effect even when the cumulative incidence in one or both of the compared groups is high. However, in this instance the OR is not a good approximation of either of the two intuitively appealing effect measures—the incidence rate ratio or the cumulative incidence ratio.

Calculation of the odds ratio is as straightforward as $\frac{x_e y_0}{x_0 y_e}$. Because lack of association implies an odds ratio equal to one, statistical significance of the deviation of the observed association from the null value can be assessed with the usual χ^2 with one degree of freedom in a fourfold table. It should be noted that continuity (Yates) correction is rarely used in the epidemiological literature,[358,466,469] whereas the finite sample correction (substitution of $N - 1$ for N in the fourfold table χ^2 formula, where $N = x_e + x_0 + y_e + y_0$) is mandatory when the χ^2 with one degree of freedom is generalized to apply to several 2 by 2 tables (the Mantel-Haenszel procedure).[326] For studies of even moderate size (N equals more than 50 individuals), the finite sample correction makes little difference *unless stratification is required for control of confounding.*

The confidence limits of an estimated odds ratio can be calculated in several ways. A straightforward way has been suggested by Woolf,[604] who has shown that the standard error of the natural logarithm of the OR approximately equals

$$\sqrt{\frac{1}{x_e} + \frac{1}{x_0} + \frac{1}{y_e} + \frac{1}{y_0}}$$

Alternatively, test-based approximate confidence limits may be derived, as suggested by Miettinen[348,349,469] and described in the chapter on cohort studies. These confidence limits are fairly accurate unless the OR deviates substantially from the null value. In the latter situation, a more accurate procedure proposed by Cornfield[75] can be used.

The data in Table 10-3 will be used to demonstrate the calculation of OR and 95 percent confidence limits in a case-control study with two levels of exposure and no allowance for confounding influences. The data are from a case-control study of the role of chronic infection with hepatitis C virus (HCV), as reflected in the presence of antibodies to HCV (anti-HCV), in the etiology of hepatocellular carcinoma (HCC). Only data concerning men are used.[241,555]

The χ^2 formula with finite sample correction in a fourfold table is:

$$\frac{(x_e y_0 - x_0 y_e)^2 (N - 1)}{(x_e + y_e)(x_0 + y_0)(x_e + x_0)(y_e + y_0)}$$

In Table 10-3, χ (i.e., the square root of χ^2) is 9.34. If the finite sample correction is not used, that is, if N, rather than $(N - 1)$, were used in the numerator of the formula, χ would be equal to 9.35. The difference is negligible because the study is fairly large *and no stratification was used*. The odds ratio is calculated as $x_e y_0 / x_0 y_e = 9.19$. Test-based 95 percent confidence limits are

Table 10-3. Number of Patients with Hepatocellular Carcinoma and Controls with Antibodies Indicating Chronic Infection with Hepatitis C Virus (anti-HCV). Males Only.

Anti-HCV	Cases	Controls	
Positive	$63 = x_e$	$24 = y_e$	
Negative	$102 = x_0$	$357 = y_0$	
Total	165	381	$546 = N$

Source: Adapted from Tzonou A, et al. Epidemiologic assessment of interactions of hepatitis-C virus with seromarkers of hepatitis-B and -D viruses, cirrhosis and tobacco smoking in hepatocellular carcinoma. *Int J Cancer* 1991;49 : 377–380.

derived by exponentiating the odds ratio to $\left(1 - \dfrac{1.96}{9.34}\right)$ and to $\left(1 + \dfrac{1.96}{9.34}\right)$ to obtain 5.77 (lower) and 14.64 (higher).

Because the OR 9.19 deviates substantially from the null value of 1, the test-based confidence limits are likely to be somewhat inaccurate in the sense that the obtained confidence interval is too narrow. Indeed, using Woolf's approach, the natural logarithm of the OR is 2.2178 with standard error equal to

$$\sqrt{\frac{1}{63} + \frac{1}{102} + \frac{1}{24} + \frac{1}{357}} \quad \text{or} \quad 0.2648$$

Adding and subtracting $1.96 \cdot 0.2648$ to and from 2.2178 and then taking antilogs give as 95 percent confidence limits 5.47 and 15.44, which define a broader and more accurate confidence interval. ORs deviating substantially from the null value are rarely encountered in epidemiology, and even when they do deviate substantially, they tend to be influenced more by subtle biases than by chance variation. It is defensible, therefore, to utilize the very simple test-based method in most instances and reserve the application of more valid but substantially more complicated methods in situations as, or more, extreme than that of the present example.

Case-Control Studies with Several Exposure Levels and No Stratification

Exposures may be expressed in more than two categories, and it is not uncommon for the categories to correspond to ordinal or quantitative variables. For instance, occupational exposures may be categorized by intensity or duration of exposure, and the same is true with respect to tobacco smoking or physical activity. Table 10-4 shows a considerable difference between patients with hepatocellular cancer unrelated to hepatitis B virus and controls in the proportion of current smokers (78% vs. 53%). In addition, within the group of current smokers, there is a difference between cases and controls according to number of cigarettes smoked.

When a study factor can be realized in several ordered categories, every effort should be made to integrate this categorization into the study design and analysis. For example, a great deal of information would be lost if the data in Table 10-4 were considered only in terms of the dichotomy of smokers to nonsmokers or another dichotomy (e.g., heavy smokers to all other smoking patterns). The consideration of a range of ordered categories of a certain exposure, as in Table 10-4, has several advantages. First,

Table 10-4. Distribution of 40 Patients with Hepatocellular Cancer with No Evidence of Chronic Infection with Hepatitis B Virus, and 204 Control Subjects by Smoking Habits

| Group | Nonsmokers | Current smokers* (cigarettes/day) | | | | All subjects |
		1–10	11–20	21–30	31+	
Cases	9	3	14	6	8	40
Controls	95	24	58	17	10	204
Odds ratio	1	1.3	2.5	3.7	8.4	
(95% CI)†	—	(0.3–5.3)	(1.1–6.1)	(1.2–11.2)	(3.0–23.8)	

Source: Adapted from Trichopoulos D, et al. Smoking and hepatitis B-negative primary hepatocellular carcinoma. *J Natl Cancer Inst* 1980;65 : 111–114.
*Including those who stopped smoking during the last 5 years
†95 percent confidence interval (test-based); there was no confounding by age or gender in this dataset

it facilitates examination of the shape of the exposure–response relationship; a monotonic relationship increases the likelihood of causality, although confounded associations can also be monotonic and even linear. Second, it reveals the rate ratio or risk ratio differentials between the more extreme exposure categories. Third, it creates conditions that usually allow the application of the test for linear trends in proportions and frequencies proposed by Armitage.[10,469] This versatile χ^2 test with one degree of freedom for a single $2 \cdot K$ table (where K is the number of ordered categories) is substantially more powerful than the χ^2 test with one degree of freedom in a fourfold table whenever there is an underlying linear component in a regular or even irregular relation between exposure and disease.[306,322] In the example of Table 10-4, the χ^2 test for the association of disease with smoking (current smokers vs. nonsmokers) is 7.90, whereas the χ^2 for linear trend across all five categories is 15.76 (in both instances with one degree of freedom). Indeed, it is possible for the χ^2 for linear trend to be statistically significant, indicating a genuine association between exposure and disease, even when the confidence intervals of the odds ratio estimates at every level of exposure straddle the null value of one. This is because the category-specific confidence intervals are inappropriately large; there is no simple way to adjust them for the underlying genuine nonzero linear trend in the proportions across exposure levels.

When dealing with quantitative variables, a comparison of distributions, such as that in Table 10-4, gives a more clear picture of the range of odds ratios associated with the variable than does a comparison in terms of means or medians. For example, in a case-control study of breast cancer in Japan,[609] the mean age at first delivery was found to be 23.8 years for the cases and 22.6 years for the controls. The difference of 1.2 years was statistically significant, but its size does not suggest any more than a tendency of breast cancer patients to have their first delivery at a later age than women without the disease. However, in the same data, comparison of the distribution of cases and controls with respect to age at first delivery showed that women who first delivered at age 35 or older had more than four times the breast cancer risk of those who first delivered under 20 years of age. The difference between the means of two distributions drawn from cases and controls will, of course, depend not only on the risk associated with being at a given level of the distribution but also on how many individuals there are at the various levels. Thus, in a comparison of means, a high risk associated with a particular level of exposure will be obscured if only a small fraction of the total population receives such exposure. The mean difference between cases and controls in age at first delivery in the study cited appeared fairly small because a relatively small proportion of women had their first deliveries in the categories that showed the greatest discrepancy in breast cancer risk, that is, under 20 and 35 and over.

A desirable and obvious characteristic of multilevel exposure tabulations without stratification is that the odds ratio contrasting any two levels of exposure can be directly derived from the odds ratios that characterize these exposure levels in comparison to the unexposed subjects. Thus, the odds ratio for hepatitis B negative hepatocellular carcinoma contrasting individuals who smoke 31 or more cigarettes per day and individuals who smoke 11–20 cigarettes per day is $8 \cdot 58 / 14 \cdot 10 = 3.3$, which is exactly equal to the ratio of 8.4/2.5, apart from rounding errors.

Occasionally, a semiquantitative or quantitative variable may be expressed in study-specific units that have limited external interpretability. This situation arises frequently in studies of nutritional epidemiology in which dietary intakes are ascertained through questionnaires covering a variable number of food items. The usual approach is to create categories of marginal quantiles (e.g., quartiles or quintiles) using the combined distribution of cases and controls.[219] This presentation allows the examination of exposure–response patterns[251] but may not be optimal for the examination of linear trends. This is because intermediate quantiles are more closely spaced than extreme ones, creating unequal increments between successive quantiles and limiting the interpretability of changes expressed "per quantile." An alternative is to use incremental units equal to the standard deviation of the distribution of the particular nutritional exposure.[243]

Occasionally, particularly in the older clinical literature, cases were compared to controls with respect to a quantitative exposure through calculation of the corresponding mean values and their standard errors. If the exposure is distributed normally, or approximately so, among both cases and controls, and the two distributions have different means μ_1 and μ_2 but the same variance (σ^2, the square of the common standard deviation), then it is possible to roughly approximate the natural logarithm of the odds ratio per unit increase in the quantitative exposure through the formula.[443]

$$\ln (\text{odds ratio per unit increase}) = \frac{\mu_1 - \mu_2}{\sigma^2}$$

If the distributions of exposure among the cases and the controls have clearly different variances, a slightly more complicated formula is required.[443]

Case-Control Studies with Two Exposure Levels and Stratification for Confounding

When there are only a few possible confounding variables, and the variability of each of them can be captured through categorization into a limited number of reasonably distinct groups (e.g., three possible confounders with two, two, and four categories, respectively), stratification and the use of specifically developed statistical techniques can adequately control confounding and summarize the evidence for association between an exposure and the study disease. As indicated in the chapter on cohort studies (see Chapter 9), the appropriate analysis depends on the existence of evidence or credible assumption that the measure of effect (the odds ratio in case-control studies) is similar (homogeneous) or different (heterogeneous, signifying interaction or effect modification) across the strata of the confounding variable(s), aside from chance variation.

First we describe the situation in which there are only two levels of exposure (unexposed, exposed) and no biomedical indication or empirical evidence (from previous investigations or from a cursory examination of the data at hand) for effect modification according to the level of the confounding variable(s). We utilize data from a case-control study by Brinton et al.[44] on the relation of menstrual factors to the risk of breast cancer, although the authors of the study have chosen to apply logistic regression modeling, a perfectly valid but more complex alternative procedure.[44] Among 2,866 women with breast cancer, 1,979 (69%) were postmenopausal, whereas 887 (31%) were still menstruating; among 3,141

Table 10-5. Distribution of Women with Incident Breast Cancer and Comparison Women by Menopausal Status and Age at Interview

Age at interview	Study group	Menstruating women	Post-menopausal women	Odds ratio	95% confidence interval
	Cases	x_e	x_o	OR =	95% CI
	Controls	y_e	y_o	$x_e y_o / x_o y_e$	(test-based)
to 44	Cases	278	65	1.13	0.79 to 1.62
	Controls	314	83		$\chi^2 = 0.44$
45–49	Cases	334	149	1.37	1.05 to 1.78
	Controls	323	197		$\chi^2 = 5.48$
50–54	Cases	240	391	1.49	1.18 to 1.87
	Controls	193	467		$\chi^2 = 11.18$
55+	Cases	35	1,374	1.02	0.64 to 1.63
	Controls	38	1,526		$\chi^2 = 0.01$
CRUDE (UNADJUSTED)					
Total	Cases	887	1,979	1.17	1.05 to 1.31
	Controls	868	2,273		$\chi^2 = 7.96$
ADJUSTED FOR AGE					
				1.33	1.15 to 1.54
					$\chi^2 = 14.21$

Source: Adapted from Brinton LA, et al. Menstrual factors and risk of breast cancer. *Cancer Invest* 1988;6 : 245–254.

comparison women (controls), the respective numbers were 2,273 (72%) and 868 (28%). Table 10-5 shows the distribution of cases and controls by age at diagnosis (cases) or interview (controls) and menopausal status (postmenopausal or menstruating). This approach for the evaluation of age at menopause (or age at menarche) as a risk factor for breast cancer (or any other disease) is based on the status quo at the time of interview, and it is more reliable than relying on the recollection of age at menopause by postmenopausal women (or age at menarche by postmenarcheal women). In the status quo approach, as applied in this example, we compare menstruating women (exposed) to postmenopausal ones (not exposed).

In the analysis of case-control studies with two exposure levels and stratification for confounding, there are several questions to be answered.

1. Is the association between exposure and disease statistically significant after accounting for the stratified, possibly confounding, variable(s)?

2. Is there, contrary to expectation, compelling evidence for heterogeneity in the association under study across the strata?

3. What is the adjusted overall odds ratio?

4. What are the confidence limits of the overall adjusted odds ratio?

Questions 1, 3, and 4 remain relevant even if the answer to question 2 is, unexpectedly, affirmative. However, in this instance, the overall odds ratio and the associated χ^2 test and confidence limits refer to an "average" or "in balance" association between the study exposure and the disease (see following discussion on analytic strategy in the presence of overt heterogeneity).

The most appropriate test for the association between a two-level exposure (unexposed, exposed) and a particular disease (absent, present) over a number of strata was introduced by Mantel and Haenszel.[326] It is a summary χ^2 with one degree of freedom. The test is easy to perform, even with a hand-held calculator. In *every stratum* (occasionally indicated as stratum i) there are $(x_e + x_0)$ cases, $(y_e + y_0)$ controls, $(x_e + y_e)$ exposed subjects, $(x_0 + y_0)$ unexposed subjects, and N subjects in general ($N = x_e + x_0 + y_e + y_0$). For the calculation of Mantel-Haenszel χ^2, the sum of x_e over all strata is taken, and from this the sum over all strata of $\dfrac{(x_e + x_0)(x_e + y_e)}{N}$ is subtracted. The difference is then squared and subsequently divided by the sum over all strata of $\dfrac{(x_e + x_0)(y_e + y_0)(x_e + y_e)(x_0 + y_0)}{N^2(N-1)}$. In essence, the Mantel-Haenszel summary χ (the square root of the corresponding χ^2) is simply the difference between the observed number of exposed cases across all strata and the expected number under the assumption of no association between exposure and disease in any of the strata divided by the standard error of the observed number of exposed cases. (The corresponding expected number has no standard error when the margins are fixed.) In Table 10-5, the crude χ^2 is 7.96 (P ~ 0.005), whereas the age-adjusted through stratification Mantel-Haenszel summary χ^2 is 14.21 (P ~ 0.0002). It can be concluded that, after controlling for age at interview, there is a highly significant association between continuation of menstruation and breast cancer risk. Moreover, in these data, age at interview was apparently a negative confounder of the association under study, having the effect of obscuring rather than exaggerating the association between menopausal status and breast cancer risk.

The data in Table 10-5 do not suggest a consistent or biologically meaningful change of the odds ratio with different age at interview. Formal statistical evaluation of heterogeneity is possible,[42,61,259,469] but it is not particularly useful unless there is reasonably strong a priori evidence that heterogeneity might be present. A simple χ^2 test for heterogeneity, with degrees of freedom equal to the number of strata minus one, has been proposed by Zelen.[610] This test is not reliable in all instances,[325] but it can be useful for a preliminary assessment of heterogeneity. It is computed by summing the simple χ^2 values from each stratum and subtracting from the sum the overall Mantel-Haenszel χ^2. For the data in Table 10-5, Zelen's χ^2 with three degrees of freedom equals

$$0.44 + 5.48 + 11.18 + 0.01 - 14.21 = 2.90$$

corresponding to P ~ 0.41, which is clearly far from significant.

The adjusted overall odds ratio, under the assumption of homogeneity across strata, has also been introduced by Mantel and Haenszel;[326] it is, in essence, a precision-weighted average of the stratum-specific estimates of the uniform odds ratio. The Mantel-Haenszel odds ratio is calculated by dividing the sum, over all strata of $x_e y_0 / N$ by the sum, over all strata of $y_e x_0 / N$. In the example of Table 10-5, the Mantel-Haenszel odds ratio is 1.33, further away from the null value than the crude odds ratio of 1.17. Again, this indicates that, in this data, age at interview is a negative confounder of the association between menopausal status and breast cancer risk.

There are several methods for the calculation of confidence limits for the Mantel-Haenszel odds ratio. A general estimator for the standard error of the natural logarithm of the Mantel-Haenszel odds ratio has been derived by Robins and colleagues,[444,445] whereas exact computation of confidence limits of the maximum likelihood pooled estimate of odds ratio is described by Thomas.[528] Simpler, but still demanding, approximation can be derived through the approach suggested by Cornfield[75] as extended by Gart.[140,141] Test-based approximate confidence limits[348,349,358,469] are reasonably accurate, unless the Mantel-Haenszel odds ratio is sharply different from the null value of one. For the data in Table 10-5, 95 percent confidence limits of the Mantel-Haenszel OR of 1.33 can be derived by exponentiating it to $\left(1 - \dfrac{1.96}{3.77}\right)$ and $\left(1 + \dfrac{1.96}{3.77}\right)$ because 3.77 is the square root of the Mantel-Haenszel $\chi^2 = 14.21$. These limits are 1.15 and 1.54.

Before turning to situations in which the odds ratio appears to vary across strata, it is essential to point out that homogeneity of effect (or, at least, of association) in stratified analysis implies that the control variable (age in Table 10-5) and the study variable (menopausal status in Table 10-5) interact in a multiplicative way. Heterogeneity in stratified analysis implies deviation from an implicitly multiplicative model of interaction. It is also important to recognize that unless there are only two strata (in which case the χ^2 for heterogeneity has just one degree of freedom) or the effect modification follows a certain meaningful pattern (e.g., the odds ratio linking a certain exposure with a certain disease declines or increases with age), it is difficult to statistically substantiate an apparent heterogeneity.

When heterogeneity is established, or is considered as likely in spite of the lack of statistical significance, the Mantel-Haenszel χ^2 is still useful as a test of the average departure from the null hypothesis, although exposed persons may be at lower relative risk in certain strata and at higher relative risk in others. However, it is no more appropriate to calculate the Mantel-Haenszel, precision-weighted estimator of a common odds ratio because there is no such entity as a "common" odds ratio. There are two options: (1) to estimate a different odds ratio for each stratum and to consider each of them as a distinct entity, or (2) to calculate a standardized odds ratio by weighting the stratum-specific odds ratios according to the distribution of either the exposed or the unexposed subjects with respect to the control variable(s).[354]

Table 10-6 is based on the same data as Table 10-3, but it examines the association of anti-HCV with hepatocellular carcinoma (HCC) in strata of individuals positive or negative for hepatitis B surface antigen in the blood, a reflection of chronic liver infection with hepatitis B virus (HBV).[555] Because HBV is an established cause of HCC, and HBV and HCV have common sources and transmission routes, HBV is likely to confound the association of HCV with HCC, described by a crude odds ratio of approximately 9.2. Moreover, there are biomedical arguments in support of an interaction between HBV and HCV viruses in the pathogenesis of HCC.[241]

The data in Table 10-6 provide a suggestion that the odds ratio linking HCV to HCC is stronger among persons chronically infected with HBV than among persons not so infected. Among HBV-positive individuals, the odds ratio is 25.9, and the natural logarithm of this is 3.25 with standard error 1.04 (Woolf's method). Among HBV-negative individuals, the odds ratio is 6.0, and the natural logarithm of this is 1.79 with standard error of 0.32. Application of a standard normal deviate test (t-test with infinite degrees of freedom) generates a P value for interaction 0.18. However, in this instance, the approach based on Woolf's method,[604] although far superior to that based on Zelen's proce-

Table 10-6. Distribution of Patients with Hepatocellular Carcinoma and Controls by Serologic Evidence of Chronic Liver Infection with Hepatitis B (HBV) and Hepatitis C (HCV) Viruses

HBV status	Group	HCV status Positive	HCV status Negative	Odds ratio (OR)	95% confidence interval
HBV (+)	Cases	37	40	25.9	3.4 to 200.0 (Woolf method)
	Controls	1	28		
HBV (−)	Cases	26	62	6.0	3.2 to 11.2 (Woolf method)
	Controls	23	329		

CRUDE (UNADJUSTED)

Total	Cases	63	102	9.2	5.5 to 15.4 (Woolf method)
	Controls	24	357		5.8 to 14.6 (test-based)

ADJUSTED FOR HBV STATUS

Mantel-Haenszel OR   8.1   4.7 to 14.0 (test-based)
Standardized (exposed) OR 10.9
Standardized (unexposed) OR 13.8

Source: Adapted from Tzonou A, et al. Epidemiologic assessment of interactions of hepatitis-C virus with seromarkers of hepatitis-B and -D viruses, cirrhosis and tobacco smoking in hepatocellular carcinoma. *Int J Cancer* 1991;49 : 377–380.

dure,[610] is still inaccurate (mainly because of the extremely small frequency of HBV-positive, HCV-positive controls, that is, just one person). An appropriate but complex likelihood ratio-based test generates a P value for interaction equal to 0.11.[42,61,469,480]

At this point, the issue becomes a matter of judgment; a statistically significant test outcome, particularly concerning interaction, may well be due to chance, and a nonsignificant outcome may reflect power limitations. One might prefer to ignore the suggestive evidence for interaction and use the Mantel-Haenszel estimator of the overall odds ratio, or one could decide that the converging biomedical and empirical evidence for effect modification is sufficiently strong and should not be ignored. In the latter instance, the standardized odds ratio should be calculated using as standard the distribution according to HBV status of either the subjects who are exposed to HCV (standardized to exposed) or those who are unexposed to HCV (standardized to unexposed).[354] For the standardized odds ratio using as standard the exposed, the sum over all strata of x_e is divided by the sum over all strata of $(y_e x_0 / y_0)$; for the standardized odds ratio using as standard the unexposed, the sum over all strata of $(x_e y_0 / y_e)$ is divided by the sum over all strata of x_0. The respective results are 10.9 and 13.8. Derivation of the confidence limits of the standardized odds ratios is fairly complicated, and the test-based procedure is not applicable. Moreover, confidence intervals around standardized odds ratios are always wider than that around the Mantel-Haenszel odds ratio because only the latter among these estimators is weighted by precision.

As discussed in the chapter on cohort studies (see Chapter 9), contemplation of the joint action of two factors under a multiplicative perspective is methodologically convenient but does not convey the essence of the effect modification that should be considered as present whenever the joint effect exceeds the sum of the effects of the individual factors. Table 10-7 demonstrates this point. It presents data from a case-control study of first venous thrombosis in relation to current oral contraceptive use and the presence of factor V Leiden mutation that has been postulated to increase susceptibility to venous thrombosis.[563] The odds ratio for venous thrombosis in relation to oral contraceptive use is 3.7 among V Leiden mutation-negative individuals and 34.7/6.9 = 5.0 among V Leiden mutation-positive individuals. Clearly, there is little evidence of effect modification in the multiplicative context. Similarly, the effect of factor V Leiden mutation on the incidence of venous thrombosis is proportionally fairly similar among nonusers of oral contraceptives (odds ratio 6.9) and among users of these compounds (odds ratio = 34.7/3.7 = 9.4). In an additive perspective, however, use of oral contraceptives alone increases the baseline incidence of venous thrombosis among V Leiden mutation-negative nonusers of these compounds by 2.7 times the baseline rate (for a total of 1 + 2.7 = 3.7), whereas presence of the V Leiden mutation alone increases the baseline incidence of venous thrombosis by 5.9 times the baseline rate (for a total

Table 10-7. Distribution of Women with Venous Thrombosis and Controls by Oral Contraceptive Use (OC) and Presence of Factor V Leiden Mutation (VL)

Group	Exposure			
	OC (−) VL(−)	OC (+) VL (−)	OC (−) VL (+)	OC (+) VL (+)
Cases	36	84	10	25
Controls	100	63	4	2
Odds ratio	baseline = 1	3.7	6.9	34.7
95% CI*	—	2.3 to 6.1	2.3 to 20.8	11.8 to 101.8
Mantel-Haenszel odds ratio for OC, controlling for VL				3.8 (2.4 to 6.1)
Mantel-Haenszel odds ratio for VL, controlling for OC				8.2 (3.5 to 19.1)

Source: Adapted from Vandenbroucke JP, et al. Increased risk of venous thrombosis in oral-contraceptive users who are carriers of factor V Leiden mutation. *Lancet* 1994;344 : 1453–1457.
*95 percent confidence interval (test-based)

of 1 + 5.9 = 6.9). Joint action of oral contraceptives and V Leiden mutation would increase the baseline rate in an additive context by 2.7 plus 5.9 times the baseline rate for a total of 1 + 2.7 + 5.9 = 9.6. This additive expectation sharply contradicts the observed odds ratio of 34.7. By contrast, the observed odds ratio is not very different from the multiplicative expectation of joint action (3.7 · 6.9 = 25.5). It can be concluded that V Leiden mutation and use of oral contraceptives interact in a way that exceeds by far the additive expectation and appears to exceed even the multiplicative expectation (although, in the latter context, not significantly so) in the causation of venous thrombosis. In more general terms, it should be clear that a judgment concerning the existence or not of interaction (effect modification) depends on the calculation of the expected joint effect on the basis of an additive or multiplicative argument. Moreover, the additive expectation generates far more sensible conclusions about the joint effect of two or more factors.

Case-Control Studies with Several Exposure Levels and Stratification for Confounding

When stratification is undertaken to control confounding of an association involving an ordinal, semiquantitative, or quantitative exposure, statistical evaluation is usually done with the Mantel extension test,[169,322] which represents a generalization, over several strata, of the Armitage test for trends in proportions.[10] The Mantel extension test shares with the Mantel-Haenszel procedure,[326] from which it was originally derived, an important property: it is valid even when there is no more than one case *and* one control per stratum, provided that the overall study size is not exceedingly small. The test statistic in the Mantel extension procedure is a χ^2 with one degree of freedom (or the corresponding χ), irrespective of the number of strata and the number of exposure levels. As with the Armitage procedure,[10] the Mantel extension test[322] assesses the straight line component of the exposure-dependent pattern in proportion of cases, and the slope of this line (the regression coefficient) can be thought of as a useful internal measure of effect. Moreover, test-based confidence limits can easily be calculated. The slope, however, has limited interpretability outside the particular study because it depends on the arbitrary cases-to-controls ratio as well as on the exposure units. Therefore, it is customary to describe the effect of the exposure at a particular level, in comparison to an arbitrary baseline level, in terms of a Mantel-Haenszel odds ratio or a standardized odds ratio. The baseline level can be that of the lowest or highest exposure (to facilitate interpretation) or a category in which there are enough cases and controls (to increase the stability of the Mantel-Haenszel odds ratio estimates at every other level). The advantages of the exposure level-specific standardized odds ratios are: (1) they do not require homogeneity (i.e., the odds ratio at a particular level of exposure does not have to be considered the same across all strata); and (2) when the same standard is used for the calculation of the standardized odds ratios at every level of exposure (usually the distribution of unexposed persons), the resulting odds ratios are internally consistent (i.e., the standardized odds ratio contrasting any two exposure levels can be immediately derived by dividing the respective standardized odds ratios versus the common baseline level, usually that of the unexposed persons). The disadvantages of standardized odds ratios are: (1) they are inefficient (imprecise) estimators in the presence of homogeneity, (2) they are inflexible in their statistical handling, and (3) their confidence intervals are both wide and difficult to estimate.[165] By contrast, the Mantel-Haenszel odds ratios are precision weighted, and their confidence intervals are as narrow as those derived from optimal maximum likelihood methods. However, these estimators are not internally consistent because they are not based on the same standard, and they are strictly valid only in the presence of homogeneity across strata.

These issues are demonstrated through data summarized in Table 10-8. They are derived from a case-control study of cancer of the urinary bladder undertaken in Athens, Greece, in the early 1980s. The data describe the empirical relation to bladder cancer of occupations a priori considered as high risk for this cancer.[430] In this study, occupational associations were not confounded by age, tobacco smoking, or coffee drinking. Among women, the trend test was statistically significant (P ~ 0.02), even though the confidence intervals of the odds ratios straddled the null value at each exposure level. Adjusting for gender reveals very little confounding (the slope changes only from $4.47 \cdot 10^{-2}$ to $5.06 \cdot 10^{-2}$), and even this confounding is negative rather than positive. The overall association is not statistically significant (P ~ 0.10), apparently because the strong association among women is diluted by the very weak association among men; however, in this instance, a one-tail interpretation of the test result might be acceptable (P ~ 0.05) because the occupational scale was a priori considered as unidirectional (from low to high risk occupations). The heterogeneity test in Table 10-8 is an extension of the Zelen test[610] and is derived by subtracting from the sum of the stratum-specific χ^2 values for trend ($0.86^2 + 2.34^2 = 6.21$) the square of the Mantel-extension χ ($1.62^2 = 2.62$). The difference 3.59 is a χ^2

Table 10-8. Distribution of Incident Cases with Cancer of the Urinary Bladder and Hospital Controls by Gender and a priori Risk of This Cancer from Main Occupation

Group		A priori occupational risk			Trend evaluation results
		Low	Undetermined	High	
Male	Cases	65	133	51	χ for trend = 0.86; P ~ 0.39
	Controls	70	137	43	slope $2.86 \cdot 10^{-2}$
	OR	1	1.05	1.28	
	(95% CI)*	baseline	(0.69, 1.58)	(0.75, 2.17)	
Female	Cases	33	13	4	χ for trend = 2.34; P ~ 0.02
	Controls	43	6	1	slope $21.25 \cdot 10^{-2}$
	OR	1	2.82	5.21	
	(95% CI)	baseline	(0.99, 8.06)	(0.67, 40.37)	
All	Cases	98	146	55	Crude χ for trend 1.52; P ~ 0.13
	Controls	113	143	44	Crude slope $4.47 \cdot 10^{-2}$
	Crude OR	1	1.18	1.44	Adjusted χ for trend 1.62; P ~ 0.10
	(95% CI)	baseline	(0.83, 1.68)	(0.89, 2.33)	Adjusted slope $5.06 \cdot 10^{-2}$
	M-H† OR	1	1.20	1.40	Heterogeneity χ^2 with 1 DF, 3.59; P ~ 0.06
	(95% CI)	baseline	(0.82, 1.76)	(0.85, 2.33)	
	Standardized OR (to unexposed)	1	1.64	2.60	

OR: Odds ratio; DF: degrees of freedom
Source: Adapted from Rebelakos A., et al. Tobacco smoking, coffee drinking and occupation as risk factors for bladder cancer in Greece. *J Natl Cancer Inst* 1985;75 : 455–461.
*95 percent confidence interval
†Mantel-Haenszel estimate of common exposure-specific odds ratio

with degrees of freedom equal to the number of strata minus 1 ($2 - 1 = 1$). χ rather than χ^2 values are preferred in the Mantel extension test because the former indicates, through its sign, the direction of the association (positive or negative). In spite of the sevenfold ratio of the slopes between women and men ($21.25/2.86 = 7.4$), the heterogeneity test is not significant at the arbitrary P $\sim$ 0.05 level. This is not surprising, given the inherently low power of most statistical procedures that probe interaction. Moreover, Zelen's test for heterogeneity is a rather poor substitute for the appropriate test for heterogeneity that is based on asymptotic likelihood ratio procedures.[42,61] If heterogeneity is indeed present, it could be attributed to the lower absolute baseline risk for bladder cancer risk among occupationally nonexposed women than among occupationally nonexposed men, because women in the population of this study are less frequently and less intensely exposed to other established or possible risk factors for bladder cancer. With respect to summary odds ratios,[354] a Mantel-Haenszel estimate of the odds ratio contrasting occupations at "high" and "undetermined" risk could *not* be derived by dividing 1.40 by 1.20 (Table 10-8), whereas the standardized odds ratio contrasting these two categories and using the distribution of unexposed persons as standard is exactly the ratio of 2.60 divided by 1.64.

Controlling for confounding influences presupposes identification and adequate categorization of confounders. Occasionally, control of confounding can be accomplished through exclusion of a certain stratum (cases as well as controls) in what has been termed matrix restriction. This procedure is acceptable only when there are very few persons in the stratum scheduled for elimination and there is no evidence for effect modification in this stratum.

In conducting stratified analyses for possible confounding variables of semiquantitative or quantitative nature, the range of measurements covered in the strata to be formed can be important, particularly when the control variable is a strong confounder. It is desirable for each stratum to contain a sufficient number of cases and controls for separate examination, but the range must not be so inclusive that the desired similarity between the compared series is not obtained. For example, if a disease is markedly related to age, the use of 20-year age groups may not eliminate the confounding effect of age because within 20-year age groups there may be sufficient age difference between cases and controls to produce appreciable confounding influences in the odds ratios. It may be difficult to decide whether the adopted grouping has been sufficiently fine to equalize the compared series effectively.

If a crude association is eliminated by holding a confounding variable constant, it may usually be assumed that the grouping was satisfactory; however, if the difference is reduced but not eliminated, the effect of finer grouping should be ascertained. If finer grouping is difficult because of inadequate numbers, and statistical modeling is considered impractical, it may be possible to estimate by indirect methods the maximum possible influence of variation within the chosen groups. Some general idea about the possible effect of finer grouping may also be obtained by noting the change in the summary odds ratio estimates that results from consideration of the strata that can be examined. Issues concerning residual confounding have been more extensively addressed in other parts of this book and by several investigators.[160,553]

Matched Case-Control Studies

Much of the original work on the methodologic properties, epidemiologic implications, and appropriate analysis of matched case-control studies was undertaken by Miettinen,[351,352,353,358] whereas other investigators have enriched the relevant literature by addressing additional important issues.[40,161,174,176,529,530,533] An "anatomy" of matched case-control studies was presented by Rothman,[466,469] and several authors have discussed stratification-based procedures for the analysis of matched case-control data with constant ($1:1$, $1:2$, $1:3$, etc.) or variable case-to-controls ratio.[40,240,259,466,469,480] Moreover, the analysis of matched case-control studies by modeling the data through conditional logistic regression[424] is covered in many moderate-to-advanced statistical and epidemiologic texts.[11,42,61,259,260,480] The overriding advantage of conditional logistic regression over the simpler stratification-based techniques is that only the former procedure allows control of additional confounders over and beyond those for which cases and controls were matched.[242]

It has already been indicated that the Mantel-Haenszel[326] and the Mantel extension procedures[322] are valid even when there are no more than one case and one control per stratum, provided that the overall study size is not very small. Moreover, Breslow[40] has shown that the Mantel-Haenszel odds ratio is almost as valid and efficient an estimate as the optimal maximum likelihood odds ratio. Therefore, statistical evaluation and odds ratio point estimation for matched case-control data can be undertaken through the Mantel-Haenszel[326] and the Mantel extension procedures[322] by considering every matched pair, triplet, quadruplet, and so forth, whether in constant or variable case-to-controls ratio, as

Table 10-9. Data Layout in a Matched Pairs
Case-Control Study with No Additional Confounding
Variables and Two Exposure Levels (Present, Absent)

	Case	
Control	Exposure present	Exposure absent
Exposure present	*r*	*s*
Exposure absent	*t*	*u*

a distinct mini-stratum. All mini-strata contribute information, except those in which the case and *all* available controls are assigned at the same exposure level. Special data layout and formulae facilitate the application of the Mantel-Haenszel and the Mantel extension procedures for the analysis of matched case-control studies.[466,469] Calculation of confidence limits for the Mantel-Haenszel odds ratio estimators can be done exactly by using the formula for standard error of the natural logarithm of the Mantel-Haenszel odds ratio described by Robins and colleagues.[444,445] An acceptable alternative is use of test-based confidence limits as suggested by Miettinen,[348,349] unless the observed data are sharply incompatible with the null hypothesis.

When the case-control study involves matched pairs (one control for every case), the study exposure has only two levels (unexposed, exposed), and there are no other confounders beyond those for which cases and controls were matched, the analysis is remarkably simple.[350] As indicated, pairs in which case and control are similar with respect to the study exposure are not considered, and estimates are based solely on pairs in which one member has and the other does not have the factor under study. Thus, Table 10-9 illustrates the distribution of all the pairs in a matched pairs case-control study. Note that presence or absence of the exposure may be defined in terms of specified levels of the exposure, as well as actual presence or absence.

In Table 10-9, *r*, *s*, *t*, and *u* are the number of pairs; that is, their sum is half the number of the individuals in the study. The appropriate test of statistical significance in such a situation is the McNemar or marginal χ^2 test,[345] where

$$\chi^2 = \frac{(t - s)^2}{t + s}$$

The Mantel-Haenszel odds ratio is estimated as $\frac{t}{s}$.

Table 10-10. Distribution of 175 Case-Control Pairs According to Whether or Not Oral Contraceptives Were Used Within 1 Month Before Admission for Thromboembolism

Oral agent used by control	Oral agent used by case		Total pairs
	Yes	No	
Yes	10	13	23
No	57	95	152
Total pairs	67	108	175

Source: Adapted from Sartwell PE, et al. Thromboembolism and oral contraceptives: an epidemiologic case-control study. *Am J Epidemiol* 1969;90 : 365–380.

These procedures are illustrated by reference to a case-control study of thromboembolism in females, in which prior use of oral contraceptives was the exposure of interest.[476] The data are shown in Table 10-10. The 10 pairs in which both case and control used the contraceptives and the 95 pairs in which neither used them provide no information on the association between pill use and thromboembolism. Such information comes only from the discordant pairs. The Mantel-Haenszel χ^2, in this instance identical to McNemar χ^2 (with one degree of freedom), is

$$\frac{(57 - 13)^2}{57 + 13} = 27.66$$

Therefore, the Mantel-Haenszel χ (the square root of χ^2) is 5.26, corresponding to $P < 10^{-6}$. The Mantel-Haenszel odds ratio is 57/13 = 4.38, with test-based 95 percent confidence limits 2.53 and 7.60.

In this particular instance, the values for the Mantel-Haenszel χ and odds ratio do not differ appreciably from those that could be calculated from the usual formulae applied to unmatched data: 5.37 and 4.10, respectively. This is a reflection of the fact that, in spite of the comprehensive matching plan used, little similarity between pair members was introduced. Given the frequency of contraceptive use by cases and controls shown in Table 10-10, one can compute that if the pairing had been random there would have been 8.8 pairs in which both members used the agents and 93.8 pairs in which neither used them. Thus, the matching plan introduced only 2 similar pairs in excess of the 103 expected by chance. The error introduced by analyzing paired data as if they were not paired is a function of the strength of the association between the exposure under study and the matching factors. When pairing has been used primarily for convenience or when the influence of matching factors is small, so that appreciable similarity within pairs with respect to study factors has not been introduced, the pairing may be ignored in the analysis. However, there is no substantial advantage to be gained by ignoring the pairing if all the confounding variables to be considered entered into the matching process. If confounding variables are to be analyzed that were not considered, or were inadequately dealt with in the matching process, it may be reasonable to treat the series in subsequent stratification as if they had not been matched.

Currently, the analysis of most matched case-control studies is undertaken by modeling the data through conditional logistic regression (see the section on multivariate analysis later in this chapter). This approach allows control of confounders that have not been matched for during data collection but, in addition, preserves the original matching and provides the versatility and flexibility of multiple regression procedures when applied to appropriately modeled data.

Multivariate Analysis and the Multiple Logistic Regression

The contents of the section introducing the principles of multivariate analysis for cohort studies are wholly transferable here, except that multiple logistic regression should be substituted for Cox regression. This is because the partial regression coefficients b_1, b_2, and so forth, in multiple logistic regression are straightforward estimators of the natural logarithms of the mutually adjusted odds ratios contrasting exposed (coded as 1) to unexposed (coded as 0) persons, or associated with a one-unit increase in an ordered, semiquantitative or quantitative exposure variable. This important property of logistic regression is illustrated here.

In a case-control study, a logical dependent variable is the probability P that a particular subject is a case rather than a control. Probabilities, however, are awkward because their values are limited between 0 and 1. A suitable transformation is to divide P by its complement (P/Q), where $Q = 1 - P$, thus creating a variable that can take values from zero to infinity. This distribution is no more limited, but it is extremely skewed and requires logarithmic transformation for normalization. Transforming P into $\ln(P/Q)$ is the logit transformation.

In multiple regression procedures, a partial regression coefficient indicates how much the dependent variable (now $\ln[P/Q]$) will change when the respective predictor variable (a certain exposure) increases by one unit (e.g., from 0 to 1, or from nonexposed to exposed status) and all other variables in the model remain constant. Algebraically, the partial regression coefficient is $\ln \left(\dfrac{P_1}{Q_1}\right) - \ln \left(\dfrac{P_0}{Q_0}\right)$, where the subfix 1 signifies exposed and the subfix 0 signifies unexposed subjects.

However,

$$\ln \left(\frac{P_1}{Q_1}\right) - \ln \left(\frac{P_0}{Q_0}\right) = \ln \left(\frac{P_1 Q_0}{P_0 Q_1}\right),$$

which is exactly the log odds ratio. Taking antilogs of the partial regression coefficients and their confidence limits provides the desired mutually adjusted odds ratios and their confidence limits. It should be obvious that multiple logistic regression is inherently multiplicative (and with respect to exposure–response pattern, inherently exponential), as are the Cox regression and the Mantel-Haenszel procedures applied to stratified data.

The analysis of matched case-control studies through multiple logistic regression requires preservation of matching, which imposes as many additional parameters in the model as there are case-control pairs (or triplets, quadruplets, etc.). In this way, a difficult situation is created because there are more parameters in the model than there are cases. A common statistical device for eliminating the nuisance parameters (i.e., the parameters that preserve the matching) without breaking the matching is to condition the likelihood process through which the model is fitted. This is the reason that conditional logistic regression is the standard procedure for analyzing matched case-control data through logistic regression modeling. It should be noted, however, that when the matching variables are of fixed nature (e.g., age, gender, race) rather than random nature (e.g., neighborhood, date, hospital ward), it is frequently acceptable to employ unconditional logistic regression, provided that the matching variables are also introduced into the model.

The use of logistic regression for the analysis of data from case-control studies is described in many textbooks[42,61,259,260,480] and reviews.[41,532]

Attributable Rates and Fractions and Their Applicability in Case-Control Studies

In the chapter on cohort studies (see Chapter 9), ratios and differences of cumulative incidence measures (mostly in closed cohorts) and incidence rates (mainly in open but also in closed cohorts) were considered, whereas in the analysis of case-control studies, the focus is on the odds ratio as an unbiased (consistent) estimate of the incidence rate ratio for any disease, or as a very good approximation of the cumulative incidence (risk) ratio for rare diseases. At this point we examine measures based on rate or risk differences, as they are formally defined in the context of cohort studies and as they are applied, whenever possible, in the analysis and interpretation of case-control investigations. We focus on rates, keeping in mind that for rare outcomes, risk-based inferences are essentially identical (although with common diseases, or very long follow up, risk differences are biased toward the zero value). Conceptual and methodological contributions in this field have been made over time by Levin,[283] MacMahon, Pugh, and Ipsen,[316] Cole and MacMahon,[67] Miettinen,[355] Walter,[579,580] Whittemore,[589,590] and several others. The relevant concepts are comprehensively presented by Kleinbaum et al.[259] and have been reviewed by Benichou[21] and Coughlin, Benichou, and Weed.[76]

The terminology for measures based on rate or risk differences is confusing. We have opted for descriptive terms that leave no doubt about their connotations. If I_e, I_o, and I_T are symbols for disease incidence rate among exposed, unexposed, and total population under study, then:

Exposed attributable rate (EAR = $I_e - I_o$) is the disease incidence rate among exposed individuals that may be attributed to the exposure under study; it is expressed in the same units as I_e and I_o.

Exposed attributable fraction $\left(\text{EAF} = \dfrac{I_e - I_o}{I_e} \right)$ is the fraction of incidence rate among exposed individuals that may be attributed to the exposure (or the proportion of exposed cases that may be attributed to the exposure); as a fraction (or proportion) it is dimensionless.

Population attributable rate (PAR = $I_T - I_o$) is the incidence rate in the total population that may be attributed to the exposure under study; it is expressed in the same units as I_T and I_o.

Population attributable fraction $\left(\text{PAF} = \dfrac{I_T - I_o}{I_T} \right)$ is the fraction of incidence rate in the total population that may be attributed to the exposure (or the proportion of all cases that may be attributed to the exposure); as a fraction (or proportion) it is dimensionless.

Several authors, notably Walker,[576] have argued that the term *attributable* that dominates the difference measures is misleading because it implies an established causal link. The argument is certainly valid; however, the term *attributable* is so widely used that a new term would be unfamiliar and possibly even more confusing. Moreover, attributable rates or fractions are regularly used either with qualifications (under the assumption of causality) or when investigators are willing to judge an association as causal. We believe also that the explanatory terms *exposed* and *population* should always precede the term attributable because they identify the referent rate (or risk). Finally, fraction may be a better expression than percentage when rates are concerned, and there is no justification for using 100 rather than 1,000 or just 1 as a basis.

When a factor prevents rather than causes a disease, conceptually similar formulations may be developed with substitution of the word "prevented" for "attributable" in the respective terminology.[259,355]

Relations of Attributable Rates and Fractions

The disease incidence among exposed (I_e) is linked to the corresponding incidence among unexposed (I_o) through the rate ratio (RR) as

$$I_e = RR \cdot I_o$$

Therefore, EAR may be expressed in terms of I_o and RR as

$$EAR = RR \cdot I_o - I_o = I_o(RR - 1)$$

EAR describes the absolute impact of a presumed causal factor among exposed persons.

Similarly, EAF can be expressed in terms of RR and independently of I_o as

$$EAF = \frac{I_e - I_o}{I_e} = \frac{RR \cdot I_o - I_o}{RR \cdot I_o} = \frac{RR - 1}{RR}$$

The overall incidence of disease (I_T) in the base population that comprises exposed and unexposed persons in proportions Π and $(1 - \Pi)$, respectively, together with the value of Π, can be directly calculated in general population cohorts (or random samples thereof) but should be obtained from outside sources when a cohort study is based on special exposure groups. In either instance, I_T is the weighted average of I_e and I_o, with "weights" equal to Π and $(1 - \Pi)$, respectively:

$$I_T = I_e \cdot \Pi + I_o \cdot (1 - \Pi)$$

and, therefore, the population attributable rate is

$$PAR = I_o \cdot RR \cdot \Pi + I_o \cdot (1 - \Pi) - I_o = I_o \cdot \Pi \cdot (RR - 1)$$

The PAR describes the limit of the beneficial impact on a certain population of the complete, irreversible, and immediate removal of an established cause of a disease. The dependence of PAR on the highly variable Π distinguishes PAR from EAR and RR. It should be noted that the two preceding equations are strictly valid only when I_T, I_e, and I_o are crude rates; when the rates are adjusted, the formulae are good approximations when the causal factor under consideration is not strongly related to the factors for which they are adjusted.

The population attributable fraction (PAF) can be reformulated on the basis of the two preceding equations as

$$PAF = \frac{\Pi \cdot (RR - 1)}{\Pi \cdot (RR - 1) + 1}$$

If π is the proportion of exposed persons among all cases, an alternative formula for PAF[355] is

$$PAF = \frac{\pi \cdot (RR - 1)}{RR} = \pi \cdot EAF$$

This last formula for PAF applies to both crude and adjusted RR.

Attributable Rates in Case-Control Studies

Incidence rates among exposed and unexposed persons may be obtained directly in cohort investigations, but they are not usually available in case-control studies that focus on the estimation of the odds ratio between exposed and unexposed individuals. Nevertheless, under certain conditions in case-control studies, estimates can be made of disease rates associated with reported exposures or other study factors.

Studies of Cases Referable to a Population

When the cases represent all cases of the disease in a defined population or a sample of such cases selected in a known way, and the control group is representative of the same population, it will be possible to estimate rates of the disease in exposed and nonexposed persons and to derive attributable rates from these estimates.

For example, the 155 women with venous thrombosis in Table 10-7 originated from a base population of about 740,000 person-years. The distribution of these person-years by current oral contraceptive use and the presence of factor V Leiden mutation can be derived from the control group, which is representative of the

Table 10-11. Estimated Incidence of First Venous Thrombosis in Women 15–49 Years Old, According to Presence of Factor V Leiden Mutation and Current Use of Oral Contraceptives (OC)

| \multicolumn{2}{c}{Category of exposure} | | Cases | Controls | Person-years | Incidence per | | Rate |
V Leiden	OCs	N	N (prevalence)	(PY)	10,000 PY		ratio
No	No	36	100 (0.592)	437,870	0.8		1.0
No	Yes	84	63 (0.373)	275,858	3.0		3.7
Yes	No	10	4 (0.024)	17,515	5.7	4.8	6.9
Yes	Yes	25	2 (0.012)	8,757	28.5		34.7
Total		155	169 (1 = 100%)	740,000	2.1		

Source: Adapted from Vandenbroucke JP, et al. Increased risk of venous thrombosis in oral-contraceptive users who are carriers of factor V Leiden mutation. *Lancet* 1994;344 : 1453–1457.

base population from which these cases originated.[563] The incidence of first venous thrombosis by categories of current oral contraceptive use and the presence of factor V Leiden mutation is shown in Table 10-11.

The exposed attributable rate is 3.0 − 0.8 = 2.2 cases of first venous thrombosis per 10,000 person-years among women who take oral contraceptives but do not have factor V Leiden mutation; the corresponding rates are 5.7 − 0.8 = 4.9 among those who have this mutation but do not take oral contraceptives, and 28.5 − 0.8 = 27.7 among those who are exposed to both this mutation and oral contraceptives. The population rate attributable to the exposure to either or both of these factors is 2.1 − 0.8 = 1.3 cases of first venous thrombosis per 10,000 person-years. The same figure (1.3) may be obtained by multiplying every exposure-specific EAR with the corresponding prevalence and summing over the three categories of exposure (0.373 · 2.2 + 0.024 · 4.9 + 0.012 · 27.7 = 1.3).

Note that in this particular example the controls were not strictly representative of the base population in that they were matched to the age distribution of the cases. If the exposures under consideration varied in frequency with age, the procedure outlined here would only provide approximations. In such circumstances, rates should be estimated within appropriate age groups, and exposed and population attributable rates should be derived by standardization to a common standard.

Indirect Estimation of Attributable Rates

Sometimes an estimate of the incidence rate of a disease is available from another source, even though it cannot be derived from the study being analyzed. Thus, the data in Table 10-3 do not supply an estimate of the incidence of hepatocellular carcinoma (HCC) among men in the study area, but on the basis of earlier work and mortality statistics this rate can be estimated as about 12 per 100,000 person-years. Given this information and the odds ratio estimate for chronic infection with hepatitis C virus (HCV) in relation to HCC, estimates of the disease incidence among HCV infected and noninfected men can be derived as explained next.

The overall incidence of a disease in a population is, as previously indicated, the weighted average of the disease incidence in the various mutually exclusive and collectively exhaustive exposure categories, weighted according to the proportion of the population in each of the exposure categories. Thus, in the simple situation where there are only two exposure categories, as in Table 10-3 (i.e., exposed and nonexposed), the overall incidence I_T is

$$I_T = I_e \cdot \Pi + I_o \cdot (1 - \Pi)$$

where, as before, I_e and I_o are the incidence rates of the disease among exposed and nonexposed persons, respectively, Π is the proportion of the population in the exposed category, and $(1 - \Pi)$ is the proportion of the population in the unexposed category.

Because $I_e = I_o \cdot OR$, where OR is the odds ratio, the formula can be written

$$I_T = I_o \cdot OR \cdot \Pi + I_o \cdot (1 - \Pi)$$

or, in terms of I_o,

$$I_o = \frac{I_T}{OR \cdot \Pi + (1 - \Pi)}$$

When I_T is in some way known, OR has been estimated, and the assumption can be made that the distribution of the controls in the study approximates the distribution of the base population with respect to exposure categories, then I_o can be estimated.

For example, in the data of Table 10-3, I_T can be considered as equal to 12 per 100,000 person-years, OR for chronic infection with HCV is 9.2, and the proportion of controls chronically infected with HCV is 0.06. Therefore,

$$I_o = \frac{12}{9.2 \cdot 0.06 + 0.94} = 8.0 \text{ per } 100,000 \text{ person-years}$$

$$I_e = 8.0 \cdot 9.2 = 73.6 \text{ per } 100,000 \text{ person-years}$$

It should again be pointed out that the basic formula $I_T = I_e \cdot \Pi + I_o \cdot (1 - \Pi)$ is strictly applicable in the absence of confounding and only if controls represent the base population. Nevertheless, even when the required conditions are not fulfilled, the crude estimates of exposure category-specific incidence rates allow an insight on the magnitude of the attributable rates that can guide public health professionals in the setting of policies and the ranking of objectives.

Attributable Fractions in Case-Control Studies

In most case-control studies, it is not possible to directly estimate disease incidence in any of the exposure categories, nor is there an incidence rate available for the relevant base population from another source. In such situations, it is not possible to derive attributable rates among the exposed or for the total population, but it is still possible to calculate the corresponding attributable fractions (EAF and PAF).

The exposure attributable fraction is simply

$$\frac{I_e - I_o}{I_e} \quad \text{or} \quad \frac{OR \cdot I_o - I_o}{OR \cdot I_o} = \frac{OR - 1}{OR}$$

Therefore, EAF can be directly calculated for any exposure level from the corresponding odds ratio, whether this OR is crude or adjusted through stratification or logistic regression modeling. Moreover, because the only source of variation in EAF is the OR, the test-based procedure can be used to set confidence limits.[348,349] Thus, in the data of Table 10-8, of the persons who developed cancer of the urinary bladder and have worked in an occupation at high risk for this cancer, 29 percent $\left(\text{because } \dfrac{1.40 - 1}{1.40} = 0.29 \right)$ could attribute their cancer to their occupational exposure(s). However, there is considerable uncertainty about this estimate; it could be as high as 57 percent $\left(\text{because } \dfrac{2.33 - 1}{2.33} = 0.57 \right)$, but it could also be as low as 0, and it is even possible (although very unlikely) that working in these presumably high-risk occupations prevents bladder cancer $\left(\text{because } \dfrac{0.85 - 1}{0.85} < 0 \right)$.

Most of the attention and a substantial amount of methodological work concerning attributable rates and fractions has focused on the population attributable fraction[67,283,316] and its derivation in case-control studies.[21,76] As indicated, PAF can be calculated as

$$\frac{\Pi \cdot (OR - 1)}{\Pi \cdot (OR - 1) + 1}$$

where Π is the proportion of exposed in the base population, or as

$$\frac{\pi \cdot (OR - 1)}{OR}$$

where π is the proportion of exposed among all cases.[355]

For the data in Table 10-3, if the distribution of controls by exposure status adequately reflects the corresponding distribution in the study base, the PAF can be estimated as

$$\frac{\Pi \cdot (OR - 1)}{\Pi \cdot (OR - 1) + 1} = \frac{0.06 \cdot 8.2}{0.06 \cdot 8.2 + 1} = 0.33 \text{ or } 33 \text{ percent}$$

The same result is obtained by using Miettinen's formula for PAF:[355]

$$\frac{\pi \cdot (OR - 1)}{OR} = \frac{0.38 \cdot 8.2}{9.2} = 0.34 \text{ or } 34 \text{ percent}$$

(The difference is due to rounding errors; 0.34 is more accurate.)

Confidence limits for PAF can be set using a simple formula proposed by Walter.[579,580] The test-based procedure[348,349] is not applicable for PAF because this measure has two sources of variation, the OR and Π, unless, of course, the proportion of exposed in the population were to be arbitrarily set.

When there are several levels of exposure (e.g., in Tables 10-4 and 10-8), it is possible to estimate the contribution to PAF from any particular exposure level and calculate the respective confidence limits.[90] However, the overall PAF due to the multilevel exposure will be identical whether the level-specific contributions to overall PAF are separately calculated and subsequently summed or all exposure levels are combined and PAF is calculated on the basis of the contrast between exposed (any level) and unexposed. The distinction in levels of exposure is more important when a public health campaign is expected to switch the distribution of an exposure toward lower levels (for an exposure that increases disease risk), even though removal of the exposure is impractical or inconceivable (e.g., most dietary exposures, blood pressure, serum cholesterol). A simple method that addresses this problem has been proposed by Wahrendorf.[573]

Several authors have examined the consequences of nondifferential exposure and outcome misclassification on PAF estimation.[218,221,566] Nondifferential exposure level misclassification *among* definitely exposed persons does not affect PAF estimation because this type of misclassification has opposing and balancing effects on the components of PAF (i.e., the level-specific ORs and the distribution of exposed subjects by level of exposure). This is the reason behind the identity of PAF estimations based on either all exposed persons taken together or level-specific proportions of exposed persons and associated odds ratios. Nondifferential misclassification between exposed and nonexposed individuals does usually bias PAF toward zero, but prevalence of exposure and sensitivity and specificity in the correct identification of exposed individuals have somewhat unexpected consequences. As pointed out by Hsieh and Walter,[221] misclassification bias tends to be larger when the prevalence of exposure is higher. More important, if the sensitivity is perfect (correct identification of all truly exposed individuals), there is no bias in the estimation of PAF even when the specificity is low (several truly unexposed individuals included among the truly exposed). This observation led Wacholder et al.[566] to recommend that exposure should be operationally defined in very broad terms whenever estimation of PAF is a research objective. For the data in Table 10-8, this reasonable recommendation would indicate the grouping together of persons who have worked in jobs with either high or undetermined a priori occupational risk for bladder cancer.

Adjustment for confounding in the estimation of PAF has been examined by several authors. The alternative formula for PAF suggested by Miettinen[355] can be used for the estimation of adjusted PAF by substituting the Mantel-Haenszel odds ratio (OR_{M-H}) for the crude odds ratio as follows:

$$\text{adjusted PAF} = \frac{\pi \cdot (OR_{M-H} - 1)}{OR_{M-H}}$$

The justification and the application of this procedure for matched and unmatched data and the estimation of appropriate confidence limits around the point estimates of adjusted PAF have been considered by Kuritz and Landis[270,271] and Greenland.[167] This approach is attractively simple, but it requires homogeneity of the odds ratio across the strata.[163] An alternative procedure developed by Whittemore[589,590] does not require homogeneity of the odds ratio.[21,76] Bruzzi et al. have employed logistic regression to obtain adjusted estimates of PAF.[46,173]

Although PAF has been extensively utilized in case-control studies,[277] there is at present considerable research activity that covers not only methodological problems but also conceptual issues surrounding PAF and its implications in science and the law.[76,180,448]

Interpretation

The basic questions likely to be asked in interpreting the results of a study are the same in a case-control as in a cohort study:

1. After control of confounding from all likely sources and careful consideration of residual confounding, do the findings indicate an association between the disease under study and the exposure of interest?
2. If an association is observed, is it likely to be due to chance?
3. Could an association that appears real and unconfounded be the result of subtle selection or information bias that was not recognized during the study design and implementation?

In attempting to answer the last question, consideration should be given to matters of comparability between cases and controls and the information provided by them or ascertained through examination of records or laboratory tests. An overview of all the items on which cases and controls differ may be revealing. When the data for cases and controls are generally similar, but clear associations are found between the disease and one or two exposures, these associations are more likely to be considered as real than if a great number of apparent associations emerges. Thus, the positive associations of cholelithiasis and diabetes mellitus with pancreatic cancer in Table 10-12 become more credible because several other medical events or conditions show no relation to this disease in the same dataset.

Results of every study should be judged in the context of the overall empirical evidence and their biomedical plausibility. Meta-analysis (i.e., systematic statistical evaluation of the results of several independent studies[166,171]) is a widely acceptable procedure for randomized trials,[273,473] but its role in observational epidemiology remains controversial.[408,490] Although it is certainly true that in observational studies residual confounding and unrecognized bias can never be excluded, there seems to be no reason to avoid the statistical formalization of a process that is informally practiced by all investigators. Nevertheless, meta-analysis of case-control or cohort studies does not carry the weight that it does in randomized clinical trials.

Biomedical plausibility is an important criterion of causality, and it assumes an overriding role when the empirical evidence for an association is inconsistent and generally weak. By contrast, a consistently demonstrated strong association may have to be considered in causal terms, even in the absence of supportive biological information.

When faced with inconclusive results, an investigator has the responsibility to judge whether the findings refute the working hypothesis or are compatible with but not strongly supportive of

Table 10-12. Frequency of Reporting of Specified Medical Events or Conditions by 181 Persons with Pancreatic Cancer and an Equal Number of Age- and Gender-Matched Controls in Each of Two Comparison Series

Event or condition	Pancreatic cancer	Hospital controls	Visitor controls	Adjusted rate ratios (95% confidence interval)*	
				Cases cf. hospital controls	Cases cf. visitor controls
Tonsillectomy	37	27	32	1.42 (0.84–2.39)	1.22 (0.70–2.11)
Appendectomy	56	63	49	0.85 (0.56–1.30)	1.22 (0.76–1.95)
Treatment for gastric ulcer	8	8	10	1.00 (0.38–2.66)	0.78 (0.29–2.09)
Treatment for duodenal ulcer	17	15	14	1.15 (0.55–2.43)	1.25 (0.59–2.67)
Treatment for gastritis	14	12	14	1.18 (0.53–2.64)	1.00 (0.48–2.10)
Treatment for hemorrhoids	34	26	22	1.44 (0.79–2.63)	1.80 (0.96–3.38)
Cholelithiasis	42	18	16	2.50 (1.40–4.46)	2.73 (1.51–4.94)
Hypertension	48	38	46	1.35 (0.83–2.18)	1.06 (0.67–1.67)
Diabetes mellitus	34	6	8	6.60 (2.58–16.91)	7.50 (2.64–21.29)
Long-term medication	104	121	106	0.67 (0.43–1.03)	0.95 (0.62–1.47)

Source: Adapted from Kalapothaki V. et al. Tobacco, ethanol, coffee, pancreatitis, diabetes mellitus, and cholelithiasis as risk factors for pancreatic carcinoma. *Cancer Causes Control* 1993;4 : 375–382.
*Adjusted for age and gender through conditional logistic regression

it. To reduce the danger of overinterpretation, the opinion has been advanced that the principal effect measure (the odds ratio) should be adjusted not only for clear confounders but also for variables with questionable, even unlikely, confounding influences. This approach may improve control of confounding, but it mainly widens the confidence interval around the point estimate of the odds ratio, thereby reducing the temptation for overinterpretation.

Case-control studies have contributed more than any other approach to the flourishing of epidemiology during the last few decades.[65,66] Methodological advances allow case-control studies to address virtually all problems that cohort studies can address, excepting the evaluation of exposures that can affect disease risk factors, which, in turn, can influence these exposures.[447] However, case-control studies require more attention and subtlety for the avoidance of selection and information bias than the more straightforward cohort studies.

References

1. The A to F of viral hepatitis. (Editorial). *Lancet* 1990;336 : 1158–1160.
2. Abelin T, Averkin JI, Egger M, et al. Thyroid cancer in Belarus post-Chernobyl: Improved detection or increased incidence? *Soz Präventiv Med* 1994;39 : 189–197.
3. Abou-Daoud KT. Epidemiology of carcinoma of the cervix uteri in Lebanese Christians and Moslems. *Cancer* 1967;20 : 1706–1714.
4. Adami H-O, Hsieh C-c, Lambe M, et al. Parity, age at first childbirth, and risk of ovarian cancer. *Lancet* 1994;344 : 1250–1254.
5. Adami H-O, Hsing AW, McLaughlin JK, et al. Alcoholism and liver cirrhosis in the etiology of primary liver cancer. *Int J Cancer* 1992;51 : 898–902.
6. Alcohol and mortality: The myth of the U-shaped curve. (Editorial). *Lancet* 1988;ii : 1292–1293.
7. American Psychiatric Association. *Diagnostic and Statistical Manual of Mental Disorders*, 3rd ed. (DSM III). Washington, DC: American Psychiatric Association, 1980.
8. American Psychiatric Association. *Diagnostic and Statistical Manual of Mental Disorders*. 4th ed. Washington, DC: American Psychiatric Association, 1994.
9. Andvord KF. What can we learn by studying tuberculosis by generations? *Norsk Mag Laegevidensk* 1930;91 : 642–660.
10. Armitage P. Tests for linear trends in proportions and frequencies. *Biometrics* 1955;11 : 375–386.
11. Armitage P, Berry G. *Statistical Methods in Medical Research*. Oxford: Blackwell Scientific Publications, 1988.
12. Armstrong B, Thériault G, Guénel P, et al. Association between exposure to pulsed electromagnetic fields and cancer in electric utility workers in Quebec, Canada, and France. *Am J Epidemiol* 1994;140 : 805–820.
13. Armstrong BG, Whittemore AS, Howe GR. Analysis of case-control data with covariate measurement error: Application to diet and colon cancer. *Stat Med* 1989;8 : 1151–1163.
14. Armstrong BK, White E, Saracci R. *Principles of Exposure Measurement in Epidemiology*. Oxford, New York, Tokyo: Oxford University Press, 1994. Monographs in Epidemiology and Biostatistics. Vol. 21.
15. Austin H, Flanders WD, Rothman KJ. Bias arising in case-control

studies from selection of controls from overlapping groups. *Int J Epidemiol* 1989;18 : 713–716.

16. Axelson O, Steenland K. Indirect methods of assessing the effects of tobacco use in occupational studies. *Am J Ind Med* 1988;13 : 105–118.

17. Aycock WL, Luther EH. The occurrence of poliomyelitis following tonsillectomy. *N Engl J Med* 1929;200 : 164–167.

18. Beasley RP, Hwang LY, Lin C-C, et al. Hepatocellular carcinoma and hepatitis B virus. A prospective study of 22,707 men in Taiwan. *Lancet* 1981;ii : 1129–1133.

19. Beebe GW. Lung cancer in World War I veterans: Possible relation to mustard-gas injury and 1918 influenza epidemic. *J Natl Cancer Inst* 1960;25 : 1231–1252.

20. Benfante R. Studies of cardiovascular disease and cause-specific mortality trends in Japanese-American men living in Hawaii and risk factor comparisons with other Japanese populations in the Pacific region: A review. *Hum Biol* 1992;64 : 791–805.

21. Benichou J. Methods of adjustment for estimating the attributable risk in case-control studies: A review. *Stat Med* 1991;10 : 1753–1773.

22. Beral V. Childhood leukemia near nuclear plants in the United Kingdom: The evolution of a systematic approach to studying rare disease in small geographic areas. *Am J Epidemiol* 1990;132 (Suppl.) : S63–S68.

23. Bergkvist L, Adami H-O, Persson I, et al. The risk of breast cancer after estrogen and estrogen-progestin replacement. *N Engl J Med* 1989;321 : 293–297.

24. Berkson J. Limitations of the application of fourfold table analysis to hospital data. *Biometrics* 1946;2 : 47–53.

25. Berkson J. The statistical interpretation of smoking and cancer of the lung. *Proc Staff Meetings Mayo Clinic* 1959;34 : 206–244.

26. Berman C. Primary carcinoma of the liver in the Bantu races of South Africa. *S Afr J Med Sc* 1940;5 : 54–72.

27. Bertazzi PA, Pesatori AC, Consonni D, et al. Cancer incidence in a population accidentally exposed to 2,3,7,8-tetrachlorodibenzo-para-dioxin. *Epidemiology* 1993;4 : 398–406.

28. Bertazzi PA, Zocchetti C, Pesatori AC, et al. Ten-year mortality study of the population involved in the Seveso incident in 1976. *Am J Epidemiol* 1989;129 : 1187–1200.

29. Bithell JF, Stone RA. On statistical methods for analyzing the geographical distribution of cancer cases near nuclear installations. *J Epidemiol Community Health* 1989;43 : 79–85.

30. Black D. *Investigation of the Possible Increased Incidence of Cancer in West Cumbria. Report of the Independent Advisory Group.* London: Her Majesty's Stationery Office, 1984.

31. Blayney JR, Hill IN. Fluorine and dental caries. *J Am Dent Ass* 1967;74 : 225–302.

32. Boffetta P, Garfinkel L. Alcohol drinking and mortality among men enrolled in an American Cancer Society prospective study. *Epidemiology* 1990;1 : 342–348.

33. Boice JD Jr, Blettner M, Kleinerman RA, et al. Radiation dose and breast cancer risk in patients treated for cancer of the cervix. *Int J Cancer* 1989;44 : 7–16.

34. Boice JD Jr, Engholm G, Kleinerman RA, et al. Radiation dose and second cancer risk in patients treated for cancer of the cervix. *Radiat Res* 1988;116 : 3–55.

35. Boring CC, Squires TS, Tong T, Montgomery S. Cancer statistics, 1994. *CA Cancer J Clin* 1994;44 : 7–26.

36. Boyle P. Relative value of incidence and mortality data in cancer research. *Recent Results Canc Res* 1989;114 : 41–63.
37. Boyle P, Robertson C. Statistical modelling of lung cancer and laryngeal cancer in Scotland, 1960–1979. *Am J Epidemiol* 1987; 125 : 731–744.
38. Boyle P, Soukop M, Scully C, et al. Improving prognosis of Hodgkin's disease in Scotland. *Eur J Cancer Clin Oncol* 1988;24 : 229–234.
39. Brenner H, Savitz DA, Jöckel K-H, et al. The effects of nondifferential misclassification in ecologic studies. *Am J Epidemiol* 1992; 135 : 85–95.
40. Breslow N. Odds ratio estimators when the data are sparse. *Bioetrika* 1981;68 : 73–84.
41. Breslow N. Design and analysis of case-control studies. *Ann Rev Public Health* 1982;3 : 29–54.
42. Breslow NE, Day NE. *Statistical Methods in Cancer Research. Volume I. The Analysis of Case-Control Studies.* Lyon: International Agency for Research on Cancer (IARC), 1980. IARC Scientific Publ. No. 32.
43. Breslow NE, Day NE. *Statistical Methods in Cancer Research. Volume II. The Design and Analysis of Cohort Studies.* Lyon: International Agency for Research on Cancer (IARC), 1987. IARC Scientific Publ. No. 82.
44. Brinton LA, Shairer C, Hoover RN, Fraumeni JF Jr. Menstrual factors and risk of breast cancer. *Cancer Invest* 1988;6 : 245–254.
45. Brunner EJ, Marmot MG, White IR, et al. Gender and employment grade differences in blood cholesterol, apolipoproteins and haemostatic factors in the Whitehall II study. *Atherosclerosis* 1993;102 : 195–207.
46. Bruzzi P, Green SB, Byar DP, et al. Estimating the population attributable risk for multiple risk factors using case-control data. *Am J Epidemiol* 1985;122 : 904–914.
47. Buck C. Popper's philosophy for epidemiologists. *Int J Epidemiol* 1975;4 : 159–168.
48. Budd W. *Typhoid Fever. Its Nature, Mode of Spreading, and Prevention.* London: 1874. Reprinted New York: American Public Health Association, 1931.
49. Caldwell GG. Twenty-two years of cancer cluster investigations at the Centers for Disease Control. *Am J Epidemiol* 1990;132 (Suppl.) : S43–S47.
50. Campion MJ, Cuzick J, McCance DJ, et al. Progressive potential of mild cervical atypia: Prospective cytological, colposcopic, and virological study. *Lancet* 1986;i : 237–240.
51. Cannell CF, Marquis KH, Laurent A. (1977). *A Summary of Studies of Interviewing Methodology.* Washington, DC: US Govt. Printing Office. DHEW Publ. No. (HRA) 77-1343.
52. Case RAM. Cohort analysis of mortality rates as an historical or narrative technique. *Br J Prev Soc Med* 1956;10 : 159–171.
53. Case RAM, Coghill C, Davies JM, et al. *Serial Mortality Tables. Neoplastic Diseases Volume 1. England and Wales, 1911–1970.* Mimeographed. London: Division of Epidemiology, Institute for Cancer Research, 1976.
54. Case RAM, Hosker ME, McDonald DB, Pearson JT. Tumours of the urinary bladder in workmen engaged in the manufacture and use of certain dyestuff intermediates in the British chemical industry. *Brit J Ind Med* 1954;11 : 75–104.
55. Castegnaro M, Pleština R, Dirheimer G, et al. (Eds.). *Mycotoxins, Endemic Nephropathy and Urinary Tract Tumours.* Lyon: Interna-

tional Agency for Research on Cancer (IARC), 1991. IARC Scientific Publ. No. 115.

56. Caverly CS. Preliminary report of an epidemic of paralytic disease, occurring in Vermont, in the summer of 1894. *Yale Med J* 1894;1 : 1–5.

57. Centers for Disease Control. Guidelines for investigating clusters of health events. *MMWR* 1990;19 : 1–23.

58. Centers for Disease Control. Proceedings of the National Conference on Clustering of Health Events, 1989. *Am J Epidemiol* 1990; 132(Suppl.).

59. Checkoway H, Pearce NE, Crawford Brown DJ. *Research Methods in Occupational Epidemiology.* New York, Oxford: Oxford University Press, 1989.

60. Chen R, Mantel N, Klingberg MA. A study of three techniques for time-space clustering in Hodgkin's disease. *Stat Med* 1984; 3 : 173–184.

61. Clayton D, Hills M. *Statistical Models in Epidemiology.* Oxford: Oxford University Press, 1993.

62. Cochran WG. Modern methods in the sampling of human populations. General principles in the selection of a sample. *Am J Public Health* 1951;41 : 647–653.

63. Coggon D, Lambert P, Langman MJ. 20 years of hospital admissions for peptic ulcer in England and Wales. *Lancet* 1981;i : 1302–1304.

64. Cohen MC, Muller JE. Onset of acute myocardial infarction—circadian variation and triggers. *Cardiovasc Res* 1992;26 : 831–838.

65. Cole P. The evolving case-control study. *J Chronic Dis* 1979; 32 : 15–27.

66. Cole P. Introduction. *In:* Breslow NE, Day NE. *Statistical Methods in Cancer Research. Volume I. The Analysis of Case-Control Studies.* Lyon: International Agency for Research on Cancer (IARC), 1980. IARC Scientific Publ. No. 32, pp. 14–40.

67. Cole P, MacMahon B. Attributable risk percent in case-control studies. *Br J Prev Soc Med* 1971;25 : 242–244.

68. Cole P, Monson RR, Haning H, Friedell GH. Smoking and cancer of the lower urinary tract. *N Engl J Med* 1971;284 : 129–134.

69. Cole P, Morrison AS. Basic issues in population screening for cancer. *J Natl Cancer Inst* 1980;64 : 1263–1272.

70. Context Software Systems, Inc. *International Classification of Diseases, 9th Rev., Clinical Modification. Vol 1. Diseases: Tabular List. Vol 2. Diseases: Alphabetic Index. Vol 3. Procedures: Tabular List and Alphabetic Index.* New York: McGraw-Hill, 1994.

71. Cook-Mozaffari PJ, Ashwood FL, Vincent T, et al. *Cancer Incidence and Mortality in the Vicinity of Nuclear Installations. England and Wales, 1959–1980.* London: Her Majesty's Stationery Office, 1987. Studies on Medical and Population Subjects, No. 51.

72. Cook-Mozaffari PJ, Darby SC, Doll R, et al. Geographical variation in mortality from leukaemia and other cancers in England and Wales in relation to proximity to nuclear installations, 1969–78. *Br J Cancer* 1989;59 : 476–485.

73. Cooper JE, Kendell RE, Gurland BJ, et al. *Psychiatric Diagnosis in New York and London.* London: Oxford University Press, 1972.

74. Cornfield J. A method of estimating comparative rates from clinical data. Applications to cancer of the lung, breast and cervix. *J Natl Cancer Inst* 1951;11 : 1269–1275.

75. Cornfield J. A statistical problem arising from retrospective studies. *In:* Neyman J. (Ed.), *Proceedings of the Third Berkeley Symposium.*

Volume IV. Berkeley: University of California Press, 1956, pp. 135–148.

76. Coughlin SS, Benichou J, Weed DL. Attributable risk estimation in case-control studies. *Epidemiol Rev* 1994;16 : 51–64.

77. Court-Brown WM, Doll R. Mortality from cancer and other causes after radiotherapy for ankylosing spondylitis. *Br Med J* 1965; 2 : 1327–1332.

78. Cox DR. Regression models and life tables (with discussion). *JR Statist Soc* Series B 1972;34 : 187–220.

79. Cullen W. *Synopsis Nosologicae Medicae (1785). Quoted by Hosack D. A System of Practical Nosology* (2nd ed.). New York: O.S. Van Winkle, 1821.

80. Cutler SJ, Ederer F. Maximum utilization of the life table method in analyzing survival. *J Chronic Dis* 1958;8 : 699–712.

81. Cuzick J, Edwards R. Spatial clustering for inhomogeneous populations. *J R Stat Soc [B]* 1990;52 : 73–104.

82. Daling JR, Malone KE, Voigt LF, et al. Risk of breast cancer among young women: Relationship to induced abortion. *J Natl Cancer Inst* 1994;86 : 1584–1592.

83. Darby SC, Doll R, Gill SK, Smith PG. Long-term mortality after a single treatment course with X-rays in patients treated for ankylosing spondylitis. *Br J Cancer* 1987;55 : 179–190.

84. David FN, Barton DE. Two time-space interaction tests for epidemicity. *Br J Prev Soc Med* 1966;20 : 44–48.

85. Dawber TR, Kannel WB, Lyell LP. An approach to longitudinal studies in a community: The Framingham study. *Ann NY Acad Sci* 1963;107 : 539–556.

86. Dawber TR, Meadors GF, Moore FE Jr. Epidemiological approaches to heart disease. The Framingham study. *Am J Public Health* 1951;41 : 279–286.

87. Day NE, Byar DP, Green SB. Overadjustment in case-control studies. *Am J Epidemiol* 1980;112 : 696–706.

88. Dean HT. Some general epidemiological considerations. *In*: Moulton FR (Ed.), *Dental Caries and Fluorine.* Washington, DC: AAAS, 1946.

89. DeBakey ME, Beebe GW. Medical follow-up studies on veterans. *JAMA* 1962;182 : 1103–1109.

90. Denman DW 3d, Schlesselman JJ. Interval estimation of the attributable risk for multiple exposure levels in case-control studies. *Biometrics* 1983;39 : 185–192.

91. de Thé G, Geser A, Day NE, et al. Epidemiological evidence for causal relationship between Epstein-Barr virus and Burkitt's lymphoma from Uganda prospective study. *Nature* 1978; 274 : 756–761.

92. Diez-Roux AV, Nieto FJ, Tyroler HA, et al. Social inequalities and atherosclerosis: The Atherosclerosis Risk in Communities study. *Am J Epidemiol* 1995;141 : 960–972.

93. Dockery DW, Pope CA III, Xu X, et al. An association between air pollution and mortality in six U.S. cities. *N Engl J Med* 1993; 329 : 1753–1759.

94. Doll R. Bronchial carcinoma: Incidence and aetiology. *Br Med J* 1953;2 : 521–527, 585–590.

95. Doll R, Evans HJ, Darby SC. Commentary. Paternal exposure not to blame. *Nature* 1994;367 : 678–680.

96. Doll R, Hill AB. A study of the aetiology of carcinoma of the lung. *Br Med J* 1952;2 : 1271–1286.

97. Doll R, Hill AB. The mortality of doctors in relation to their smoking habits. A preliminary report. *Br Med J* 1954;1 : 1451–1455.

98. Doll R, Hill AB. Lung cancer and other causes of death in relation to smoking. A second report on the mortality of British doctors. *Br Med J* 1956;2 : 1071–1081.

99. Doll R, Hill AB. Mortality in relation to smoking: Ten years' observations of British doctors. *Br Med J* 1964;1 : 1399–1410, 1460–1467.

100. Doll R, Payne P, Waterhouse J (Eds.). *Cancer Incidence in Five Continents. A Technical Report.* Berlin, Heidelberg, New York: Springer-Verlag, 1966.

101. Doll R, Peto R. Mortality in relation to smoking: 20 years' observations on male British doctors. *Br Med J* 1976;ii : 1525–1536.

102. Dorn HF. Tobacco consumption and mortality from cancer and other diseases. *Public Health Rep* 1959;74 : 581–593.

103. Dorn HF, Cutler SJ. *Morbidity from Cancer in the United States. Part 1. Variations in Incidence by Age, Sex, Race, Marital Status, and Geographic Region.* Washington, DC: U.S. Govt. Printing Office, 1955. Public Health Monograph No. 29. Public Health Service Publ. No. 418.

104. Dorn HF, Cutler SJ. *Morbidity from Cancer in the United States.* Washington, DC: U.S. Govt. Printing Office, 1959. Publ. Health Monograph No. 56.

105. Dosemeci M, Wacholder S, Lubin JH. Does non-differential misclassification of exposure always bias a true effect toward the null value? *Am J Epidemiol* 1990;132 : 746–748.

106. Drews CD, Kraus JF, Greenland S. Recall bias in a case-control study of sudden infant death syndrome. *Int J Epidemiol* 1990; 19 : 405–411.

107. Driscoll RJ, Mulligan WJ, Schultz D, Candelaria A. Malignant mesothelioma. A cluster in a Native American pueblo. *N Engl J Med* 1988;318 : 1437–1438.

108. Dunn JE Jr, Buell P. Association of cervical cancer with circumcision of sexual partner. *J Natl Cancer Inst* 1959; 22 : 749–764.

109. Dunn JE Jr, Martin PL. Morphogenesis of cervical cancer. Findings from the San Diego County cytology registry. *Cancer* 1967; 20 : 1899–1906.

110. Eaton JW, Weil RJ. *Culture and Mental Disorders.* Glencoe, Ill: Free Press, 1955.

111. Ederer F, Axtell LM, Cuttler SJ. The relative survival rate. A statistical methodology. *Natl Cancer Inst Monogr* 1961;6 : 101–121.

112. Editorial Committee, the National Cancer Control Office of the Ministry of Health, and Nanjing Institute of Geography of Academia Sinica. *Atlas of Cancer Mortality in the People's Republic of China.* Beijing: China Map Press, 1980.

113. Edwards JH. The recognition and estimation of cyclic trends. *Ann Human Genet* 1961;25 : 83–87.

114. Ehrlich PR, Holm RW. Patterns and populations. *Science* 1962; 137 : 652–657.

115. Ekbom A, Hsieh C-c, Yuen J, et al. Risk of extrahepatic bile duct cancer after cholecystectomy. *Lancet* 1993;342 : 1262–1265.

116. Elandt-Johnson RC. Various estimators of conditional probabilities of death in follow-up studies: summary of results. *J Chronic Dis* 1977;30 : 247–256.

117. Elley WB, Irving JC. Revised socioeconomic index for New Zealand. *NZ J Econ Studies* 1976;11 : 25–30.

118. Enstrom JE. Health practices and cancer mortality among active California Mormons. *J Natl Cancer Inst* 1989;81 : 1807–1814.

119. Estève J, Benhamou E, Raymond L. *Statistical Methods in Cancer Research. Volume IV. Descriptive Epidemiology.* Lyon: International

Agency for Research on Cancer (IARC), 1994. IARC Scientific Publ. No. 128.

120. Evans AS. *Causation and Disease. A Chronological Journey.* New York: Plenum, 1993.

121. Evans AS, Mueller NE. Malignant lymphomas. *In*: Evans AS (Ed.). *Viral Infections of Humans: Epidemiology and Control.* 4th ed. New York: Plenum Medical, in press.

122. Feinleib M. Breast cancer and artificial menopause: A cohort study. *J Natl Cancer Inst* 1968;41 : 315–329.

123. Feinleib M. Counting isn't easy. (Editorial). *Epidemiology* 1995; 6 : 343–345.

124. Feinstein AR. Methodologic problems and standards in case-control research. *J Chronic Dis* 1979;32 : 35–41.

125. Finlay C. Yellow fever: Its transmission by means of the *Culex* mosquito. *Am J Med Sci* 1886;92 : 395–409.

126. Flanders WD. Limitations of the case-exposure study. *Epidemiology* 1990;1 : 34–38.

127. Flanders WD, Austin H. Possibility of selection bias in matched case-control studies using friend controls. *Am J Epidemiol* 1986;124 : 150–153.

128. Fleiss JL. *Statistical Methods for Rates and Proportions.* New York: Wiley, 1973.

129. Fletcher W. Rice and beri-beri: Preliminary report of an experiment conducted at the Kuala Lumpur Lunatic Asylum. *Lancet* 1907; i : 1776–1779.

130. Fonnebo V. Mortality in Norwegian Seventh-Day Adventists 1962–1986. *J Clin Epidemiol* 1992;45 : 157–167.

131. Forman D, Cook-Mozaffari P, Darby S. Commentary. Cancer near nuclear installations. *Nature* 1987;329 : 499–505.

132. Fox SH, Koepsell TD, Daling JR. Birth weight and smoking during pregnancy-effect modification by maternal age. *Am J Epidemiol* 1994;139 : 1008–1015.

133. Francis T Jr., Epstein FH. Survey methods in general populations. I. Studies of a total community. Tecumseh, Michigan. *In*: Acheson R.M. (Ed.), *Comparability in International Epidemiology.* New York: Milbank Memorial Fund, 1965.

134. Fraumeni JF Jr. Etiologic clues from cancer mapping in the United States. *Gann Monograph on Cancer Research* 1987;33 : 171–179.

135. Freeman J, Hutchison GB. Prevalence, incidence and duration. *Am J Epidemiol* 1980;112 : 707–723.

136. Friedenreich CM, Howe GR, Miller AB. An investigation of recall bias in the reporting of past food intake among breast cancer cases and controls. *Ann Epidemiol* 1991;1 : 439–453.

137. Friedman M, Rosenman RH, Carroll V. Changes in the serum cholesterol and blood clotting time in men subjected to cyclic variation of occupational stress. *Circulation* 1958;17 : 852–861.

138. Frost WH. The age selection of mortality from tuberculosis in successive decades. *Am J Hygiene Sect A* 1939;30 : 91–96.

139. Galen RS, Gambino SR. *Beyond normality. The Predictive Value and Efficiency of Medical Diagnoses.* New York: Wiley, 1975.

140. Gart JJ. Point and interval estimation of the common odds ratio in the combination of 2×2 tables with fixed marginals. *Biometrika* 1970;57 : 471–475.

141. Gart JJ. The comparison of proportions: A review of significance tests, confidence intervals and adjustments for stratification. *Rev Int Stat Inst* 1971;39 : 148–169.

142. Gaziano JM, Buring JE, Breslow JL, et al. Moderate alcohol intake, increased levels of high-density lipoprotein and its subfractions,

and decreased risk of myocardial infarction. *N Engl J Med* 1993;329 : 1829–1834.

143. Geddes M, Balzi D, Buiatti E, et al. Cancer mortality in Italian migrants to Canada. *Tumori* 1994;80 : 19–23.

144. Geddes M, Parkin DM, Khlat M, et al. (Eds.). *Cancer in Italian Migrant Populations.* Lyon: International Agency for Research on Cancer (IARC), 1993. IARC Scientific Publ. No. 123.

145. Gilliam AG. A note on evidence relating to the incidence of primary liver cancer among the Bantu. *J Natl Cancer Inst* 1954;15 : 195–199.

146. Gilliam AG. Trends of mortality attributed to carcinoma of the lung: Possible effects of faulty certification of deaths to other respiratory disease. *Cancer* 1955;8 : 1130–1136.

147. Giovannucci E, Ascherio A, Rimm EB, et al. A prospective cohort study of vasectomy and prostate cancer in U.S. men. *JAMA* 1993;269 : 873–877.

148. Giovannucci E, Stampfer MJ, Colditz GA, et al. A comparison of prospective and retrospective assessments of diet in the study of breast cancer. *Am J Epidemiol* 1993;137 : 502–511.

149. Glass AG, Hill JA, Miller RW. Significance of leukemia clusters. *J Pediatr* 1968;73 : 101–107.

150. Goldacre MJ. Space-time and family characteristics of meningococcal disease and haemophilus meningitis. *Int J Epidemiol* 1977; 6 : 101–105.

151. Goldberger J. The etiology of pellagra. The significance of certain epidemiological observations with respect thereto. *Publ Health Rep* 1914;29 : 1683–1686. Reprinted in Terris M. (Ed.), *Goldberger on Pellagra.* Baton Rouge: Louisiana State University Press, 1964.

152. Goldberger J, Wheeler GA. The experimental production of pellagra in human subjects by means of diet. *Hyg Lab Bull* 1920;120 : 7–116. Reprinted in Terris M. (Ed.), *Goldberger on Pellagra.* Baton Rouge: Louisiana State University Press, 1964.

153. Goldblatt P. Changes in social class between 1971 and 1981: Could these affect mortality differentials among men of working age? *Popul Trends* 1988;51 : 9–17.

154. Gordis L. Should dead cases be matched to dead controls? *Am J Epidemiol* 1982;115 : 1–5.

155. Gordon T, Garcia-Palmieri MR, Kagan A, et al. Differences in coronary heart disease mortality in Framingham, Honolulu and Puerto Rico. *J Chronic Dis* 1974;27 : 329–344.

156. Gould SJ. Why we should not name human races: A biological view. *In*: Gould SJ. (Ed.), *Ever Since Darwin.* New York: WW Norton, 1977, pp. 231–236.

157. Gove PB. (Ed.). *Webster's Third New International Dictionary of the English Language Unabridged.* Springfield, MA: G & C Merriam, 14th ed., 1963.

158. Graunt J. *Natural and Political Observations Made upon the Bills of Mortality.* London, John Martin, James Allestry, and Thomas Dicas, 1662. Republished Baltimore: The Johns Hopkins Press, 1939.

159. Greenberg ER. Random digit dialing for control selection. A review and a caution on its use in studies of childhood cancer. *Am J Epidemiol* 1990;131 : 1–5.

160. Greenland S. The effect of misclassification in the presence of covariates. *Am J Epidemiol* 1980;112 : 564–569.

161. Greenland S. The effect of misclassification in matched-pair case-control studies. *Am J Epidemiol* 1982;116 : 402–406.

162. Greenland S. Tests for interaction in epidemiologic studies: A review and a study of power. *Stat Med* 1983;2 : 243–251.
163. Greenland S. Bias in methods for deriving standardized morbidity ratio and attributable fraction estimates. *Stat Med* 1984;3 : 131–141.
164. Greenland S. Elementary models for biological interaction. *J Hazardous Materials* 1985;10 : 449–454.
165. Greenland S. Estimating variances of standardized estimators in case-control studies and sparse data. *J Chronic Dis* 1986;39 : 473–477.
166. Greenland S. Quantitative methods in the review of epidemiologic literature. *Epidemiol Rev* 1987;9 : 1–30.
167. Greenland S. Variance estimators for attributable fraction estimates consistent in both large strata and sparse data. *Stat Med* 1987;6 : 701–708.
168. Greenland S. Statistical uncertainty due to misclassification: Implications for validation substudies. *J Clin Epidemiol* 1988; 41 : 1167–1174.
169. Greenland S. Generalized Mantel-Haenszel estimators for K 2 × J tables. *Biometrics* 1989;45 : 183–191.
170. Greenland S. Basic problems in interaction assessment. *Environmental Health Perspect* 1993;101, Suppl. 4 : 59–66.
171. Greenland S. Invited commentary: A critical look at some popular meta-analytic methods. *Am J Epidemiol* 1994;140 : 290–296.
172. Greenland S. Dose-response and trend analysis in epidemiology: Alternatives to categorical analysis. *Epidemiology* 1995;6 : 356–365.
173. Greenland S, Drescher K. Maximum-likelihood estimation of the attributable fraction from logistic models. *Biometrics* 1993; 49 : 865–872.
174. Greenland S, Kleinbaum DG. Correcting for misclassification in two-way tables and matched-pair studies. *Int J Epidemiol* 1983; 12 : 93–97.
175. Greenland S, Morgenstern H. Matching and efficiency in cohort studies. *Am J Epidemiol* 1990;131 : 151–159.
176. Greenland S, Morgenstern H, Thomas DC. Considerations in determining matching criteria and stratum sizes for case-control studies. *Int J Epidemiol* 1981;10 : 389–392.
177. Greenland S, Neutra R. Control of confounding in the assessment of medical technology. *Int J Epidemiol* 1980; 9 : 361–367.
178. Greenland S, Robins JM. Confounding and misclassification. *Am J Epidemiol* 1985;122 : 495–506.
179. Greenland S, Robins JM. Estimation of a common effect parameter from sparse follow-up data. *Biometrics* 1985;41 : 55–68.
180. Greenland S, Robins JM. Conceptual problems in the definition and interpretation of attributable fractions. *Am J Epidemiol* 1988;128 : 1185–1197.
181. Greenland S, Schlesselman JJ, Criqui MH. The fallacy of employing standardized regression coefficients and correlations as measures of effect. *Am J Epidemiol* 1986; 123 : 203–208.
182. Greenland S, Thomas DC. On the need for the rare disease assumption in case-control studies. *Am J Epidemiol* 1982;116 : 547–553.
183. Greenland S, Thomas DC, Morgenstern H. The rare-disease assumption revisited. A critique of "Estimators of relative risk for case-control studies." *Am J Epidemiol* 1986;124 : 869–883.
184. Greenwood M. *The Natural Duration of Cancer.* London: His Majesty's Stationery Office, 1926: Rep. Publ. Health Med. Subj. No. 33.

185. Greenwood M. *Epidemics and Crowd-Diseases. An Introduction to the Study of Epidemiology.* New York: Macmillan, 1935.
186. Grumet RF, MacMahon B. Trends in mortality from neoplasms of the testis. *Cancer* 1958;11 : 790–797.
187. Hadley JN. Health conditions among Navajo Indians. *Pub Health Rep* 1955;70 : 831–836.
188. Hadziyannis S, Tabor E, Kaklamani E, et al. A case-control study of hepatitis B and C virus infections in the etiology of hepatocellular carcinoma. *Int J Cancer* 1995;60 : 627–631.
189. Haenszel W, Kurihara M. Studies of Japanese migrants. I. Mortality from cancer and other diseases among Japanese in the United States. *J Natl Cancer Inst* 1968;40 : 43–68.
190. Hahn RA. The state of Federal health statistics on racial and ethnic groups. *JAMA* 1992;267 : 268–271.
191. Hahn RA, Eberhardt S. Life expectancy in four U.S. racial/ethnic populations: 1990. *Epidemiology* 1995;6 : 350–355.
192. Hahn RA, Mulinare J, Teutsch SM. Inconsistencies in coding of race and ethnicity between birth and death in US infants. A new look at infant mortality, 1983 through 1985. *JAMA* 1992; 267 : 259–263.
193. Hahn RA, Stroup DF. Race and ethnicity in public health surveillance: Criteria for the scientific use of social categories. *Pub Health Rep* 1994;109 : 7–15.
194. Hammond EC. Smoking in relation to the death rates of one million men and women. *Natl Cancer Inst Monogr* 1966;19 : 127–204.
195. Hammond EC, Garfinkel L. Coronary heart disease, stroke and aortic aneurysm. Factors in the etiology. *Arch Environ Health* 1969;19 : 167–182.
196. Hammond EC, Horn D. Smoking and death rates—Report on forty-four months of follow-up of 187,783 men. *JAMA* 1958;166 : 1159–1172,1294–1308.
197. Harlow BL, Davis S. Two one-step methods for household screening and interviewing using random digit dialing. *Am J Epidemiol* 1988;127 : 857–863.
198. Hartge P, Brinton LA, Rosenthal JF, et al. Random digit dialing in selecting a population-based control group. *Am J Epidemiol* 1984;120 : 825–833.
199. Hatch M, Thomas D. Measurement issues in environmental epidemiology. *Environ Health Perspect* 1993;101(Suppl. 4) : 49–57.
200. Hatten J. Medicare's common denominator: The covered population. *Health Care Financing Rev* 1980;2 : 53–64.
201. Heasman MA, Urquhart JD, Black RJ, et al. Leukaemia in young persons in Scotland: A study of its geographical distribution and relationship to nuclear installations. *Health Bull* (Edinb.) 1987; 45 : 147–151.
202. Heath CW Jr, Hasterlik RJ. Leukemia among children in a suburban community. *Am J Med* 1963;34 : 796–812.
203. Hein HO, Suadicani P, Gyntelberg F. Ischaemic heart disease incidence by social class and form of smoking: The Copenhagen Male Study—17 years' follow-up. *J Intern Med* 1992;231 : 477–483.
204. Hempel CG. Introduction to problems of taxonomy. *In*: Zubin J. (Ed.), *Field Studies in the Mental Disorders.* New York: Grune & Stratton, 1961.
205. Henderson DA. The aetiology of chronic nephritis in Queensland. *Med J Australia* 1958;1 : 377–386.
206. Henle W, Henle G, Lennette ET. The Epstein-Barr virus. *Sci Am* 1979;241 : 48–59.
206a. Hernberg S, Partanen T, Nordman C-H, Sumari P. Coronary heart

disease among workers exposed to carbon disulphide. *Br J Ind Med* 1970;27 : 313–325.

207. Hill AB. Observation and experiment. *N Engl J Med* 1953; 248 : 995–1001.

208. Hill AB. The environment and disease: association or causation? *Proc Roy Soc Med* 1965;58 : 295–300.

209. Hill C, Laplanche A. Overall mortality and cancer mortality around French nuclear sites. *Nature* 1990;347 : 755–757.

210. Hippocrates. *On Airs, Waters, and Places*. Translated and published in *Med Classics* 1938;3 : 19–42.

211. Hirayama T. Non-smoking wives of heavy smokers have a higher risk of lung cancer: A study from Japan. *Br Med J (Clin Res Ed)* 1981;282 : 183–185.

212. Hirsch A. *Handbook of Geographical and Historical Pathology. Vols. I–II*. Translated from the Second German Edition by Creighton C. London: The New Sydenham Society, 1883–1886.

213. Hobbs MST, Woodward SD, Murphy B, et al. The incidence of pneumoconiosis, mesothelioma and other respiratory cancer in men engaged in mining and milling crocidolite in Western Australia. *In*: Wagner JC. (Ed.), *Biological Effects of Mineral Fibers*. Lyon: International Agency for Research on Cancer (IARC), 1980 : 615–625.

214. Holford TR. The estimation of age, period and cohort effects for vital rates. *Biometrics* 1983;39 : 311–324.

215. Hollingshead AB, Redlich FC. *Social Class and Mental Illness. A Community Study*. New York: Wiley, 1958.

216. Horwitz RI. Selected annotated bibliography of case-control studies. *J Chronic Dis* 1979;32 : Appendix i–iv.

217. Horwitz RI, Horwitz SM, Feinstein AR, et al. Necropsy diagnosis of endometrial cancer and detection-bias in case-control studies. *Lancet* 1981:ii : 66–68.

218. Hsieh C-c. The effect of nondifferential outcome misclassification on estimates of the attributable and prevented fraction. *Stat Med* 1991;10 : 361–373.

219. Hsieh C-c, Maisonneuve P, Boyle P, et al. Analysis of quantitative data by quantiles in epidemiologic studies: Classification according to cases, noncases, or all subjects? *Epidemiology* 1991;2 : 137–140.

220. Hsieh C-c, Trichopoulos D, Katsouyanni K, et al. Age at menarche, age at menopause, height and obesity as risk factors for breast cancer: Associations and interactions in an international case-control study. *Int J Cancer* 1990;46 : 796–800.

221. Hsieh C-c, Walter SD. The effect of nondifferential exposure misclassification on estimates of the attributable and prevented fraction. *Stat Med* 1988;7 : 1073–1085.

222. Hubert HB, Feinleib M, McNamara PM, et al. Obesity as an independent risk factor for cardiovascular disease: 26-year follow-up of participants in the Framingham Heart Study. *Circulation* 1983; 67 : 968–977.

223. Hume D. *Treatise of Human Nature*. 1739. Reproduced by Selby-Bigge (Ed.). Oxford, Eng: Clarendon, 1896.

224. Humphreys NA (Ed.). *Vital Statistics: A Memorial Volume of Selections from the Reports and Writings of William Farr, 1807–1883*. London: The Sanitary Institute of Great Britain, 1885.

225. Hunter DJ, Willett WC. Diet, body size, and breast cancer. *Epidemiol Rev* 1993;15 : 110–132.

226. Hutchison GB. Leukemia in patients with cancer of the cervix uteri

treated with radiation. A report covering the first 5 years of an international study. *J Natl Cancer Inst* 1968;40 : 951–982.

227. Hutchison GB, Shapiro S. Lead time gained by diagnostic screening for breast cancer. *J Natl Cancer Inst* 1968;41 : 665–681.

228. Hypertension Detection and Follow-up Program Cooperative Group. Five-year findings of the Hypertension and Detection Follow-up Program. *JAMA* 1979;242 : 2562–2571.

229. Ibrahim MA, Spitzer WO. The case-control study: The problem and the prospect. *J Chronic Dis* 1979;32 : 139–144.

230. International Agency for Research on Cancer. *Chromium, Nickel and Welding.* Lyon: International Agency for Research on Cancer (IARC), 1990. IARC Monographs on the Evaluation of Carcinogenic Risks to Humans, Vol. 49.

231. Israel RA, Rosenberg HM, Curtin LR. Analytical potential for multiple cause-of-death data. *Am J Epidemiol* 1986;124 : 161–179.

232. Jablon S, Hrubec Z, Boice JD Jr. Cancer in populations living near nuclear facilities. A survey of mortality nationwide and incidence in two states. *JAMA* 1991;265 : 1403–1408.

233. Jacquez GM. Cuzick and Edwards' test when exact location are unknown. *Am J Epidemiol* 1994;140 : 58–64.

234. Jacquez GM. (Ed.). Proceedings of the Workshop on Statistics and Computing in Disease Clustering. *Stat Med* 1993;12 : 19–20.

235. Jaglal SB, Goel V. Social inequity in risk of coronary artery disease in Ontario. *Can J Cardiol* 1994;10 : 439–443.

236. Jenner E. *An Inquiry into the Causes and Effects of the Variola Vaccinae.* London: Law, 1798.

237. Jick SS, Perera DR, Walker AM, Jick H. Non-steroidal anti-inflammatory drugs and hospital admission for perforated peptic ulcer. *Lancet* 1987;ii : 380–382.

238. Johnson CC Jr. *Consistency of Reporting of Ethnic Origin in the Current Population Survey.* Washington, DC: U.S. Bureau of the Census, 1974. Technical paper No. 31.

239. Kahn HA. The Dorn study of smoking and mortality among U.S. veterans: Report on eight and one-half years of observation. *In:* Haenszel W. (Ed.), *Epidemiological Approaches to the Study of Cancer and Other Chronic Diseases.* Washington, DC: U.S. Govt. Printing Office, 1966. Natl Cancer Inst. Monograph 19.

240. Kahn HA, Sempos CT. *Statistical Methods in Epidemiology.* New York: Oxford University Press, 1984.

241. Kaklamani E, Trichopoulos D, Tzonou A, et al. Hepatitis B and C viruses and their interaction in the origin of hepatocellular carcinoma. *JAMA* 1991;265 : 1974–1976.

242. Kalandidi A, Doulgerakis M, Tzonou A, et al. Induced abortions, contraceptive practices, and tobacco smoking as risk factors for ectopic pregnancy in Athens, Greece. *Br J Obstet Gynaec* 1991;98: 207–213.

243. Kalapothaki V, Tzonou A, Hsieh C-c, et al. Nutrient intake and cancer of the pancreas: A case-control study in Athens, Greece. *Cancer Causes and Control* 1993;4 : 383–389.

244. Kalapothaki V, Tzonou A, Hsieh C-c, et al. Tobacco, ethanol, coffee, pancreatitis, diabetes mellitus, and cholelithiasis as risk factors for pancreatic carcinoma. *Cancer Causes Control* 1993;4 : 375–382.

245. Kaplan EL, Meier P. Nonparametric estimation from incomplete observations. *J Amer Statist Assoc* 1958;53 : 457–481.

246. Karhausen LR. Re: "Popperian refutation in epidemiology." (Letter to the Editor). *Am J Epidemiol* 1986;123 : 199.

247. Kashgarian M. The concepts of prevalence and incidence as applied

to the study of development and duration of disease. *Meth Inform Med* 1968;7 : 111–117.

248. Kassirer JP. Diagnostic reasoning. *Ann Intern Med* 1989; 110 : 893–900.

249. Kato H, Schull WJ. Studies of the A-bomb survivors. 7. Mortality, 1950–1978. Part I. Cancer mortality. *Radiat Res* 1982;90 : 395–432.

250. Katsouyanni K, Karakatsani A, Messari J, et al. Air pollution and cause specific mortality in Athens. *J Epidemiol Community Health* 1990;44 : 321–324.

251. Katsouyanni K, Trichopoulos D, Stuver S, et al. The association of fat and other macronutrients with breast cancer: A case-control study from Greece. *Br J Cancer* 1994;70 : 537–541.

252. Kawachi I, Marshall S, Pearce N. Social class inequalities in the decline of coronary heart disease among New Zealand men, 1975–1977 to 1985–1987. *Int J Epidemiol* 1991;20 : 393–398.

253. Kemp I, Boyle P, Smans M, Muir C. *Atlas of Cancer in Scotland, 1974–1980. Incidence and Epidemiological Perspective.* Lyon: International Agency for Research on Cancer (IARC), 1985. IARC Scientific Publ. No. 72.

254. Keys A. *Seven Countries: A Multivariate Analysis of Death and Coronary Heart Disease.* Cambridge: Harvard University Press, 1980.

255. Keys A. (Ed.). *Coronary Heart Disease in Seven Countries.* New York: American Heart Foundation Inc., 1970. American Heart Foundation Monograph No. 29. (Circulation 1970;41: Suppl. 1).

256. Khlat M, Vail A, Parkin M, Green A. Mortality from melanoma in migrants to Australia: Variation by age at arrival and duration of stay. *Am J Epidemiol* 1992;135 : 1103–1113.

257. Kingsley LA, Detels R, Kaslow R, et al. Risk factors for seroconversion to human immunodeficiency virus among male homosexuals. *Lancet* 1987;i : 345–349.

258. Klatsky AL, Armstrong MA, Friedman GD. Risk of cardiovascular mortality in alcohol drinkers, ex-drinkers and nondrinkers. *Am J Cardiol* 1990;66 : 1237–1242.

259. Kleinbaum DG, Kupper LL, Morgenstern H. *Epidemiologic Research: Principles and Quantitative Methods.* London: Lifetime Learning Publications, 1982.

260. Kleinbaum DG, Kupper LL, Muller KE. *Applied Regression Analysis and Other Multivariable Methods.* (2nd ed.). Belmont, CA: PWS-Kent Publishing Company, 1988.

261. Knox G. Detection of low intensity epidemicity. Application to cleft lip and palate. *Br J Prev Soc Med* 1963;17 : 121–127.

262. Knox G. The detection of space-time interactions. *Appl Statist* 1964;13 : 25–29.

263. Knox G. Epidemiology of childhood leukaemia in Northumberland and Durham. *Br J Prev Soc Med* 1964;18 : 17–24.

264. Koch R. The aetiology of tuberculosis. *Berlin Klin Wschr* 1882; 19 : 221. Translated and reprinted in Pinner M. (Trans). *The Aetiology of Tuberculosis.* New York: National Tuberculosis Association, 1932.

265. Koopman JS. Causal models and sources of interaction. *Am J Epidemiol* 1977;106 : 439–444.

266. Kramer M. *Some Problems for International Research Suggested by Observations on Differences in First Admission Rates to Mental Hospitals of England and Wales and of the United States.* Proceedings of the Third World Congress of Psychiatry. Montreal: University of Toronto Press and McGill University Press, 1961.

267. Kreiss K, Wasserman S, Mroz MM, et al. Beryllium disease screening in the ceramics industry. *J Occup Med* 1993;35 : 267–274.

268. Kupper LL, McMichael AJ, Spirtas R. A hybrid epidemiologic study design useful in estimating relative risk. *J Am Stat Assoc* 1975;70 : 524–528.

269. Kupper LL, McMichael AJ, Symons MJ, Most BM. On the utility of proportional mortality analysis. *J Chronic Dis* 1978;31 : 15–22.

270. Kuritz SJ, Landis JR. Attributable risk ratio estimation from matched-pairs case-control data. *Am J Epidemiol* 1987;125 : 324–328.

271. Kuritz SJ, Landis JR. Summary attributable risk estimation from unmatched case-control data. *Stat Med* 1988;7 : 507–517.

272. Kutz FW, Wood PH, Bottimore DP. Organochlorine pesticides and polychlorinated biphenyls in human adipose tissue. *Rev Environ Contam Toxicol* 1991;120 : 1–82.

273. L'Abbé KA, Detsky AS, O'Rourke K. Meta-analysis in clinical research. *Ann Intern Med* 1987;107 : 224–233.

274. Lancaster HO. Deafness as an epidemic disease in Australia. *Br Med J* 1951;2 : 1429–1432.

275. Lanes SF. The logic of causal inference in medicine. *In*: Rothman K.J. (Ed.), *Causal Inference*. Chestnut Hill, MA: Epidemiology Resources Inc., 1988.

276. Lasky T, Stolley PD. Selection of cases and controls. *Epidemiol Rev* 1994;16 : 6–17.

277. La Vecchia C, D'Avanzo B, Negri E, et al. Attributable risks for stomach cancer in Northern Italy. *Int J Cancer* 1995;60 : 748–752.

278. Lee I-M, Paffenbarger RS Jr., Hsieh C-c. Physical activity and risk of prostatic cancer among college alumni. *Am J Epidemiol* 1992;135 : 169–179.

279. Leger AS, Cochrane AL, Mooer F. Factors associated with cardiac mortality in developed countries with particular reference to the consumption of wine. *Lancet* 1979;1 : 1017–1020.

280. Lenz W. Thalidomide and congenital abnormalities. (Letter to the Editor). *Lancet* 1962;1 : 45.

281. Lepage P, Van de Perre P, Msellati P, et al. Mother-to-child transmission of human immunodeficiency virus type 1 (HIV-1) and its determinants: A cohort study in Kigali, Rwanda. *Am J Epidemiol* 1993;137 : 589–599.

282. Lerchen ML, Samet JM. An assessment of questionnaire responses provided by a surviving spouse. *Am J Epidemiol* 1986;123 : 481–489.

283. Levin ML. The occurrence of lung cancer in man. *Acta Unio Internat Contra Cancrum* 1953;9 : 531–541.

284. Lewontin RC. The apportionment of human diversity. *Evol Biol* 1972;6 : 381–398.

285. Li JY, Liu BQ, Li GY, et al. Atlas of cancer mortality in the People's Republic of China. An aid for cancer control and research. *Int J Epidemiol* 1981;10 : 127–133.

286. Lilienfeld AM. *Foundations of Epidemiology*. New York: Oxford University Press, 1976.

287. Lilienfeld AM, Levin ML, Kessler II. Mortality among the foreign-born in their countries of origin. *In*: Lee HP, Lilienfeld AM, Levin ML, Kessler II (Eds.), *Cancer in the United States*. Cambridge, MA: Harvard University Press, 1972, pp. 233–278.

288. Lilienfeld AM, Lilienfeld DE. A century of case-control studies: Progress? *J Chronic Dis* 1979;32 : 5–13.

289. Lind J. *A Treatise of the Scurvy*. Edinburgh: Kincaird & Donalson,

1753. Reprinted in Steward CP, Guthrie D (Eds.), *Lind's Treatise on Scurvy*. Edinburgh: University Press, 1953.

290. Linder FE, Grove RD. *Vital Statistics Rates in the United States, 1900–1940*. Washington, DC: U.S. Govt. Printing Office, 1943.

291. Linet MS, Brookmeyer R. Use of cancer controls in case-control cancer studies. *Am J Epidemiol* 1987;125 : 1–11.

292. Lipworth L, Katsouyanni K, Ekbom A, et al. Abortion and the risk of breast cancer: A case-control study in Greece. *Int J Cancer* 1995;61 : 181–184.

293. Littell AS. Estimation of the T-year survival rate from follow-up studies over a limited period of time. *Human Biology* 1952;24 : 87–116.

294. Lombard HC. Observations suggested by a comparison of the post mortem appearances produced by typhous fever in Dublin, Paris and Geneva. *Dublin J Med Sci* 1836;10 : 17–24.

295. Longnecker MP. Alcoholic beverage consumption in relation to risk of breast cancer: Meta-analysis and review. *Cancer Causes Control* 1994;5 : 73–82.

296. Longnecker MP, Berlin JA, Orza MJ, Chalmers TC. A meta-analysis of alcohol consumption in relation to risk of breast cancer. *JAMA* 1988;260 : 652–656.

297. Longnecker MP, Newcomb PA, Mittendorf R, et al. Risk of breast cancer in relation to lifetime alcohol consumption. *J Natl Cancer Inst* 1995;87 : 923–929.

298. Lubin JH, Boice JD Jr, Edling C, et al. Lung cancer in radon-exposed miners and estimation of risk from indoor exposure. *J Natl Cancer Inst* 1995;87 : 817–827.

299. Lubin JH, Hartge P. Excluding controls: Misapplications in case-control studies. *Am J Epidemiol* 1984;120 : 791–793.

300. Lyon JL, Gardner K, Gress RE. Cancer incidence among Mormons and non-Mormons in Utah. *Cancer Causes Control* 1994;5 : 149–156.

301. MacFarlane GJ, Boyle P. Scottish Mortality Data, 1911–1985. Mimeographed. Personal communication, 1987.

302. Mackenzie SG, Lippman A. An investigation of report bias in a case-control study of pregnancy outcome. *Am J Epidemiol* 1989;129 : 65–75.

303. Maclure KM, MacMahon B. An epidemiologic perspective of environmental carcinogenesis. *Epidemiol Rev* 1980;2 : 19–48.

304. Maclure M. Popperian refutation in epidemiology. *Am J Epidemiol* 1985;121 : 343–350.

305. Maclure M. The case-crossover design: A method for studying transient effects on the risk of acute events. *Am J Epidemiol* 1991;133 : 144–153.

306. Maclure M, Greenland S. Tests for trend and dose response: Misinterpretations and alternatives. *Am J Epidemiol* 1992;135 : 96–104.

307. MacMahon B. Epidemiologic evidence on the nature of Hodgkin's disease. *Cancer* 1957;10 : 1045–1054.

308. MacMahon B. Perspective. Leukemia clusters around nuclear facilities in Britain. *Cancer Causes Control* 1992;3 : 283–288.

309. MacMahon B. The quantification of alcohol-caused morbidity and mortality in Australia—A critique. *Med J Aust* 1992;157 : 557–560.

310. MacMahon B, Kovar MG, Feldman JJ. *Infant Mortality Rates: Socioeconomic Factors*. Washington, DC: National Center for Health Statistics. Vital and Health Statistics. Series 22, No. 14. U.S. Govt. Printing Office, 1972.

311. MacMahon B, et al. Lactation and cancer of the breast. Summary of an international study. *Bull WHO* 1970;42 : 185–194.

312. MacMahon B, Monson RR. Mortality in the US rayon industry. *J Occup Med* 1988;30 : 698–705.

313. MacMahon B, Newill VA. Birth characteristics of children dying of malignant neoplasms. *J Natl Cancer Inst* 1962;28 : 231–244.

314. MacMahon B, Pugh TF. *Epidemiology: Principles and Methods.* Boston: Little, Brown, 1970.

315. MacMahon B, Pugh TF, Ingalls TH. Anencephalus, spina bifida and hydrocephalus. Incidence related to sex, race, and season of birth, and incidence in siblings. *Br J Prev Soc Med* 1953;7 : 211–219.

316. MacMahon B, Pugh TF, Ipsen J. *Epidemiologic Methods.* Boston: Little, Brown, 1960.

317. MacMahon B, Worcester J. *Age at Menopause. United States. 1960–1962.* Washington, DC: U.S. Govt. Printing Office, 1966. National Center for Health Statistics, Series 11, No. 19.

318. MacMahon B, Yen S. Unrecognized epidemic of anencephaly and spina bifida. *Lancet* 1971;i : 31–33.

319. MacMahon K. Short-term fluctuations in the frequency of suicide, United States, 1972–1978. *Am J Epidemiol* 1983;117 : 744–750.

320. Mainland D. Chance and random sampling. *Meth Med Res* 1954;6 : 127–137.

321. Mangoud A, Hillier VF, Leck I, Thomas RW. Space-time interaction in Hodgkin's disease in Greater Manchester. *J Epidemiol Community Health* 1985;39 : 58–62.

322. Mantel N. Chi-square tests with one degree of freedom: Extensions of the Mantel-Haenszel procedure. *J Am Stat Assoc* 1963;59 : 690–700.

323. Mantel N. Evaluation of survival data and two new rank order statistics arising in its consideration. *Cancer Chemother Rep* 1966;50 : 163–170.

324. Mantel N. The detection of disease clustering and a generalized regression approach. *Cancer Res* 1967;27 : 209–220.

325. Mantel N, Brown C, Byar DP. Tests for homogeneity of effect in an epidemiologic investigation. *Am J Epidemiol* 1977;106 : 125–129.

326. Mantel N, Haenszel W. Statistical aspects of the analysis of data from retrospective studies of disease. *J Natl Cancer Inst* 1959; 22 : 719–748.

327. Marler AR, Price TR, Clark GL, et al. Morning increase in onset of ischemic stroke. *Stroke* 1989;20 : 473–476.

328. Marmot M. Epidemiological approach to the explanation of social differentiation in mortality: The Whitehall studies. *Soz Präventiv Med* 1993;38 : 271–279.

329. Marmot MG, Adelstein AM, Robinson N, Rose GA. Changing social-class distribution of heart disease. *Br Med J* 1978;2 : 1109–1112.

330. Marmot MG, McDowall ME. Mortality decline and widening social inequalities. *Lancet* 1986;ii : 274–276.

331. Marmot MG, Rose G, Shipley MJ, Thomas BJ. Alcohol and mortality: A U-shaped curve. *Lancet* 1981;1 : 580–583.

332. Marmot MG, Smith GD, Stansfeld S, et al. Health inequalities among British civil servants: The Whitehall II study. *Lancet* 1991;337 : 1387–1393.

333. Marshall RJ. A review of methods for the statistical analysis of spatial patterns of disease. *J R Stat Soc [A]* 1991;154 : 421–441.

334. Mason TJ, Fraumeni JF Jr, Hoover R, Blot WJ. *An Atlas of Mortality from Selected Diseases.* Washington, DC: U.S. Govt. Printing Office, 1981. DHEW Publ. No. (NIH) 81-2397.

335. Mason TJ, McKay FW. *U.S. Cancer Mortality by County: 1950–1969*. Washington, DC: U.S. Govt. Printing Office, 1974. DHEW Publ. No. (NIH) 74-615.

336. Mason TJ, McKay FW, Hoover R, et al. *Atlas of Cancer Mortality for U.S. Counties: 1950–69*. Washington, DC: U.S. Govt. Printing Office, 1975. DHEW Publ. No. (NIH) 75-780.

337. Mason TJ, McKay FW, Hoover R, et al. *Atlas of Cancer Mortality among U.S. Nonwhites: 1950–69*. Washington, DC: U.S. Govt. Printing Office, 1976. DHEW Publ. No. (NIH) 76-1204.

338. Matanoski GM, Sartwell P, Elliott E, et al. Cancer risks in radiologists and radiation workers. *In*: Boice JD Jr, Fraumeni JF Jr (Eds.). *Carcinogenesis: Epidemiology and Biological Significance*. New York: Raven, 1984, pp. 83–96.

339. Mathews JD, Glasse R, Lindenbaum S. Kuru and cannibalism. *Lancet* 1968;2 : 449–452.

340. Matos EL, Khlat M, Loria DI, et al. Cancer in migrants to Argentina. *Int J Cancer* 1991;49 : 805–811.

341. McLaughlin JK, Blot WJ, Mehl ES, Mandel JS. Problems in the use of dead controls in case-control studies. I. General results. *Am J Epidemiol* 1985;121 : 131–139.

342. McLaughlin JK, Blot WJ, Mehl ES, Mandel JS. Problems in the use of dead controls in case-control studies. II. Effect of excluding certain causes of death. *Am J Epidemiol* 1985;122 : 485–494.

343. McMichael AJ. Molecular epidemiology: New pathway or new travelling companion? (Invited Commentary). *Am J Epidemiol* 1994; 14 : 1–11.

344. McMichael AJ, McCall MG, Hartshorne JM, Woodings TL. Patterns of gastro-intestinal cancer in European migrants to Australia: The role of dietary change. *Int J Cancer* 1980;25 : 431–437.

345. McNemar Q. Note on the sampling of the difference between corrected proportions or percentages. *Psychometrika* 1947;12 : 153–157.

346. Merletti F, Cole P. Detection bias and endometrial cancer. *Lancet* 1981;ii : 579–580.

347. Miettinen OS. Confounding and effect modification. *Am J Epidemiol* 1974;100 : 350–353.

348. Miettinen O. Simple interval estimation of risk ratio. *Am J Epidemiol* 1974;100 : 515–516.

349. Miettinen O. Estimability and estimation in case-referent studies. *Am J Epidemiol* 1976;103 : 226–235.

350. Miettinen OS. The matched pairs design in the case of all-or-none responses. *Biometrics* 1968;24 : 339–352.

351. Miettinen OS. Individual matching with multiple controls in the case of all-or-none responses. *Biometrics* 1969;25 : 339–355.

352. Miettinen OS. Estimation of relative risk from individually matched series. *Biometrics* 1970;26 : 75–86.

353. Miettinen OS. Matching and design efficiency in retrospective studies. *Am J Epidemiol* 1970;91 : 111–118.

354. Miettinen OS. Standardization of risk ratios. *Am J Epidemiol* 1972;96 : 383–388.

355. Miettinen OS. Proportion of disease caused or prevented by a given exposure, trait or intervention. *Am J Epidemiol* 1974;99 : 325–332.

356. Miettinen OS. Public health policy on coronary heart disease. *Hart Bull* 1979;10 : 165–167.

357. Miettinen OS. The "case-control" study: Valid selection of subjects. *J Chronic Dis* 1985;38 : 543–548.

358. Miettinen OS. *Theoretical Epidemiology: Principles of Occurrence Research in Medicine*. New York: Wiley, 1985.

359. Miettinen OS, Cook EF. Confounding: Essence and detection. *Am J Epidemiol* 1981;114 : 593–603.

360. Miettinen OS, Wang J-D. An alternative to the proportionate mortality ratio. *Am J Epidemiol* 1981;114 : 144–148.

361. Mill JS. *A System of Logic, Ratiocinative and Inductive.* 5th ed. London: Parker, Son & Bowin, 1862.

362. Ministry of Health. *Mortality and Morbidity During the London Fog of December, 1952.* London: Her Majesty's Stationery Office, 1954. Reports on Public Health and Medical Subjects No. 95.

363. Monson RR. *Occupational Epidemiology* (2nd ed.). Boca Raton, FL: CRC Press, 1990.

364. Monson RR, MacMahon B. Prenatal x-ray exposure and cancer in children. *In*: Boice JD Jr, Fraumeni JF Jr. (Eds.), *Radiation Carcinogenesis: Epidemiology and Biological Significance.* New York: Raven, 1984.

365. Montagu A. *The Idea of Race.* Lincoln: Univ Nebraska Press, 1965.

366. Moore RD, Pearson TA. Moderate alcohol consumption and coronary artery disease: A review. *Medicine* (Baltimore) 1986;65 : 242–267.

367. Morabia A. On the origin of Hill's causal criteria. *Epidemiology* 1991;2 : 367–369.

368. Morrison AS. Sequential pathogenic components of rates. *Am J Epidemiol* 1979;109 : 709–718.

369. Morrison AS. *Screening in Chronic Disease.* (2nd ed.). New York, Oxford: Oxford University Press, 1992.

370. Mueller N. The epidemiology of HTLV-I infection. *Cancer Causes & Control* 1991;2 : 37–52.

371. Mueller NE, Evans AS, Harris N, et al. Hodgkins' disease and Epstein-Barr virus. Altered antibody pattern before diagnosis. *N Engl J Med* 1989;320 : 689–695.

372. Muller JE, Ludmer PL, Willich SN, et al. Circadian variation in the frequency of sudden cardiac death. *Circulation* 1987;75 : 131–138.

373. Muller JE, Stone PH, Turi ZG, et al. Circadian variation in the frequency of onset of acute myocardial infarction. *N Engl J Med* 1985;313 : 1315–1322.

374. Muller JE, Toffler GH, Stone PH. Circadian variation and triggers of onset of acute cardiovascular disease. *Circulation* 1989; 79 : 733–743.

375. Nathanson N, Langmuir AD. The Cutter incident. Poliomyelitis following formaldehyde-inactivated poliovirus vaccination in the United States during the spring of 1955. Parts I, II and III. *Am J Epidemiol* 1963;78 : 16–28, 29–60, 61–81.

376. National Center for Health Statistics. *National Death Index Users Manual.* Hyattsville, MD: National Center for Health Statistics, 1990. DHHS Publ. No. (PHS) 90–1148.

377. National Center for Health Statistics. *Current Estimates from the National Health Interview Survey, 1993.* Hyattsville, MD: National Center for Health Statistics, 1994. DHHS Publ. No. (PHS) 95-1518.

378. National Center For Health Statistics. *Vital Statistics of the United States 1990. Volume II: Mortality. Part A.* Hyattsville, MD: National Center for Health Statistics, 1994. DHHS Publ. No. (PHS) 94-1100.

379. National Center for Health Statistics. *Health, United States, 1993.* Hyattsville, MD: Public Health Service, 1994. DHHS Publ. No. (PHS) 94-1232.

380. National Center for Health Statistics. *Health, United States, 1995.* Hyattsville, MD: Public Health Service, 1994. DHHS Publ. No. (PHS) 95-1232.

381. Neutel CI, Quinn A, Brancker A. Brain tumour mortality in immigrants. *Int J Epidemiol* 1989;18 : 60–66.

382. Newell DJ. Errors in the interpretation of errors in epidemiology. *Am J Public Health* 1962;52 : 1925–1928.

383. Newell GR, Cole SR, Miettinen OS, MacMahon B. Age differences in the histology of Hodgkin's disease. *J Natl Cancer Inst* 1970; 45 : 311–317.

384. Newill VA. Distribution of cancer mortality among ethnic subgroups of the white population of New York City, 1953–58. *J Natl Cancer Inst* 1961;26 : 405–417.

385. New Zealand Contraception and Health Study Group. The prevalence of abnormal cervical cytology in a group of New Zealand women using contraception: A preliminary report. *NZ Med J* 1989;102 : 369–371.

386. New Zealand Contraception and Health Study Group. History of long-term use of depot-medroxyprogesterone acetate in patients with cervical dysplasia; case-control analysis nested in a cohort study. *Contraception* 1994;50 : 443–449.

387. New Zealand Contraception and Health Study Group. An attempt to estimate the incidence of cervical dysplasia in a group of New Zealand women using contraception. *Epidemiology* 1995;6 : 121–126.

388. Nilsson B, Gustavson-Kadaka E, Rotstein S, et al. Cancer incidence in Estonian migrants to Sweden. *Int J Cancer* 1993;55 : 190–195.

389. Oleinick A, Mantel N. Family studies in systemic lupus erythematosus. II. Mortality among siblings and offspring of index cases with a statistical appendix concerning life table analysis. *J Chronic Dis* 1970;22 : 617–625.

390. Olsen J. Causes and prevention. *Scand J Soc Med* 1991;19 : 1–6.

391. Osler W. *The Principles and Practice of Medicine* (7th ed.). New York, London: Appleton, 1909, p. 364.

392. Paffenbarger RS Jr, Hale WE. Work activity and coronary heart mortality. *N Engl J Med* 1975;292 : 545–550.

393. Paffenbarger RS Jr, Hyde RT, Wing AL, et al. The association of changes in physical activity and other lifestyle characteristics with mortality among men. *N Engl J Med* 1993;328 : 538–545.

394. Paffenbarger RS Jr, Wolf PA, Notkin J, et al. Chronic disease in former college students. I. Early precursors of fatal coronary heart disease. *Am J Epidemiol* 1986;83 : 314–328.

395. Panayotou P, Kaskarelis D, Miettinen O, et al. Induced abortion and ectopic pregnancy. *Am J Obstet Gynec* 1972;114 : 507–510.

396. Panum PL. *Observations Made During the Epidemic of Measles on the Faroe Islands in the Year 1846.* Reproduced New York: American Public Health Association, 1940.

397. Papaevangelou G, Trichopoulos D, Kremastinou T, Papoutsakis G. Prevalence of hepatitis B antigen and antibody in prostitutes. *Br Med J* 1974;2 : 256–258.

398. Parkin DM. Studies of cancer in migrant populations. *Rev Epidémiol Santé Publique* 1992;40 : 410–424.

399. Parkin DM, Muir CS, Whelan SL, et al. *Cancer Incidence in Five Continents.* Volume VI. Lyon: International Agency for Research on Cancer (IARC), 1992. IARC Scientific Publications No. 120.

400. Parkin DM, Steinitz R, Khlat M, et al. Cancer in Jewish migrants to Israel. *Int J Cancer* 1990;45 : 614–621.

401. Paul JR, White L. (Eds.). *Serological Epidemiology.* New York: Academic Press, 1973.

402. Pearce N. White swans, black ravens, and lame ducks: Necessary

and sufficient causes in epidemiology. *Epidemiology* 1990; 1 : 47–50.

403. Pearce N, Crawford-Brown D. Critical discussion in epidemiology: Problems with the Popperian approach. *J Clin Epidemiol* 1989; 42 : 177–184.

404. Pearce N, de Sanjose S, Boffetta P, et al. Limitations of biomarkers of exposure in cancer epidemiology. *Epidemiology* 1995;6 : 190–194.

405. Percy C, Holten VV, Muir C (Eds.). *ICD-O: International Classification of Diseases for Oncology*, 2nd ed. Geneva, Switzerland: World Health Organization, 1990.

406. Perera FP, Weinstein IB. Molecular epidemiology and carcinogen-DNA adduct detection: New approaches to studies of human cancer causation. *J Chronic Dis* 1982;35 : 581–600.

407. Petitti DB. Associations are not effects. (Editorial). *Am J Epidemiol* 1991;133 : 101–102.

408. Petitti DB. *Meta-Analysis, Decision Analysis and Cost-Effectiveness Analysis in Medicine: Methods for Quantitative Synthesis in Medicine*. New York: Oxford University Press, 1994.

409. Peto J. Some problems in dose-response estimation of cancer epidemiology. *In: Methods for Estimating Risk of Chemical Injury: Human and Non-human Biota and Ecosystems*. Vouk VB, Butler GC, Hoel DG, Peakall DB (Eds.). New York: Wiley, 1985.

410. Peto R, Pike MC, Armitage P, et al. Design and analysis of randomized clinical trials requiring prolonged observation of each patient. I. Introduction and design. *Br J Cancer* 1976;34 : 585–612. II. Analysis and examples. *Br J Cancer* 1977;35 : 1–39.

411. Petrakis NL, King MC. Genetic markers and cancer epidemiology. *Cancer* 1977;39 (Suppl.) : 1861–1866.

412. Pickle LM, Mason TJ, Howard N, et al. Atlas of U.S. Cancer Mortality among Whites: 1950–69. Washington, DC: U.S. Govt. Printing Office, 1987. DHEW Publ. No. (NIH) 87-2900.

413. Pifer JW, Toyooka ET, Murray RW, et al. Neoplasms in children treated with X-rays for thymic enlargement. I. Neoplasms and mortality. *J Natl Cancer Inst* 1963;31 : 1333–1356.

414. Pike MC, Bull D. Knox test for space-time clustering in epidemiology. *Appl Statist* 1974;23 : 92–95.

415. Pinkel D, Dowd JE, Bross IDJ. Some epidemiological features of malignant solid tumors of children in the Buffalo, N.Y. area. *Cancer* 1963;16 : 28–33.

416. Poole C. Exposure opportunity in case-control studies. *Am J Epidemiol* 1986;123 : 352–358.

417. Poole C, Trichopoulos D. Extremely low-frequency electric and magnetic fields and cancer. *Cancer Causes and Control* 1991; 2 : 267–276.

418. Popper KR. *The Logic of Scientific Discovery*, 2nd ed. New York: Harper & Row, 1968.

419. Popper KR. *Conjectures and Refutations*, 4th ed. London: Routledge & Kegan Paul, 1972.

420. Popper KR. *Objective Knowledge: An Evolutionary Approach*. London: Oxford University Press, 1972.

421. Poskanzer DC, Schapira K, Miller H. Multiple sclerosis and poliomyelitis. *Lancet* 1963;2 : 917–921.

422. Poskanzer DC, Schwab RS. Cohort analysis of Parkinson's syndrome. *J Chronic Dis* 1963;16 : 961–973.

423. Prentice RL. A case-cohort design for epidemiologic cohort studies and disease prevention trials. *Biometrika* 1986;73 : 1–11.

424. Prentice RL, Breslow NE. Retrospective studies and failure time models. *Biometrika* 1978;65 : 153–158.

425. Prentice RL, Thomas D. Methodologic research needs in environmental epidemiology: Data analysis. *Environmental Health Perspectives* 1993;101(Suppl. 4) : 39–48.

426. Preston DL, Kato H, Kopecky KJ, Fujita S. Studies of the mortality of A-bomb survivors. 8. Cancer mortality, 1950–1982. *Radiat Res* 1987;111 : 151–178.

427. Preston-Martin S, Bernstein L, Maldonado AA, et al. A dental x-ray validation study. Comparison of information from patient interviews and dental charts. *Am J Epidemiol* 1985;121 : 430–439.

428. Pukkala E, Gustavsson N, Teppo L. *Atlas of Cancer Incidence in Finland.* Helsinki: Finnish Cancer Registry, 1987. Cancer Society of Finland Publ. No. 37.

429. Raffle PAB, Adams PH, Baxter PJ, Lee WR. *Hunter's Diseases of Occupations.* 8th ed. London, Boston: Edward Arnold Publ., 1994.

430. Rebelakos A, Trichopoulos D, Tzonou A, et al. Tobacco smoking, coffee drinking and occupation as risk factors for bladder cancer in Greece. *J Natl Cancer Inst* 1985;75 : 455–461.

431. Reed W, Carroll J, Agramonte A, et al. The etiology of yellow fever. A preliminary note. *Phil Med J* 1900;6 : 790–796.

432. Reeves WC, Brinton LA, Garcia M, et al. Human papillomavirus infection and cervical cancer in Latin America. *N Engl J Med* 1989;320 : 1437–1441.

433. Reeves WC, Caussy D, Brinton LA, et al. Case-control study of human papillomaviruses and cervical cancer in Latin America. *Int J Cancer* 1987;40 : 450–454.

434. Registrar General for England and Wales. *The Registrar General's Decennial Supplement, England and Wales, 1931. Part IIa. Occupational Mortality.* London: Her (His) Majesty's Stationery Office, 1938.

435. Registrar General for England and Wales. *The Registrar General's Decennial Supplement, England and Wales, 1951. Occupational Mortality, Part II. Vol. 1, Commentary. Vol. 2, Tables.* London: Her Majesty's Stationery Office, 1958 and 1957. Table 5.

436. Reid DD, Brett GZ, Hamilton PJS, et al. Cardiorespiratory disease and diabetes among middle-aged male Civil Servants. A study of screening and intervention. *Lancet* 1974;i : 469–473.

437. Renton A, Whitaker L. Proof of causation and relative risk (Letter). *Lancet* 1992;339 : 1058.

438. Riboli E. Nutrition and cancer: Background and rationale of the European Prospective Investigation into Cancer and Nutrition (EPIC). *Annals of Oncology* 1992;3 : 783–791.

439. Rich-Edwards JW, Corsano KA, Stampfer MJ. Test of the National Death Index and Equifax Nationwide Death Search. *Am J Epidemiol* 1994;140 : 1016–1019.

440. Rimm EB, Giovannucci EL, Stampfer MJ, et al. Reproducibility and validity of an expanded self-administered semiquantitative food frequency questionnaire among male health professionals. *Am J Epidemiol* 1992;135 : 1114–1126.

441. Rimm EB, Stampfer MJ, Ascherio A, et al. Vitamin E consumption and the risk of coronary heart disease in men. *N Engl J Med* 1993;328 : 1450–1456.

442. Rizzi DA, Pedersen SA. Causality in medicine: towards a theory and terminology. *Theor Med* 1992;13 : 233–254.

443. Robertson C, Boyle P, Hsieh C-c, et al. Some statistical considerations in the analysis of case-control studies when the exposure variables are continuous measurements. *Epidemiology* 1994;5 : 164–170.

444. Robins J, Breslow NE, Greenland S. Estimators of the Mantel-Haenszel variance consistent in both sparse-data and large-stratum limiting models. *Biometrics* 1986;42 : 311–323.

445. Robins J, Greenland S, Breslow NE. A general estimator for the variance of the Mantel-Haenszel odds ratio. *Am J Epidemiol* 1986;124 : 719–723.

446. Robins J, Pike M. The validity of case-control studies with nonrandom selection of controls. *Epidemiology* 1990;1 : 273–284.

447. Robins JM. A new approach to causal inference in mortality studies with sustained exposure periods—Application to control of the healthy worker survivor effect. *Math Modelling* 1986;7 : 1393–1512.

448. Robins JM, Greenland S. Estimability and estimation of excess and etiologic fractions. *Stat Med* 1989;8 : 845–859.

449. Robins LN, Helzer JE, Croughan J, et al. National Institute of Mental Health Diagnostic Interview Schedule. Its history, characteristics, and validity. *Arch Gen Psychiatry* 1981;38 : 381–389.

450. Robins LN, Helzer JE, Weissman MN, et al. Lifetime prevalence of specific psychiatric disorders in three sites. *Arch Gen Psychiatry* 1984;41 : 949–958.

451. Rogentine GN, Trapani RJ, Yankee RA, Henderson ES. HL-A antigens and acute lymphocytic leukemia: The nature of the HL-A2 association. *Tissue Antigens* 1973;3 : 470–476.

452. Rogot E. A note on measurement errors and detecting real differences. *J Am Stat Assoc* 1961;56 : 314–319.

453. Rogot E, Sorlie PD, Johnson NJ, Schmitt C. *A Mortality Study of 1.3 Million Persons by Demographic, Social, and Economic Factors: 1979–1985 Follow-Up.* Bethesda, MD, National Institutes of Health, 1992. NIH Publ. No. 92-3297.

454. Rom WN, Renzetti AD Jr, Lee JS, Archer VE. *Environmental and Occupational Medicine.* Boston: Little, Brown, 1983.

455. Rose G, Barker DJP. Epidemiology for the uninitiated. Observer variation. *Br Med J* 1978;2 : 1006–1007.

456. Rose G, Barker DJP. Epidemiology for the uninitiated. Repeatability and validity. *Br Med J* 1978;2 : 1070–1071.

457. Rose G, Marmot MG. Social class and coronary heart disease. *Br Heart J* 1981;45 : 13–19.

458. Rosenbaum PR. Case definition and power in case-control studies. *Stat Med* 1984;3 : 27–34.

459. Rosner B, Spiegelman D, Willett WC. Correction of logistic regression relative risk estimates and confidence intervals for measurement error: The case of multiple covariates measured with error. *Am J Epidemiol* 1990;132 : 734–745.

460. Rosner B, Spiegelman D, Willett WC. Correction of logistic regression relative risk estimates and confidence intervals for random within-person measurement error. *Am J Epidemiol* 1992;136 : 1400–1413.

461. Rosner B, Willett WC, Spiegelman D. Correction of logistic regression relative risk estimates and confidence intervals for systematic within-person measurement error. *Stat Med* 1989;8 : 1051–1069.

462. Rothman KJ. Synergy and antagonism in cause-effect relationships. *Am J Epidemiol* 1974;99 : 385–388.

463. Rothman KJ. Causes. *Am J Epidemiol* 1976;104 : 587–592.

464. Rothman KJ. The estimation of synergy or antagonism. *Am J Epidemiol* 1976;103 : 506–511.

465. Rothman KJ. Estimation of confidence limits for the cumulative probability of survival in life table analysis. *J Chronic Dis* 1978;31 : 557–560.
466. Rothman KJ. *Modern Epidemiology*. Boston: Little, Brown, 1986.
467. Rothman KJ. A sobering start for the cluster busters' conference. *Am J Epidemiol* 1990;132(Suppl.) : S6–13.
468. Rothman KJ. (Ed.). *Causal Inference*. Chestnut Hill, MA: Epidemiology Resources Inc., 1988.
469. Rothman KJ, Boice JD. *Epidemiologic Analysis with a Programmable Calculator*. Washington, DC: Government Printing Office, 1979. NIH Publ. No. 79-1649.
470. Rothman KJ, Greenland S, Walker AM. Concepts of interaction. *Am J Epidemiol* 1980;112 : 467–470.
471. Ryder RW, Nsa W, Hassig SE, et al. Perinatal transmission of the human immunodeficiency virus type 1 to infants of seropositive women in Zaire. *N Engl J Med* 1989;320 : 1637–1642.
472. Sackett DL. Bias in analytic research. *J Chronic Dis* 1979;32 : 51–63.
473. Sacks HS, Berrier J, Reitman D, et al. Meta-analyses of randomized controlled trials. *N Engl J Med* 1987;316 : 450–455.
474. Saracci R. Interaction and synergism. *Am J Epidemiol* 1980; 112 : 465–466.
475. Saracci R, Simonato L, Artvinli M, Skidmore J. The age-mortality curve of endemic pleural mesothelioma in Karain, Central Turkey. *Br J Cancer* 1982;45 : 147–149.
476. Sartwell PE, Masi AT, Arthes FG, et al. Thromboembolism and oral contraceptives: An epidemiologic case-control study. *Am J Epidemiol* 1969;90 : 365–380.
477. Savitz DA, Pearce N. Control selection with incomplete case ascertainment. *Am J Epidemiol* 1988;127 : 1109–1117.
478. Sawyer WA, Meyer KF, Eaton MD, et al. Jaundice in army personnel in the Western Region of the United States and its relation to vaccination against yellow fever. *Am J Hyg* 1944;39 : 337–430.
479. Schlesselman JJ. Sample size requirements in cohort and case-control studies of disease. *Am J Epidemiol* 1974;99 : 381–384.
480. Schlesselman JJ. *Case-Control Studies: Design, Conduct and Analysis*. New York: Oxford University Press, 1982.
481. Schmauz R, de Villiers E-M, Dennin R, et al. Multiple infections in cases of cervical cancer from a high-incidence area in tropical Africa. *Int J Cancer* 1989;43 : 805–809.
482. Schrenk HH, Heimann H, Clayton GD, et al. *Air Pollution in Donora, Pa: Epidemiology of the Unusual Smog Episode of October, 1948*. Washington, DC: Federal Security Agency, 1949. Public Health Bulletin No. 306.
483. Segi M. *Cancer Mortality for Selected Sites in 24 Countries. (1950–1957)*. Sendai, Japan: Tohoku University School of Medicine, 1962.
484. Segi M, Fukushima I, Fujisaku S, et al. Cancer morbidity in Myagi Prefecture Japan, and a comparison with morbidity in the United States. *J Natl Cancer Inst* 1957;18 : 373–383.
485. Segi M, Kurihara M. *Cancer Mortality for Selected Sites in 24 Countries. No.2 (1958–59). No.3 (1960–61)*. Sendai, Japan: Department of Public Health, Tohoku University School of Medicine, 1962, 1964.
486. Selikoff IJ, Hammond EC, Churg J. Asbestos exposure, smoking, and neoplasia. *JAMA* 1968;204 : 106–112.
487. Seltser R, Sartwell PE. The influence of occupational exposure to radiation on the mortality of American radiologists and other medical specialists. *Am J Epidemiol* 1965;81 : 2–22.

488. Semmelweis IP. The Etiology, the Concept and the Prophylaxis of Childbed Fever. 1861. Translated and republished in *Med Classics* 1941;5 : 350–773.

489. Shaper AG, Wannamethee G, Walker M. Alcohol and mortality in British men: Explaining the U-shaped curve. *Lancet* 1988;2 : 1267–1273.

490. Shapiro S. Meta-analysis/Shmeta-analysis. *Am J Epidemiol* 1994;140 : 771–778.

491. Shapiro S, Weinblatt E, Frank CW, Sager RV. Incidence of coronary heart disease in a population insured for medical care (HIP). *Am J Public Health* 1969;59(Suppl. June) : 1–101.

492. Shepard O. (Ed.). *The Heart of Thoreau's Journals.* New York: Dover, 1961. pp. 20, 30 January 1841.

493. Shimizu Y, Kato H, Schull WJ. Studies of the mortality of A-bomb survivors. IX. Mortality, 1950–1985; Part 2. Cancer mortality based on the recently revised doses (DS86). *Radiat Res* 1990;121 : 120–141.

494. Shore RE, Pasternak BS, Curnen MG. Relating influenza epidemics to childhood leukemia in tumor registries without a defined population base: A critique with suggestions for improved methods. *Am J Epidemiol* 1976;103 : 527–535.

495. Siemiatycki J, Wacholder S, Dewar R, et al. Degree of confounding bias related to smoking, ethnic group, and socioeconomic status in estimates of the associations between occupation and cancer. *J Occup Med* 1988;30 : 617–625.

496. Simpson CL, Hempelmann LH, Fuller LM. Neoplasia in children treated with X-rays in infancy for thymic enlargement. *Radiology* 1955;64 : 840–845.

497. Simpson REH. Infectiousness of communicable diseases in the household (measles, chickenpox, and mumps). *Lancet* 1952; ii : 549–554.

498. Smans M, Muir CS, Boyle P. *Atlas of Cancer Mortality in the European Economic Community.* Lyon: International Agency for Research on Cancer (IARC), 1992. IARC Scientific Publ. No.107.

499. Smith GD, Shipley MJ, Rose G. Magnitude and causes of socioeconomic differentials in mortality: Further evidence from the Whitehall Study. *J Epidemiol Community Health* 1990;44 : 265–270.

500. Smith PG. Spatial and temporal clustering. *In*: Schottenfeld D, Fraumeni JF Jr. (Eds.). *Cancer Epidemiology and Prevention.* Philadelphia: Saunders, 1982, pp. 391–407.

501. Smith RL. Recorded and expected mortality among the Japanese of the United States and Hawaii, with special reference to cancer. *J Natl Cancer Inst* 1956;17 : 459–473.

502. Smith RL. Recorded and expected mortality among the Chinese of Hawaii and the United States, with special reference to cancer. *J Natl Cancer Inst* 1956;17 : 667–676.

503. Smith RL, Salsbury CG, Gilliam AG. Recorded and expected mortality among the Navajo, with special reference to cancer. *J Natl Cancer Inst* 1956;17 : 77–89.

504. Smith WC, Crombie IK, Tavendale R, et al. The Scottish Heart Health Study: Objectives and development of methods. *Health Bull (Edinb)* 1987;45 : 211–217.

505. Snedecor GW, Cochran WG. *Statistical Methods* (6th ed.). Ames: Iowa State University Press, 1967.

506. Snedecor GW, Cochran WG. *Statistical Methods* (7th ed). Ames: Iowa State University Press, 1980.

507. Snipp CM, Passel JS. Who are American Indians? Some observations about the perils and pitfalls for data for race and ethnicity. *Pop Res Policy Rev* 1986;5 : 237–252.

508. Snow J. *On the Mode of Communication of Cholera* (2nd ed.). London: Churchill, 1855. Reproduced in Snow J. *Snow on Cholera*. New York: Commonwealth Fund, 1936. Reprinted New York: Hafner, 1965.

509. Sorlie PD, Backlund E, Keller JB. US mortality by economic, demographic, and social characteristics: The National Longitudinal Mortality Study. *Am J Public Health* 1995;85 : 949–956.

510. Stampfer MJ, Colditz GA, Willett WC, et al. A prospective study of moderate alcohol consumption and the risk of coronary disease and stroke in women. *N Engl J Med* 1988;319 : 267–273.

511. Stampfer MJ, Hennekens CH, Manson JE, et al. Vitamin E consumption and the risk of coronary heart disease in women. *N Engl J Med* 1993;328 : 1444–1449.

512. Stampfer MJ, Willett WC, Colditz GA, et al. A prospective study of postmenopausal estrogen therapy and coronary heart disease. *N Engl J Med* 1985;313 : 1044–1049.

513. Stampfer MJ, Willett WC, Speizer FE. A test of the National Death Index. *Am J Epidemiol* 1984;119 : 837–839.

514. Staszewski J, Haenszel W. Cancer mortality among the Polish-born in the United States. *J Natl Cancer Inst* 1965;35 : 291–297.

515. Stebbing LS. *Philosophy and the Physicists*. 2nd ed. New York: Dover, 1958. Chapter III.

516. Steering Committee of the Physicians' Health Study Research Group. Final report on the aspirin component of the ongoing Physicians' Health Study. *N Engl J Med* 1989;321 : 129–135.

517. Steinitz R, Parkin DM, Young JL, et al. (Eds.). *Cancer Incidence in Jewish Migrants to Israel, 1961–1981*. Lyon: International Agency for Research on Cancer (IARC), 1989. IARC Scientific Publ. No. 98.

518. Stevens RG, Moolgavkar SH, Lee JAH. Temporal trends in breast cancer. *Am J Epidemiol* 1982;115 : 759–777.

519. Stokes J, Kannel WB, Wolf PA, et al. Blood pressure as a risk factor for cardiovascular disease. *Hypertension* 1989;13(suppl. I) : 113–118.

520. Susser M. The logic of Sir Karl Popper and the practice of epidemiology. *Am J Epidemiology* 1986;124 : 711–718.

521. Susser M. Falsification, verification and causal inference in epidemiology: Reconsiderations in the light of Sir Karl Popper's philosophy. *In*: Rothman KJ (Ed.). *Causal Inference*. Chestnut Hill, MA: Epidemiology Resources Inc., 1988.

522. Susser M. What is a cause and how do we know one? A grammar for pragmatic epidemiology. *Am J Epidemiol* 1991;133 : 635–648.

523. Susser MW, Watson W, Hopper K. *Sociology in Medicine*. 3rd ed. New York: Oxford University Press, 1985.

524. Sutton E. *Human Genetics*. 4th ed. San Diego: Harcourt Brace Javanovich, 1988.

525. Tagnon I, Blot WJ, Stroube RB, et al. Mesothelioma associated with the shipbuilding industry in coastal Virginia. *Cancer Res* 1980;40 : 3875–3879.

526. Tarone RE, Chu KC. Implications of birth cohort patterns in interpreting trends in breast cancer rates. *J Natl Cancer Inst* 1992; 84 : 1402–1410.

527. Tetlow C. Psychoses of childbearing. *J Ment Sci* 1955;101 : 629–639.

528. Thomas DG. Exact and asymptotic methods for the combination of 2 times 2 tables. *Comput Biomed Res* 1975;8 : 423–446.

529. Thomas DC, Greenland S. The relative efficiencies of matched and independent sample designs for case-control studies. *J Chronic Dis* 1983;36 : 685–697.

530. Thomas DC, Greenland S. The efficiency of matching in case-control studies of risk-factor interactions. *J Chronic Dis* 1985; 38 : 569–574.

531. Thompson MW, McInnes RR, Willard HF. *Genetics in Medicine.* 5th ed. Philadelphia: Saunders, 1991.

532. Thompson WD. Statistical analysis of case-control studies. *Epidemiol Rev* 1994;16 : 33–50.

533. Thompson WD, Kelsey JL, Walter SD. Cost and efficiency in the choice of matched and unmatched case-control studies. *Am J Epidemiol* 1982;116 : 840–851.

534. Tofler GH, Brezinski D, Schafer AI, et al. Concurrent morning increase in platelet aggregability and the risk of myocardial infarction and sudden cardiac death. *N Engl J Med* 1987;316 : 1514–1518.

535. Topley WWC, Wilson GS. *The Principles of Bacteriology and Immunity* (2nd ed.). Baltimore: Wood, 1936.

536. Townsend P, Phillimore P, Beattie A. *Health and Deprivation: Inequality and the North.* London: Croom Helm, 1988.

537. Trichopoulos D. Risk of lung cancer from passive smoking. *Principles and Practices of Oncology: PPO Updates* 1994;8 : 1–8.

538. Trichopoulos D, Desmond L, Yen S, MacMahon B. A study of time-place clustering in anencephaly and spina bifida. *Am J Epidemiol* 1971;94 : 26–30.

539. Trichopoulos D, Kalandidi A, Sparros L. Lung cancer and passive smoking. *Int J Cancer* 1981;27 : 1–4.

540. Trichopoulos D, Katsouyanni K, Zavisanos X, et al. Psychological stress and fatal heart attack: The Athens (1981) earthquake natural experiment. *Lancet* 1983;1 : 441–444.

541. Trichopoulos D, MacMahon B, Sparros L, Merikas G. Smoking and hepatitis B-negative primary hepatocellular carcinoma. *J Natl Cancer Inst* 1980;65 : 111–114.

542. Trichopoulos D, Ouranos G, Day N, et al. Diet and cancer of the stomach: A case-control study in Greece. *Int J Cancer* 1985; 36 : 291–297.

543. Trichopoulos D, Petridou E. Epidemiologic studies and cancer etiology in humans. *Med Exerc Nutr Health* 1994;3 : 206–225.

544. Trichopoulos D, Tabor E, Gerety R, et al. Hepatitis B and primary hepatocellular carcinoma in a European population. *Lancet* 1978; 2 : 1217–1219.

545. Trichopoulos D, Tzonou A, Katsouyanni K, Trichopoulou A. Diet and cancer: The role of case-control studies. *Ann Nutr Metab* 1991;35(Suppl. 1) : 89–92.

546. Trichopoulou A, Kouris-Blazos A, Vassilakou T, et al. Diet and survival of elderly Greeks: A link to the past. *Am J Clin Nutr* 1995; 61(suppl) : 1346S–1350S.

547. Troisi RJ, Speizer FE, Rosner B, et al. Cigarette smoking and incidence of chronic bronchitis and asthma in women. Chest 1995; 108 : 1557–1561.

548. Tsementzis SA, Gill JS, Hitchcock ER, et al. Diurnal variation of and activity during the onset of stroke. *Neurosurgery* 1985; 17 : 901–904.

549. Tsuang MT, Hsieh C-c, Fleming JA. Group comparison approaches in psychiatric research. *In*: Hsu LKG, Hersen M. (Eds.). *Research in Psychiatry: Issues, Strategies and Methods.* New York: Plenum Press, 1992, pp. 107–132.

550. Tsuang MT, Tohen M, Murphy JM. Psychiatric epidemiology. *In*:

Nicholi A Jr (Ed.). *The Harvard Guide to Modern Psychiatry.* Cambridge: Belknap Harvard, 1988.

551. Tunstall-Pedoe H, Smith WCS, Crombie IK, Tavendale R. Coronary risk factor and lifestyle variation across Scotland: Results from the Scottish Heart Health Study. *Scot Med J* 1989;34 : 556–560.

552. Tyczynski J, Parkin D, Zatonski W, Tarkowski W. Cancer mortality among Polish migrants to France. *Bull Cancer* 1992;79 : 789–800.

553. Tzonou A, Kaldor J, Smith P, et al. Misclassification in case-control studies with two dichotomous risk factors. *Rev Epidemiol Santé Publ* 1986;34 : 10–17.

554. Tzonou A, Maragoudakis G, Trichopoulos D, et al. Urban living, tobacco smoking, and chronic obstructive pulmonary disease: A study in Athens. *Epidemiology* 1992;3 : 57–60

555. Tzonou A, Trichopoulos D, Kaklamani E, et al. Epidemiologic assessment of interactions of hepatitis-C virus with seromarkers of hepatitis-B and -D viruses, cirrhosis and tobacco smoking in hepatocellular carcinoma. *Int J Cancer* 1991;49 : 377–380.

556. U.S. Bureau of the Census. *Statistical Abstract of the United States: 1966.* (87th ed.). Washington, DC: U.S. Govt. Printing Office, 1966.

557. U.S. Bureau of the Census. *The Current Population Survey: Design and Methodology.* Washington, DC: US Bureau of the Census, 1978. Technical Paper 40.

558. U.S. Bureau of the Census. *1980 Census of Population. Ancestry of the Population by State: 1980.* Current Population Reports, 1983 (PC80-S1-10).

559. U.S. Bureau of the Census. *Statistical Abstract of the United States: 1993.* (113th ed.) Washington, DC: U.S. Govt Printing Office, 1993.

560. U.S. Bureau of the Census. *Statistical Abstract of the United States, 1994.* Washington, D.C.: U.S. Department of Commerce, 1994.

561. Van den Brandt PA, Goldbohm RA, Van't Veer P, et al. A large-scale prospective cohort study on diet and cancer in The Netherlands. *J Clin Epidemiol* 1990;45 : 285–295.

562. Van den Brandt PA, Schouten LJ, Goldbohm RA, et al. Development of a record linkage protocol for use in the Dutch Cancer Registry for epidemiological research. *Int J Epidemiol* 1990;19 : 553–558.

563. Vandenbroucke JP, Koster T, Briët E, et al. Increased risk of venous thrombosis in oral-contraceptive users who are carriers of factor V Leiden mutation. *Lancet* 1994;344 : 1453–1457.

564. Vecchio TJ. Predictive value of a single diagnostic test in unselected populations. *N Engl J Med* 1966;274 : 1171–1173.

565. Wacholder S. When measurement errors correlate with truth: Surprising effects of non-differential misclassification. *Epidemiology* 1995;6 : 157–161.

566. Wacholder S, Benichou J, Heineman EF, et al. Attributable risk: Advantages of a broad definition of exposure. *Am J Epidemiol* 1994;140 : 303–309.

567. Wacholder S, Boivin JF. External comparisons with the case-cohort design. *Am J Epidemiol* 1987;126 : 1198–1209.

568. Wacholder S, McLaughlin JK, Silverman DT, Mandel JS. Selection of controls in case-control studies. I. Principles. *Am J Epidemiol* 1992; 135 : 1019–1028.

569. Wacholder S, Silverman DT, McLaughlin JK, Mandel JS. Selection of controls in case-control studies: II. Types of controls. *Am J Epidemiol* 1992;135 : 1029–1041.

570. Wacholder S, Silverman DT, McLaughlin JK, Mandel JS. Selection

Index